Introductory
Clinical
Pharmacology

JEANNE C. SCHERER, R.N., M.S.

Assistant Director and
Medical-Surgical Coordinator,
Sisters of Charity Hospital
School of Nursing, Buffalo, N.Y.

Introductory Clinical Pharmacology

J. B. LIPPINCOTT COMPANY PHILADELPHIA / NEW YORK / TORONTO

Copyright © 1975 by J. B. Lippincott Company

This book is fully protected by copyright and, with
the exception of brief excerpts for review, no part of
it may be reproduced in any form, by print, photoprint,
microfilm, or any other means, without the written
permission of the publisher.

Distributed in Great Britain by Blackwell Scientific Publications
Oxford, London, and Edinburgh

ISBN 0-397-54168-6

Library of Congress Catalog Card Number 75-4606

Printed in the United States of America

3 5 7 9 8 6 4 2

Library of Congress Cataloging in Publication Data
Scherer, Jeanne C.
    Introductory clinical pharmacology.

    1. Pharmacology. I. Title. DNLM: 1. Drug
therapy—Nursing texts. 2. Pharmacology—Nursing texts.
QV4 S326i
RM300.S264   615'.1   75-4606
ISBN 0-397-54168-6

I owe the idea for this text to the students who participated in my classes in pharmacology. Their questions led to marginal notations on lecture material, which ultimately became an outline and, finally, after several transitions, a manuscript. If a dedication of this text were to be made, it would be to the students of the Sisters of Charity Hospital School of Nursing, especially the class of 1974; and to the physicians, nurses, and other health professionals who attended my seminars and challenged me to present the principles of pharmacology in clear and relevant terms.

Behind the scenes there are many people who contribute to a textbook. Paul A. Young, Ph.D., of Canisius College, worked with me on the original draft of the manuscript. Sister Geraldine P. Coleman, B.S. in Pharmacy, M.P.H., the administrative assistant of Sisters of Charity Hospital, painstakingly read the completed manuscript and made many valuable suggestions. Antoinette DeMarco was an ever-patient typist.

My thanks also go to Mary Dennesaites Morgan and David T. Miller of the J. B. Lippincott Company, especially for their invaluable editorial assistance and encouragement. The thoughtful attention of copy editor Joyce Mkitarian is especially appreciated.

Without the help of all these individuals, those marginal notes would most probably still be in my lecture file.

Acknowledgments

v

This text is designed for students and practitioners who wish a concise, clear introduction to pharmacology. However, the basic explanations presented here should not lead anyone to the conclusion that pharmacology is a simple subject. Drug therapy is one of the most important treatment modalities in modern health care. Because of its importance and complexity, and the ever-increasing new knowledge in the field, it is imperative that all health professionals develop a system of study to help them cope with drug information. This book is designed to aid the student and practitioner in that study.

Each chapter is followed by a table which summarizes the clinical considerations of the specific drugs discussed in that chapter.* An attempt has been made to use charts and tables wherever possible for quick and easy reference; key points are highlighted in color, and material on patient education is discussed. An appendix, covering basic mathematics related to drug administration, has been included for review.

Preface vii

* The only exception is Chapter 35, Anesthetic Agents; the wide variations in uses, dosages, etc. encountered with this group of drugs would make such a summary impractical.

The drugs and dosages listed in this text have been compiled from several references. The reader should keep in mind, however, that drug therapy is constantly being revised; that new products are continuously being marketed and older ones withdrawn; and that the Food and Drug Administration (FDA) often orders changes in labeling on the basis of ongoing research in safety and effectiveness. Therefore it is advisable that current references be consulted. Periodic supplements are issued by the *Hospital Formulary* and the *Physicians' Desk Reference* (PDR); manufacturers' package inserts should also be checked for changes. Some drugs have a wide dose range, indicating that different doses are advised for specific disease conditions and/or degrees of severity.

If official references are not available or if there appears to be a discrepancy between the dose ordered and the reference consulted, the hospital pharmacist should be contacted for updated information. No health professional should administer, or permit a patient to take, a medication when there is doubt as to the correct dosage.

1 Introduction 1

2 Adrenergic Drugs 7

3 Adrenergic Blocking Agents 17

4 Cholinergic Drugs 23

5 Cholinergic Blocking Agents 29

6 The Narcotic Analgesics and the Narcotic Antagonists 35

7 Non-Narcotic Analgesics 47

8 Sedatives and Hypnotics 55

9 Drug Abuse 63

10 The Cardiotonics and the Cardiac Depressants 71

Contents

ix

11 Anticoagulant Drugs 85

12 Vasodilating Agents 93

13 Management of Body Fluids 97

14 Diuretics and Antihypertensive Agents 103

15 Central Nervous System Stimulants 115

16 Insulin and Oral Hypoglycemic Agents 121

17 The Sulfonamides 131

18 Penicillin, Broad-Spectrum Antibiotics, and Antifungal Agents 135

19 Drugs Used in the Treatment of Tuberculosis 159

20 Drugs Used in the Treatment of Parasitic Diseases 165

21 Pituitary Hormones and Adrenal Cortical Hormones 177

22 Male and Female Hormones 191

23 Thyroid and Antithyroid Agents 203

24 Drugs That Act on the Uterus 209

25 Antineoplastic Agents 215

26 Drugs Used in the Treatment of Convulsive Disorders 227

27 Agents Used in the Treatment of Parkinson's Disease 235

28 Psychotherapeutic Agents 241

29 Histamine and Antihistamines, Antitussives and Mucolytics 259

30 Agents Used in the Management of Gastrointestinal Disorders 267

31 Heavy Metals and Heavy Metal Antagonists 281

32 Vitamins and Drugs Used in the Treatment of Anemias 285

33 Immunological Agents 293

34 Antiseptics, Disinfectants, and Other Locally Acting Agents 301

35 Anesthetic Agents 309

 36 Drugs Used in the Management of Musculoskeletal Disorders 317

Appendix 327

Index 353

Throughout the ages man has used drugs to produce desired changes in the body, but the exact science of the study of drugs—**pharmacology**—is relatively recent when considered in light of the number of years drugs have been used. Yet even with the advancement of modern science the exact mechanism of action of many pharmacological agents is not well understood. Physical differences among individual patients also influence the action of any one drug; these factors must be taken into consideration when drugs are administered.

Factors Influencing Drug Action

The **age** of the patient may influence the action of drugs. Children almost always require smaller doses of a drug than adults. Elderly patients also may require smaller doses, although this may well depend on the type of drug administered. As an example, the elderly patient may be given the same amount of an antibiotic as a younger adult, but may not require the usual adult dose of a sedative or a hypnotic.

Drugs for children may be calculated on a weight basis; however, drugs for the adult patient may also be calculated in this manner. For example, the recommended dosage

Chapter **1**

Introduction

for a drug may be stated as 20 mg./Kg./day (20 milligrams per Kilogram of body weight per day). This particular drug may also be given in equally divided doses several times per day. An example of this is shown below.

DRUG DOSE: 20 mg./Kg./day in 3 equally divided doses

WEIGHT OF PATIENT (child): 39 pounds or 17.7 Kilograms

(2.2 pounds = 1 Kilogram;
39 ÷ 2.2 = 17.7 Kilograms)

20 milligrams per Kilogram equals 354 milligrams *per day* (20 × 17.7). Since this drug is to be administered in 3 equally divided doses, then *each dose* is 118 milligrams (354 ÷ 3).

Body size influences the action of some drugs. For example, a common dose of meperidine (Demerol), a synthetic narcotic agent, is 75 milligrams. This dose may produce the desired effect, relief of pain, in most adult patients, but a very large patient may require a larger dose and a slender patient may require a smaller dose to produce the desired effect.

The **sex** of the individual may also influence the action of some drugs. Women may require a smaller dose of some drugs than men. This is based on the fact that many women are smaller than men and have a different ratio of fat and body water than males. Sex is not so great a factor as age and body size.

The **presence of disease** may influence the action of some drugs and in some instances may be an indication for omitting one drug and possibly using others in its stead. The patient with liver disease for example might have an impaired ability to metabolize a specific type of drug. If the average or normal dose of the drug is given, the liver will be unable to metabolize it; consequently lower doses may be required or other drugs not metabolized or detoxified by the liver may be necessary. The package insert, the *Physicians' Desk Reference*, the *Hospital Formulary*, and other drug references should be consulted concerning cautions or contraindications of drugs, as certain diseases or conditions may warrant the withholding of a drug until the physician is consulted.

Adverse Drug Reactions

Along with factors discussed above that may influence the action of a drug, the possibility of an untoward response of the patient to a pharmacological agent is also important. An **adverse reaction** to a drug is unpredictable and sometimes unexplainable. An adverse reaction may occur the first time a drug is given or after several and even many doses.

Drug allergy appears to occur after more than 1 dose of the drug has been given. The individual becomes *sensitized* to the drug; that is, the drug has become an *antigen* which stimulates the body to produce *antibodies*. If the patient takes the drug again after the antigen/antibody response has occurred, an allergic reaction will result. This can be compared to an allergy to ragweed pollen ("hay fever"). The ragweed pollen is the antigen; the response of an individual allergic to ragweed pollen usually includes itching and watering of the eyes, increased nasal discharge, swollen nasal membranes, and sneezing.

Allergic reactions to drugs can be mild or extremely serious and may be manifested by a variety of symptoms and complaints. Even a mild reaction can become serious if it goes unnoticed and the drug is repeated. It is possible, then, for a mild reaction to be followed by an extremely serious reaction. This is why even the most mild reaction should be detected early and reported to the physician before the next dose is administered.

Drug allergic reactions may occur immediately, within minutes (and even seconds) after administration, or they may be delayed, occurring hours or days later. In many instances, immediate reactions are the most serious. **Anaphylactic reactions** usually occur shortly after the administration of the drug to which the individual is sensitive (or allergic) and they are extremely serious and require immediate medical intervention. Shock, bronchospasm, loss of consciousness, cyanosis, dyspnea (due to the severe bronchospasm), convulsions, and cardiac arrest are signs of an anaphylactic reaction. It is believed that this type of reaction is due to the sudden release of histamine. (See Chapter 29.)

Milder drug reactions include rashes of varying types, urticaria (hives), itching, and nasal stuffiness. *Any* patient complaint or overt symptom should be considered as a warning that a drug reaction *may* be occurring, and the drug should be stopped until the

physician has been notified and a decision made as to the cause of the complaint or symptom.

Drug idiosyncrasy is a term usually used to describe any unusual or abnormal reaction to a drug, that is, any reaction that is different from the one normally expected of a specific drug and dose. For example, a patient may receive a normal dose of secobarbital (Seconal), a sedative/hypnotic barbiturate, and still be unable to sleep or show evidence of drowsiness. This is an *underresponse* and is abnormal. Another patient may receive the same drug and dose, sleep 8 hours, and find it extremely difficult to waken from sleep. This is an *overresponse* and is also abnormal. It is believed that drug idiosyncrasies occur because of a genetic deficiency wherein the patient is unable to tolerate certain chemicals.

Other Responses to Drugs

Besides those factors which influence drug action and adverse drug reactions, there are other factors that must be considered regarding the administration of drugs. **Drug tolerance** is a term used to describe a *decreased* response to the dose of the drug, usually requiring an increase in dosage to elicit the desired effect. Drug tolerance may be seen in the patient taking a barbiturate every night for sleep. After a period of time, which may vary, the individual may find that 1 capsule no longer produces sleep and that 2 capsules are now required. Not all pharmacological agents are capable of creating drug tolerance.

A cumulative effect may be seen in some patients. This effect occurs when the body is unable to metabolize and excrete 1 dose of a drug before the next dose is administered. Below is a hypothetical example of the course of a narcotic dose during normal metabolic breakdown and excretion.

NORMAL METABOLISM

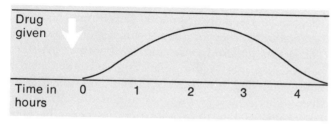

Note that at the end of 4 hours there is very little drug left in the body of this patient. Compare this with a patient with severe cirrhosis of the liver receiving the same drug and dose.

ABNORMAL METABOLISM

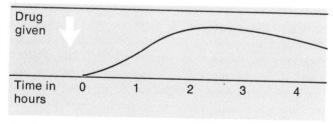

At the end of 4 hours very little of the drug has been metabolized and excreted. If a second dose of the drug were given, the patient would most likely experience toxic drug effects, namely symptoms of narcotic overdose, even though normal doses were given both times.

Drug interaction is another factor that must be considered during drug administration. Some drugs may interact with other drugs, foods, or chemicals, producing an *antagonistic* (or opposing) *effect*. In some instances an antagonistic drug effect may be extremely serious. On the other hand, drug *synergism* may occur. Drug synergism is an effect *greater than* the sum of the separate actions of two (or more) drugs. Depending on the agents involved, synergism can be serious.

An illustration of drug synergism is seen in the individual using secobarbital (Seconal) indiscriminately, taking more of the drug than is ordered by the physician. If whiskey is also taken at the same time, the action of the barbiturate may be potentiated and the individual will most likely obtain a greater response from the combination of the two agents than from either of the agents taken singly. For example, the ordinary effect of 1 ounce of whiskey is a slightly elevated feeling; that of 1 capsule of Seconal is sleep. Taken together, however, these agents may produce *deep* sleep. On occasion, the results of a combination such as this can be extremely serious and even fatal.

The **route of administration** is another consideration that may influence drug action. The intravenous route of administration almost always produces the most rapid drug effect, whereas the oral route almost always produces the slowest. Some drugs may be manufactured to be absorbed slowly or to have a delayed absorption. Examples of these products are enteric coated aspirin, procaine penicillin, and protamine zinc insulin.

It must be remembered that all drugs administered orally, parenterally, or sublingually will not produce the desired results in exactly the same time. For example, an intravenous short-acting barbiturate produces its effect in a matter of seconds, whereas an intravenously administered diuretic may require 3, 4, or even more minutes to produce diuresis. Similarly, an oral drug may work faster when the stomach is empty rather than full.

Drugs are complex chemicals producing a variety of effects on the body. No drug is absolutely safe, and all drugs appear to be capable of producing serious adverse effects, at least in some individuals.

The **autonomic nervous system** is one part of the peripheral nervous system. The autonomic nervous system has two divisions: the *sympathetic nervous system* and the *parasympathetic nervous system*.

The sympathetic nervous system tends to regulate the expenditure of energy and is operative when the organism is confronted with stressful situations such as danger or intense emotion. The parasympathetic nervous system works to help conserve body energy; it is partly responsible for such activities as slowing the heart, digestion of food, and elimination of body wastes.

There are two neurohormones of the sympathetic nervous system that are of clinical significance as adrenergic drugs: **epinephrine** (also called adrenaline) and **norepinephrine** (also called noradrenaline). Epinephrine is secreted by the medulla (central portion) of the adrenal gland. Norepinephrine is mainly found at the nerve endings of sympathetic (also called adrenergic) nerve fibers.

Types of Adrenergic Drugs

There are two types of adrenergic drugs: **catecholamines** and **noncatecholamines.** The catecholamines, organic compounds normally found in the sympathetic nervous sys-

Chapter 2

Adrenergic Drugs

tem, are the neurohormones epinephrine and norepinephrine. When manufactured and used as drugs they are the most potent of the adrenergic agents. The noncatecholamines lack catechol, hence the name NONcatecholamines. This group of drugs usually has a longer and less intense action than the catecholamines.

THE CATECHOLAMINES

Catecholamines usually affect alpha and beta receptors. One profound effect is on the blood vessels (which have mainly alpha receptors) resulting in **vasoconstriction** of peripheral blood vessels and **slight vasodilatation** of coronary arteries (which have mainly beta receptors). When peripheral blood vessels constrict, blood from these smaller vessels is shunted to larger blood vessels such as the aorta, vena cava, and renal arteries. This vasoconstricting action, also called a **vasopressor effect,** results in a *rise* in blood pressure.

Catecholamines also affect the heart and are sometimes referred to as cardiac stimulants, since they not only increase the pulse rate but may also increase cardiac output (the amount of blood pumped during each contraction of the heart).

Catecholamines have a short-acting effect on the respiratory system, namely dilatation of the bronchi and stimulation of the medulla of the spinal cord resulting in an increase in the respiratory rate.

Pharmaceutical companies manufacture synthetic catecholamines, for example epinephrine (Adrenalin), levarterenol (Levophed), and isoproterenol (Isuprel).

THE NONCATECHOLAMINES

The noncatecholamines act in two ways. They may stimulate the release of norepinephrine at adrenergic nerve endings or may act directly on alpha and/or beta receptors. Usually, the effect of these drugs on body organs and structures is less intense and of a somewhat longer duration than the catecholamines. In some instances these drugs do appear to be greater central nervous system stimulants ·than the catecholamines.

Two noncatecholamines, dextroamphetamine and methamphetamine, have limited use because of their drug abuse potential. There are times when the use of these drugs appears to be warranted, for example in the treatment of narcolepsy. Presently, most physicians prefer to use other types of central nervous system stimulants.

Metaraminol (Aramine), mephentermine (Wyamine), methoxamine (Vasoxyl), and phenylephrine (Neo-Synephrine) are noncatecholamines used for their vasopressor effect.

General Drug Action

Adrenergic drugs (also called sympathomimetic drugs) act like or "mimic" the actions of the sympathetic nervous system, producing the following responses:

CENTRAL NERVOUS SYSTEM—wakefulness; quick reaction to stimuli; quickened reflexes

Table 2-1.

ACTION OF THE AUTONOMIC NERVOUS SYSTEM ON BODY ORGANS AND STRUCTURES

Organs and Structures	Sympathetic (Adrenergic) Effects	Type of Adrenergic Receptor	Parasympathetic (Cholinergic) Effects
HEART	increase in: pulse, muscle contractility, speed of electrical conduction	Beta	decrease in: pulse, muscle contractility, and A-V conduction
BLOOD VESSELS			
1. skin, mucous membrane	constriction	Alpha	dilatation
2. skeletal muscle	dilatation (usually)	Alpha, Beta	dilatation
3. coronary	dilatation + occasional constriction	Alpha, Beta	dilatation
BRONCHIAL MUSCLES	relaxation	Beta	contraction
GASTROINTESTINAL			
Stomach			
Motility	decrease (usually)	Beta	increase (usually)
Sphincters	contraction (usually)	Alpha	relaxation (usually)
Intestine			
Motility	decrease	Alpha, Beta	increase
Sphincters	contraction (usually)	Alpha	relaxation (usually)
Gallbladder	relaxation	?	contraction
BLADDER			
detrusor	relaxation	Beta	contraction
trigone, sphincter	contraction	Alpha	relaxation
EYE			
radial muscles of iris	contraction	Alpha	—
sphincter muscle of iris	—	?	contraction
ciliary muscle	relaxation	Beta	contraction

Table 2-1. (Continued)

ORGANS AND STRUCTURES	SYMPATHETIC (ADRENERGIC) EFFECTS	TYPE OF ADRENERGIC RECEPTOR	PARASYMPATHETIC (CHOLINERGIC) EFFECTS
SKIN			
sweat glands	increased activity in localized areas	Alpha	generalized increase in sweating
pilomotor muscles	contraction	Alpha	—
UTERUS	variable response depending on menstrual cycle, pregnancy	Alpha, Beta	variable response depending on menstrual cycle, pregnancy
SALIVARY GLANDS	thickened secretions	Alpha	copious, watery secretions
LACRIMAL GLANDS, NASOPHARYNGEAL GLANDS	—	?	increased secretions
LIVER	glycogenolysis	?	—

PERIPHERY—relaxation of smooth muscles of the bronchi; constriction of blood vessels, sphincters of the stomach; dilatation of coronary blood vessels; decrease in stomach motility

HEART—increase in the heart rate

METABOLISM—increased use of sugar plus liberation of fatty acids from adipose tissue

Adrenergic drugs may evoke one or more of the above responses to a greater degree than other responses to be discussed, since adrenergic nerves may have alpha receptors only; beta receptors only; *or* both alpha and beta receptors.

Alpha receptors are **excitatory** (or stimulating) and beta receptors are **inhibitory** (or relaxing). Some adrenergic drugs act chiefly on alpha receptors with minimal action on beta receptors, whereas others act chiefly on beta receptors with minimal action on alpha receptors. Other adrenergic drugs may act on both alpha and beta receptors.

Refer to Table 2-1. Various body organs and structures are listed along with sympathetic (adrenergic) and parasympathetic (cholinergic) effects and the type of adrenergic receptor. If an adrenergic nerve fiber has *beta* receptors, the effect is one of relaxation or decreased activity. If an adrenergic nerve fiber has *alpha* receptors, the effect is one of constriction, contraction, or increased activity. Adrenergic drugs will produce their effects depending on whether they affect alpha receptors, beta receptors, or both alpha and beta receptors. For example, if an adrenergic drug acts chiefly on beta receptors, it will *dilate* (relax) the bronchi, but if an adrenergic drug acts chiefly on alpha receptors, its effect on the bronchi would be negligible. In the heart, however, beta receptors are *not* inhibitory but are excitatory (see again Table 2-1).

Uses of Adrenergic Drugs

Adrenergic drugs have a variety of uses, depending on the type of drug (catecholamine or noncatecholamine) and the receptors (alpha, beta, or both) affected by the drug. Such drugs are used in

1. moderate to severe episodes of hypotension
2. control of superficial bleeding during surgical procedures of the mouth, nose, throat, skin
3. bronchial asthma
4. cardiac arrest
5. allergic reactions to drugs (anaphylactic shock, angioneurotic edema)
6. heart block
7. nasal congestion (applied topically) and
8. in conjunction with local anesthetics to control bleeding.

Side Effects of Adrenergic Drugs

The side effects of adrenergic drugs depend on the type of drug used and the dose administered. Below is a summary of the side effects that may be encountered. Side effects for specific adrenergic drugs are listed in Table 2-3 at the end of this chapter.

CATECHOLAMINES: tachycardia, cardiac arrhythmias, bradycardia, increase in blood pressure (which may reach dangerously high levels), headache

NONCATECHOLAMINES: insomnia, nervousness, headache, increase in blood pressure, tachycardia, anorexia

Table 2-2.
ROUTES OF ADMINISTRATION OF ADRENERGIC VASOPRESSORS

DRUG	I.V.	I.M.	S.C.	TOPICAL	ORAL
epinephrine (Adrenalin)*	√	√	√	√	
levarterenol (Levophed)	√				
mephentermine (Wyamine)	√	√			√
metaraminol (Aramine)	√	√	√		
methoxamine (Vasoxyl)	√	√			
phenylephrine (Neo-Synephrine)	√	√	√	√	√

* also given intracardially.

Clinical Considerations

When a patient has marked hypotension and requires a vasopressor, the physician first determines the cause of the hypotensive episode and then selects the best method of treatment. Some situations require the use of a less potent vasopressor, such as metaraminol (Aramine), while others require the use of a potent vasopressor such as levarterenol (Levophed).

Table 2-2 shows the routes of administration of various adrenergic vasopressors.

POINTS TO REMEMBER DURING THE ADMINISTRATION
OF LEVARTERENOL (LEVOPHED)

[Note that levarterenol (Levophed) is administered only by the *intravenous* route and that great care must be taken when this drug is administered.]

1. the drug is given in *diluted* form, that is, the drug is added to 500-1000 ml. of an intravenous solution
2. the blood pressure and pulse must be taken *frequently,* usually every 2-5 minutes
3. the rate of the intravenous administration (that is, drops per minute) is adjusted according to the patient's blood pressure
4. the site of the intravenous infusion (where the needle enters the skin) and the surrounding areas must be inspected for leakage (extravasation).

The physician will usually order a specific systolic pressure to be maintained during the administration of levarterenol, as shown in this example:

> 5/24
> Add 4 mg. of levophed to 1000 ml. of 5% dextrose in water. Maintain blood pressure between 100 and 110 systolic.
> Dr. Greene

The rate of flow of the intravenous solution must be adjusted in order to maintain the patient's blood pressure at the level stated by the physician. (NOTE: If the physician does not designate the desirable blood pressure, he should be requested to do so.) The rate of intravenous flow, as well as the patient's blood pressure, should be recorded on the patient's chart.

The time interval between blood pressure and pulse determinations depends, in part, on clinical judgment. If the blood pressure fluctuates widely, it may be necessary to take the blood pressure and pulse every 1-1½ minutes. AT NO TIME MUST THE PATIENT RECEIVING LEVARTERENOL BE LEFT UNATTENDED.

Levarterenol may be harmful to the tissues surrounding the vein, should the intravenous solution leak (extravasate) into them. Necrosis and sloughing can occur. If extravasation does occur, the physician must be contacted *immediately* and the I.V. infusion started in another vein by appropriate hospital personnel.

OTHER ADRENERGIC AGENTS

The noncatecholamine vasopressors, for example metaraminol (Aramine), also require close supervision during administration by the intravenous, intramuscular, or subcutaneous route. The same procedure as that for the administration of levarterenol (Levophed) is followed; however, blood pressure and pulse determinations may be required less frequently. Sound clinical judgment should always be used, since there are no absolute minimum or maximum time limits between determinations.

Other adrenergic agents have specific uses. Isoproterenol (Isuprel) may be used for its bronchodilating properties, or epinephrine (Adrenalin) to treat asthma. Points to remember are:

1. observe the effect of the drug. Example: Is the breathing of an asthmatic patient improved after the administration of the drug?
2. *record* the effect of the drug on the patient's chart

3. observe the patient for the appearance of side effects
4. report side effects to the attending physician.

Adrenergic drugs are, in most instances, potent and potentially dangerous drugs; therefore great care should be exercised in the measurement of the dose and the administration of the drug. All side effects should be reported to the attending physician, but here again judgment is necessary. Some side effects, such as the development of cardiac arrhythmias, must be reported immediately, regardless of the time of day or night. Other side effects, such as anorexia, should be reported but usually are not of an emergency nature.

Any complaint the patient may have should also be reported, for occasionally unusual side effects can occur during the administration of *any* drug.

Although adrenergic drugs are potentially dangerous, proper supervision and management during administration will usually minimize the occurrence of serious side effects.

Table 2-3.
ADRENERGIC DRUGS

Generic Name	Trade Name	Uses	Side Effects	Dose Ranges
CATECHOLAMINES				
epinephrine	Adrenalin	angioneurotic edema, anaphylactic shock, cardiac arrest, status asthmaticus. Also used topically to control capillary bleeding	marked elevation of blood pressure, cardiac arrhythmias	0.1-1.0 ml. of 1:1000 aqueous solution I.M., S.C.; CHILD: 0.05-0.3 ml. S.C. For intravenous use: 0.05-0.1 ml. Intracardiac dose: 1 ml. of 1:1000 aqueous solution
isoproterenol	Isuprel	bronchodilator, shock, Adams-Stokes syndrome	tachycardia, insomnia, nervousness, headache, vertigo, coronary insufficiency	1 mg. diluted in 500 ml. of 5% dextrose (higher concentrations may be necessary) I.V.; 10-20 mg. sublingually; 200 mcg.-1 mg. I.M.; 200 mcg. S.C.
levarterenol	Levophed	severe hypotensive episodes	same as epinephrine plus headache, bradycardia	1 or more ampuls diluted in 5% dextrose I.V. ONLY
NONCATECHOLAMINES				
ephedrine		treatment of enuresis, narcolepsy, carotid sinus syncope	insomnia, nervousness, palpitations, vertigo, sweating, headache, nausea	25-50 mg. orally; 15-50 mg. I.M., S.C.

Generic Name	Trade Name	Uses	Side Effects	Dose Ranges
mephentermine	Wyamine	cardiogenic shock, used prophylactically during spinal, general, epidural anesthesia, treatment of extra systoles	headache, tachycardia	15-30 mg. I.M., I.V.; 25 mg. orally
metaraminol	Aramine, Pressonex	shock, prophylactically during spinal or general anesthesia	headache, tachycardia, hypertension	2-10 mg. I.M., S.C.; 15-100 mg. diluted in 500 ml. of 5% dextrose or saline I.V.; 500 mcg.-5 mg. undiluted I.V. as an emergency measure
methoxamine	Vasoxyl	same as metaraminol	same as metaraminol	10-30 mg. I.M.; 5 mg. by slow I.V. injection; 35 mg. in 250 ml. 5% dextrose I.V.
phenylephrine	Neo-Synephrine	treatment of nasal congestion (as a spray or drops), hay fever, also to prevent or treat shock during and after anesthesia, especially spinal anesthesia	cardiac arrhythmias, sensation of fullness in the head, tingling of extremities	1-10 mg. I.M., S.C.; 25-150 mg. daily orally; 100-500 mcg. I.V.

Adrenergic blocking agents (also called sympathomimetic blocking agents) may be divided into three groups:

1. those which block alpha receptors (alpha adrenergic blocking agents)
2. those which block beta receptors (beta adrenergic blocking agents)
3. those which block adrenergic nerves (antiadrenergic or adrenergic neuron blocking agents)

Types of Adrenergic Blocking Agents

THE ALPHA ADRENERGIC BLOCKING AGENTS

The alpha adrenergic blocking agents produce their greatest effect on alpha receptors of the vascular system, with resultant **vasodilatation.** This is directly opposite to the effect of an adrenergic drug, which has a vasoconstrictor effect.

Drugs such as tolazoline (Priscoline), phenoxybenzamine (Dibenzyline), and phentolamine (Regitine) are used for their vasodilating properties.

THE BETA ADRENERGIC BLOCKING AGENTS

Stimulation of beta receptors of the heart results in a rise in the pulse. Consequently, a drug that **blocks** this effect would slow the heart's rate and decrease the pulse.

Propranolol (Inderal) is a drug of this kind.

Chapter 3

Adrenergic Blocking Agents

The adrenergic neuron blocking agents appear to act on adrenergic (sympathetic) nerve fibers. Although responses to these drugs are variable, they are chiefly used as **antihypertensive** agents, since they are capable of lowering the blood pressure.

General Drug Action

Adrenergic blocking agents prevent norepinephrine, epinephrine, and adrenergic drugs from producing a response in adrenergic nerve fibers.

Although adrenergic blocking agents would appear to be effective, few of these drugs are used in medicine for these reasons: first, the amount (dose) of the drug necessary to produce *effective* blocking activity often must be so high that undesirable side effects occur; secondly, these drugs do not block *all* adrenergic receptors.

Uses of Adrenergic Blocking Agents

Adrenergic blocking agents have a variety of uses, depending on the *type* of blocking agents used, that is, alpha blocking, beta blocking, or neuron blocking.

As indicated above, the alpha adrenergic blocking agents are mainly used for their vasodilating effects and therefore are beneficial in the treatment of peripheral vascular diseases such as Raynaud's disease. In conditions such as these, there is a reduced blood supply to an extremity. By means of a vasodilating action, these drugs increase the amount of blood in the extremities and are also capable of reducing the blood pressure.

Unfortunately, the vasodilating effect of these drugs has been disappointing. In some cases, there are beneficial results for a time, but in other cases the drugs appear to produce little, if any, effect.

Phentolamine (Regitine) has been useful in the diagnosis and treatment of pheochromocytoma—a catecholamine-secreting tumor of the adrenal gland. This drug may also be added to an intravenous solution containing levarterenol (Levophed) in order to prevent extravasation (leakage) of the intravenous solution into the surrounding tissues. The dose used is not large enough, when diluted in an intravenous solution, to block the effects of levarterenol on peripheral blood vessels. Instead, the drug appears to act locally, around the needle site.

The beta adrenergic blocking agent propranolol (Inderal) is useful in treating cardiac arrhythmias such as extrasystoles, paroxysmal atrial tachycardia, and atrial fibrillation. This drug has also proved useful in the treatment of ventricular tachycardia, a life-threatening arrhythmia, when cardioversion methods are not available.

The adrenergic neuron blocking agents guanethidine (Ismelin) and methyldopa (Aldomet) are used only to treat hypertension. The rauwolfia alkaloids are used in the treatment of hypertension and have also proved of value in the treatment of some mild forms of anxiety and some psychoses, although other agents, such as the tranquilizers, are generally used in psychiatry.

Side Effects of Adrenergic Blocking Agents

The side effects of the adrenergic blocking agents depend on the type of drug used.

ALPHA ADRENERGIC BLOCKING AGENTS: nausea, vomiting, tachycardia, diarrhea, postural hypotension

BETA ADRENERGIC BLOCKING AGENTS: bradycardia, respiratory difficulty in patients with asthma or a history of asthma, nausea, vomiting, diarrhea

ADRENERGIC NEURON BLOCKING AGENTS: orthostatic and postural hypotension, diarrhea, sedation; mental depression and nasal stuffiness may occur during administration of rauwolfia alkaloids.

Clinical Considerations

As with any drug, side effects must be reported to the attending physician. Orthostatic and postural hypotension (see below) may disappear with continued therapy. The physician may wish to continue drug therapy despite the appearance of these side effects. However, proper measures should be taken to eliminate, as much as possible, any danger.

Orthostatic and postural *hypo*tension occur when the patient arises suddenly from a sitting or lying position or shifts position after standing in one place for a prolonged period. The cause may be drugs or some physiological mechanism.

In order to minimize these symptoms:

1. instruct the patient to rise from a sitting or lying position *slowly*. Patients should avoid standing for long periods. This is rarely a problem in the hospital setting, but should be included in discharge teaching plans.
2. place the call bell nearby, and instruct the patient to call for assistance in getting in and out of bed or chair.
3. have the patient sit on the edge of the bed for a short period of time before standing. This will often alleviate these side effects during ambulation. If lightheadedness persists, the patient should not be allowed to walk unless assisted by hospital personnel. In rising from a chair, the patient should stand for the time necessary for the symptoms to disappear.
4. the patient should receive adequate instruction regarding drugs that can cause orthostatic and/or postural hypotension. This includes warnings about sudden exercise, prolonged periods of standing, and sudden changes in the posture.

It may also be necessary to take the blood pressure and pulse when the patient is sitting on the edge of the bed or standing erect, especially if the symptoms persist.

Patients receiving adrenergic neuron blocking agents for the control of hypertension should have their blood pressure and pulse checked. The frequency depends on dose, drug, route, and the patient's response to therapy. Other factors may also alter the number of times this nursing measure is performed. Patients receiving antihypertensive drugs for the first time may require blood pressure and pulse determinations every 2-6 hours, whereas patients who have attained a relatively stable condition might require these measurements only once or twice a day, unless ordered otherwise by the physician. Here again, clinical judgment is important, since it may be necessary to increase the frequency should the patient begin to develop side effects or show a change (increase or decrease) in these vital signs.

Patients receiving alpha adrenergic blocking agents for peripheral vascular diseases should be observed for increased warmth, improvement in color, and relief of pain in the extremities affected by the disease. Since relief may be only temporary, the patient should be observed for a return of symptoms, that is, complaints of pain or discomfort, as well as pale, cool extremities. Since an increase or decrease of symptoms during drug therapy is, in most instances, gradual, the patient's judgment is of greatest importance. Most patients are aware of obvious changes in their condition, and if the patient appears reliable he should be asked about the color and temperature (warmth, coolness) of the involved extremities at least once a day. Clinical judgment is important, since some patients may be upset by questions regarding pain, discomfort, color, and temperature whereas others are cooperative in answering questions and appreciate interest in their problems.

Patients receiving a beta adrenergic blocking agent for the treatment of cardiac arrhythmias are usually placed in specialized units such as a coronary care unit. When a patient receives propranolol (Inderal) intravenously, cardiac monitoring is advisable during administration. When the drug is given orally for a less serious cardiac arrhythmia, cardiac monitoring usually is not necessary, but the patient should be carefully observed for the appearance of side effects, as well as for changes in pulse rate and quality.

The rauwolfia alkaloids and methyldopa (Aldomet) may cause sedation in some patients. It is possible to anticipate the problems that can occur by first noting the degree of sedation and then taking steps to prevent accidents. Depending on the degree of sedation the patient may require:

1. assistance in and out of bed
2. supervision while smoking (if smoking is allowed)
3. removal of obstacles (chairs, footstools, slippers, etc.) around or near the bed

These drugs are also capable of causing mental depression in some individuals. Should this be apparent, the physician should be informed immediately and this fact documented in the patient's record. Severe mental depression may require *frequent* observation of the patient.

Table 3-1.

ADRENERGIC BLOCKING AGENTS

Generic Name	Trade Name	Uses	Side Effects	Dose Ranges
guanethidine	Ismelin	moderate to severe hypertension	dizziness, weakness, orthostatic and postural hypotension, bradycardia, diarrhea, edema, nausea, vomiting	10-50 mg. daily orally
methyldopa	Aldomet	same as guanethidine	same as guanethidine	250 mg.-2 Grams daily, orally; 250-500 mg. q6h I.V.
phenoxybenzamine	Dibenzyline	peripheral vascular diseases	nasal congestion, postural hypotension, dizziness, tachycardia, dryness of the mouth	10-60 mg. daily orally in single or divided doses
phentolamine	Regitine	diagnosis and medical management of pheochromocytoma, prevention of necrosis and severe vasoconstriction during administration of levarterenol (Levophed)	hypotension, tachycardia, nausea, nasal congestion, vomiting	for pheochromocytoma: 50 mg. 4-6 times daily orally. May also be administered before and during surgical removal. For infusions of levarterenol: 5 mg. added to the infusion
propranolol	Inderal	cardiac arrhythmias	hypotension, asystole, bradycardia, circulatory collapse, bronchospasm, dyspnea, nausea, vomiting, vertigo, mental confusion	10-40 mg. T.I.D., Q.I.D. orally; 1-3 mg. I.V. PATIENT SHOULD BE MONITORED DURING AND AFTER I.V. ADMINISTRATION
rauwolfia	Raudixin, Rautina	mild hypertension, mild anxiety states	nausea, fatigue, nasal congestion, diarrhea, headache, bradycardia, weight gain, muscular pain	50-400 mg. daily orally in single or divided doses

Table 3-1. (*Continued*)

Generic Name	Trade Name	Uses	Side Effects ♣	Dose Ranges
rescinnamine	Moderil	same as rauwolfia	same as rauwolfia	250-500 mcg. daily orally
reserpine	Serpasil, Rau-sed	same as rauwolfia	same as rauwolfia	100 mcg.-1 mg. daily orally in 2-3 divided doses
syrosingopine	Singoserp	same as rauwolfia	same as rauwolfia	500 mcg.-3 mg. daily orally
tolazoline	Priscoline	peripheral vascular disorders	flushing, tachycardia, nausea, tingling of extremities	25-50 mg. 4-6 times daily orally; 25-75 mg. Q.I.D. I.M., S.C., I.V.

Cholinergic drugs **mimic** the actions of the parasympathetic nervous system. They are also called **parasympathomimetic** drugs.

Types of Cholinergic Drugs

There are two types of cholinergic drugs:

1. those which act like (or mimic the action of) the neurohormone acetylcholine. These are called **direct-acting** cholinergic drugs
2. those which inhibit or inactivate acetylcholinesterase. These are called **indirect-acting** cholinergic drugs.

The direct-acting cholinergic drugs, for example bethanechol (Urecholine), act like the neurohormone acetylcholine. The indirect-acting cholinergic drugs, for example neostigmine (Prostigmin), prevent acetylcholinesterase from inactivating acetylcholine. Regardless of the type of cholinergic drug used, the results will basically be the same.

General Drug Action

There are two neurohormones released at nerve endings of (1) parasympathetic nerve fibers, (2) some nerve endings in the sympathetic nervous system, and (3) skeletal muscles. These neurohormones are **acetyl-**

Chapter 4

Cholinergic Drugs

choline and **acetylcholinesterase.** Acetylcholine is abbreviated as ACh and acetylcholinesterase as AChE.

High-powered (electron) microscopes have revealed an infinitesimal space between nerve endings and between nerve endings and effector organs (muscles, cells, glands). In order for a nerve impulse to be transmitted across this "space," a substance called a **neurohumoral transmitter** is needed. In the sympathetic nervous system norepinephrine and epinephrine are neurohumoral transmitters; in the parasympathetic nervous system the neurohumoral transmitter is acetylcholine.

Acetylcholine (ACh) and acetylcholinesterase (AChE) are found at the junctions between nerve endings or nerve endings and effector organs. It is believed that these neurohormones are manufactured by special cells located in the nerve ending. Without acetylcholine, a nerve impulse cannot pass *from* the nerve ending *to* the effector organ or structure. After the impulse has crossed over to the effector organ, acetylcholine is *inactivated* by acetylcholinesterase. When the next impulse travels along the nerve fiber, acetylcholine is again released and then inactivated by acetylcholinesterase.

Uses of Cholinergic Drugs

Generally, cholinergic drugs have a limited use in medicine due to the side effects that occur during their administration. However, there are diseases or conditions for which this class of drugs is either definitely indicated or may be of value.

Myasthenia gravis, a disease involving rapid fatigue of the skeletal muscles, may be treated with pyridostigmine (Mestinon) or ambenonium (Mytelase). The dose of these preparations must be adjusted to the patient's need. Neostigmine (Prostigmin), used to diagnose myasthenia gravis, produces a dramatic (though brief) change in the patient's condition *if* the disease is present. Due to the relatively brief duration of action, this drug is not used for daily treatment of this disease.

Cholinergic drugs may also be used to treat paralytic ileus and postoperative atony of the bowel when caused by inadequate parasympathetic stimulation. These drugs are *never* used when the obstruction is thought to be, or is definitely diagnosed as, a mechanical obstruction. After surgery the bowel may lack peristalsis (wave-like motions); gas as well as other products undergoing digestion and absorption are trapped. This results in abdominal distention, pain, and/or tenderness. Since the bowel is under the control of the parasympathetic nervous system (see Table 2-1, pages 9-10), administration of a cholinergic drug, such as bethanechol (Urecholine) *may* relieve this condition.

Urinary retention may also be treated with cholinergic drugs, providing this condition is *not* caused by a mechanical obstruction, for example enlargement of the prostate. Urinary retention may occur in postoperative and postpartum patients; the physician may elect to use drugs, such as bethanechol (Urecholine) or neostigmine (Prostigmin), rather than bladder catheterization.

The parasympathetic nervous system partly controls the process of micturition (which is both voluntary and involuntary) by constricting the detrusor muscle and relaxing the bladder sphincter (see Table 2-1, pages 9-10). Administration of a cholinergic drug *may* result in the spontaneous passage of urine.

Natural cholinergic alkaloids, for example pilocarpine and physostigmine (Eserine), are used to produce *miosis* or contraction of the pupil of the eye. This is useful in the treatment of glaucoma and in counteracting the mydriatic (dilating) effect of atropine, when atropine is used for eye examinations.

Side Effects of Cholinergic Drugs

Cholinergic drugs do not affect one specific area of the body, that is, they are not selective in action. Instead, they affect many organs and structures and cause a variety of side effects, namely: nausea, vomiting, diarrhea, abdominal cramping, bradycardia, diaphoresis, and dilatation of blood vessels. Also, flushing, a feeling of warmth, salivation, difficulty in breathing, and miosis may be seen. These side effects, which will appear along with the beneficial effects, limit the usefulness of cholinergic agents.

Clinical Considerations

When a cholinergic drug, such as pyridostigmine (Mestinon), is given to a patient with myasthenia gravis, the patient must be observed for drug effects, that is, the patient's response to the drug. This will indicate whether the dose is too large, too small, or correct. Regulation of dosage is important to keep the disease symptoms from incapacitating the patient.

Although this is not possible in all cases, symptoms of many patients are fairly well controlled, once the optimum drug dose is reached. In many patients the drug must be regulated throughout their lifetime. At the beginning, it may be difficult to achieve optimum results with drug therapy; consequently signs of drug overdose or underdose may be seen. Signs of overdose are muscle rigidity and spasm, salivation, and clenching of the jaw. Signs of underdose are the signs of the disease itself, namely rapid fatigability of muscles, ptosis of the eyelids, and difficulty in breathing. If *any* of these symptoms occur, the physician should be notified, as an antidote might be necessary in cases of drug overdose, or more medication and other measures may be required for drug underdose. In order to aid the physician in determining the dose that will relieve the symptoms of disease, an accurate record of the patient's response to the drug should be kept.

When a cholinergic drug is administered to treat paralytic ileus or postoperative atony of the bowel, the patient should be observed for drug effects, namely passage of flatus, decrease in size of the abdomen, and decrease in abdominal tenderness. These facts are important since if the drug does not produce results, it may be necessary to try other measures.

After administration of the drug the patient should be checked in one-half hour, and hourly thereafter. In some instances, more frequent observations may be necessary. Any increase in pain and abdominal rigidity must be reported to the physician *at once*, since a more serious problem may be present.

If a patient receives a cholinergic drug for the treatment of urinary retention, it should be remembered that spontaneous micturition may occur in 5-15 minutes after parenteral administration. Consequently, the call light should be within easy reach and the urinal or bedpan nearby. If the patient is able to secure these utensils from the bedside stand, it is important that they can be obtained easily and safely. Other patients may not be able to reach these utensils, requiring prompt answering of the call light. In some instances it may be necessary to stay with the patient. The same measures apply to patients receiving an oral form of the drug; drug response usually occurs in 30+ minutes.

In all cases, the amount of urine of each voiding should be measured, and the patient placed on a measured intake and output.

If cholinergic drugs are given by the subcutaneous route, the patient should be observed for bradycardia, hypotension, abdominal cramps, sweating, and flushing of the skin. Appearance of these side effects should be reported to the physician *at once*. Severe episodes of hypotension, diarrhea, and abdominal cramps may require the administration of a cholinergic blocking agent—such as atropine—to abolish parasympathetic stimulation. Oral administration of these drugs is less likely to cause side effects.

Ophthalmic preparations, such as pilocarpine, may be administered to the hospitalized patient by the nurse or by the patient himself. In some instances the patient may have been using the drug for months or years and the physician may approve of self-administration. When this is so stated on the order sheet, the medication can be left at the patient's bedside. At other times the nurse will be responsible for administration. Great care must be taken that the proper dose (usually expressed in drops) is administered and that the drug is placed in the conjunctival sac. The hand holding the eyedropper should be supported against the patient's forehead. The tip of the dropper must *never* touch any part of the patient's eye.

Even though the patient is allowed to administer his own eye medication, he should be checked to be sure the medication is taken properly and at the right time.

Discharge Teaching
Discharge teaching should include:

1. teaching the patient the signs of drug overdose and underdose
2. showing the patient how to keep a record of his response to the drug
3. indicating to the patient the importance of keeping clinic or office appointments

Table 4-1.
CHOLINERGIC DRUGS

Generic Name	Trade Name	Uses	Side Effects	Dose Ranges
ambenonium	Mytelase	myasthenia gravis	signs of cholinergic stimulation: nausea, vomiting, abdominal cramps, urinary urgency, miosis, sweating, muscular weakness, salivation	DOSE INDIVIDUALIZED: 5-200 mg. or more daily orally
bethanechol	Urecholine	postoperative abdominal distention, urinary retention	abdominal cramps, flushing of skin, sweating, diarrhea, headache, hypotension	10-30 mg. T.I.D., Q.I.D. orally; 2.5-5 mg. S.C. DO NOT give I.M.
edrophonium	Tensilon	antidote for curariform drugs, diagnosis of myasthenia gravis	bronchospasm, salivation, bradycardia	10 mg. I.V. as antidote for curariform drugs, diagnostic agent for myasthenia gravis
neostigmine	Prostigmin	screening test for early pregnancy, treatment of delayed menses, myasthenia gravis, postoperative distention, urinary retention	same as ambenonium	myasthenia gravis: 15-30 mg. T.I.D. orally; postoperative distention: 1 ml. 1:4000 S.C., I.M.; urinary retention: 1-2 ml. 1:2000 S.C., I.M.; amenorrhea: 2 ml. 1:2000 S.C. daily × 3
physostigmine	Eserine	glaucoma, antagonize mydriatic effect of atropine		1-2 gtt. of ½% solution into conjunctival sac several times daily. Ointment form may be used h.s.
pilocarpine		same as physostigmine		1-2 gtt. of 1% or 2% solution into conjunctival sac several times daily
pyridostigmine	Mestinon	myasthenia gravis	epigastric distress, abdominal or muscle cramps, muscular weakness, diarrhea	DOSE INDIVIDUALIZED: 360 mg.-1.5 Grams daily in divided doses orally

Cholinergic blocking agents are also called **parasympathomimetic blocking agents.** Some of these drugs were known to the ancient Greeks and Hindus, who used them for relieving abdominal pain and discomfort. Medieval women used belladonna drops in their eyes to enlarge the pupils—a sign of beauty. This is most probably the origin of the name of the drug, since in Italian, belladonna means "beautiful lady."

Types of Cholinergic Blocking Agents

Cholinergic blocking agents may be natural (that is, obtained from plants), semisynthetic, or synthetic.

Belladonna (also called "deadly nightshade") is a plant of the nightshade (Solanaceae) family which also includes potatoes and eggplants. The drug is prepared from the leaves of the plant in the form of an extract or tincture. Belladonna contains **atropine** and **scopolamine,** which are alkaloids (chemicals that have been extracted from part of the plant) of belladonna. Scopolamine is also obtained from other members of the solanaceae family, such as henbane.

In order to decrease some of the undesirable side effects of atropine and scopolamine, semisynthetic derivatives were developed.

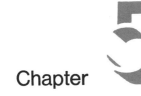

Chapter

Cholinergic Blocking Agents

An example of this type of cholinergic blocking agent is atropine methylnitrate.

The synthetic cholinergic blocking agents were developed to produce drugs with more *selective* action, rather than the *generalized* action of the naturally occurring alkaloids. Examples of synthetic cholinergic blocking agents are pipenzolate (Piptal) and oxyphencyclimine (Daricon).

A drug having selective action is one which acts in one or two areas or structures of the body, such as the gastrointestinal tract. A drug with generalized action affects many organs and structures of the body.

General Drug Action

Cholinergic blocking agents **inhibit** the action of acetylcholine, therefore nerve impulses cannot be transmitted from nerve fibers to other nerve fibers or effector organs. These drugs are also capable of reversing the action of cholinergic drugs.

Cholinergic blocking agents produce the following responses:

CENTRAL NERVOUS SYSTEM—dreamless sleep, drowsiness. Atropine *may* produce mild stimulation

EYE—mydriasis (dilatation of the pupil) and cycloplegia (paralysis of accommodation or ability to focus the eye) when applied topically. This effect is minimal when these drugs are administered by the oral or parenteral routes

RESPIRATORY TRACT—dry secretions of the mouth, nose, throat, bronchi; relax smooth muscles of the bronchi with slight bronchodilatation

GASTROINTESTINAL TRACT—inhibit secretions of the stomach, decrease gastric motility

URINARY TRACT—dilate smooth muscles of the ureters and kidney pelvis

HEART—increase in pulse rate (atropine)

These responses may vary, according to the dose and route. Occasionally scopolamine may cause excitement, restlessness, and delirium, which are thought to be drug idiosyncrasies.

Uses of Cholinergic Blocking Agents

Atropine and scopolamine may be used as preoperative preparations for general anesthesia because of their effect on the respiratory tract. These drugs inhibit the formation of excessive secretions that occurs during the administration of gas anesthetics, which are irritating to the respiratory tract. Since the anesthetized patient cannot swallow or cough (these reflexes disappear during general anesthesia) to clear the bronchi and trachea, these secretions would flow into the lungs, thus blocking the small air sacs (alveoli) where oxygen is exchanged for carbon dioxide.

These drugs are sometimes included in OTC (*over-the-counter* or nonprescription) products available for the relief of colds or seasonal allergies.

Cholinergic blocking agents are used in the form of

ophthalmic solutions prior to examination of the eyes. Mydriasis (dilatation of the pupil) allows examination of the retina and other structures of the eye. These drugs may also be used in the treatment of keratitis and acute iritis. In some instances, they may be alternated with miotic agents (drugs that decrease the pupil size) for preventing or breaking adhesions between the iris and the lens.

Atropine may be administered to cardiac patients with bradycardia and associated hypotension that may occur after an acute myocardial infarction. Atropine will usually increase the heart rate, followed by a rise in blood pressure.

Atropine is used in the treatment of poisoning with insecticides containing organophosphorus compounds. This drug is also indicated in the reversal of the effects of cholinergic agents.

Cholinergic blocking agents are frequently used in the treatment of gastrointestinal diseases and disorders such as peptic ulcer, spastic colon, pylorospasm, gastritis, and ulcerative colitis. These drugs may be used in conjunction with other medical management including dietary restrictions, adequate rest, and other drugs such as barbiturates, tranquilizers, and antacids.

Cholinergic blocking agents may be used in the treatment of enuresis (bedwetting) in children, as well as in the treatment of renal colic. By themselves they are of little value for relieving the pain of renal colic, but administered with a narcotic they may contribute to the alleviation of symptoms. These drugs have also been used in the treatment of dysmenorrhea (painful menses), but consistent use for dysmenorrhea has been disappointing.

Side Effects of Cholinergic Blocking Agents

Dryness of the mouth with resultant difficulty in swallowing, blurred vision, and an aversion to light (photophobia) are the most common side effects of cholinergic blocking agents. In normal doses, some degree of dryness of the mouth almost always occurs.

Constipation may occur in those patients taking the drug on a regular basis. This side effect does not occur in patients receiving the drug on a one-time basis, such as part of preoperative medication.

Drowsiness may occur, but there are times when this effect may be desirable, such as after the administration of preoperative medications.

Patients with prostatic hypertrophy should be given these drugs with caution, since urinary retention can occur. This caution also applies to OTC preparations containing atropine, scopolamine, or other cholinergic blocking agents. This precaution is on the label of OTC products, but unfortunately few people read the labels of drugs purchased without a prescription.

Cholinergic blocking agents are contraindicated in patients with glaucoma, since continued use of preparations containing atropine and scopolamine may lead to attacks of acute glaucoma. This precaution is also stated on the label of OTC's. Unfortunately, glaucoma in its early stages may go unnoticed and the individual may be unaware of the disease.

Clinical Considerations

The dose of cholinergic blocking agents, especially those in liquid form, must be measured *accurately*. This is especially important when these drugs are prepared for administration to children.

```
5/24
H. Atropine sulfate gr. 1/200
Stat.
                    Dr. Greene
```

```
9/12
H. Atropine sulfate 0.004 mg.
7.30 a.m.
                    Dr. James
```

```
11/26  Tincture of belladonna
gtt. X T.I.D., p.c.
                    Dr. Case
```

Some of the side effects that may be bothersome for some patients can be relieved. For the patients taking these drugs several times a day, frequent sips of cool water, hard candy slowly dissolved in the mouth, and the frequent use of mouthwash will help relieve the dry mouth often experienced. (However, there may be instances when excessive fluids or candy may not be allowed.) To relieve photophobia, dark glasses may be worn. Drapes or venetian blinds can be partly closed and overhead lights turned off. Soft, indirect lighting or well-shaded lamps are usually well tolerated.

Episodes of constipation should be reported, since a mild laxative or stool softener may be necessary. The patient should be encouraged to discuss any discomforts or complaints with his physician. The physician will then be able to judge the emotional impact (if present) of these side effects on the particular patient, and decide whether or not therapy with a particular drug should be continued.

The cardiac patient receiving atropine for episodes of bradycardia and associated hypotension should be placed on a cardiac monitor during and after administration of the drug. The monitor should be watched for a change in pulse rate. Tachycardia and/or other arrhythmias must be reported *at once*, since other drugs or medical management may be necessary on an emergency basis.

Children who receive *normal* doses of scopolamine, for example as part of preoperative medication, may show signs of dilated pupils, slight fever, and a flushing of the skin, sometimes referred to as a "scopolamine flush." When this occurs, the surgeon or anesthetist should be notified. These symptoms are usually transitory and do not necessarily require cancellation of surgery.

Discharge Teaching

Patients taking these medications after discharge from the hospital should have drug side effects fully explained. Failure to explain drug side effects may promote undue worry in the uninformed patient!

Patients should be warned of the drowsiness that may occur during the use of these drugs, and that the operation of a motor vehicle or heavy machinery may be hazardous. Elderly patients using the ophthalmic form should be warned of the hazards of the impairment of vision that may be present. Blurring of vision could be an added danger when the patient is walking, using stairs, etc.

Although the belladonna alkaloids have a fairly wide margin of safety when taken as directed, overdose and/or drug idiosyncrasy can occur. Overdose, sometimes referred to as "atropine poisoning," occasionally happens. Young children may be given an accidental overdose by parents who either increase the dose prescribed or inaccurately measure the dose. Elderly patients may experience difficulty in measuring liquid medications. And, as with any substance, young children may accidentally find and ingest medications that are not kept in a secure place.

The signs of atropine poisoning are:

1. dryness and burning of the mouth; marked thirst
2. hot, dry, and flushed skin
3. rash
4. rise in body temperature
5. weak and rapid pulse
6. restlessness, weakness, mental confusion
7. urinary urgency, urinary retention, difficulty in voiding

Table 5-1.
CHOLINERGIC BLOCKING AGENTS

GENERIC NAME	TRADE NAME	USES	SIDE EFFECTS	DOSE RANGES
atropine		eye examinations; treatment of: peptic ulcer, eye disorders, urinary frequency, ureteral colic, bladder spasms; preoperative preparation for anesthesia; treatment of insecticide poisoning	dryness of mouth, constipation, C.N.S. stimulation, flushing of skin, urinary retention, tachycardia, mydriasis and cycloplegia when applied topically	0.4-0.6 mg. S.C., I.M., I.V.; 250 mcg. orally
belladonna		disorders of the G.I. and G.U. tracts	same as atropine but less intense	belladonna tincture: 0.3-1.0 ml. orally (may be ordered in drops)
dicyclomine	Bentyl	G.I. disorders such as irritable colon, peptic ulcer, ulcerative colitis	euphoria, dizziness	20-40 mg. orally, I.M., T.I.D., Q.I.D.; CHILD: 5 mg. 3-4 times daily I.M., orally

Table 5-1. (*Continued*)

Generic Name	Trade Name	Uses	Side Effects	Dose Ranges
diphemanil	Prantal	same as dicyclomine	dryness of mouth, urinary retention, blurred vision, constipation, tachycardia, dizziness	100 mg. q4-6h orally (between meals); 0.5 mg./Kg. S.C., I.M.
hexocyclium	Tral	same as dicyclomine	same as diphemanil	25 mg. Q.I.D. orally
homatropine	Novatrin	gastrointestinal spasm, hyperchlorhydria	diarrhea, visual disturbances, dryness of mouth and other atropine-like effects	2.5-5 mg. T.I.D., a.c. orally
isopropamide	Darbid	peptic ulcer, hyperchlorhydria	dryness of mouth, urinary retention, blurred vision	5 mg. q12h orally
methantheline	Banthine	same as dicyclomine plus treatment of urinary frequency and enuresis	same as diphemanil	50-100 mg. T.I.D., Q.I.D. orally; 50 mg. I.M., I.V.
methscopolamine	Pamine	same as dicyclomine	same as diphemanil	12.5-20 mg. a.c. and h.s. orally; 250 mcg.-1 mg. q6-8h I.M., S.C.
methylatropine nitrate	Metropine	gastrointestinal hypermotility	same as atropine	1-2.5 mg. q3-4h orally
oxyphencyclimine	Daricon, Setrol	same as dicyclomine	same as diphemanil	20-50 mg. daily in divided doses orally
pipenzolate	Piptal	same as dicyclomine	same as diphemanil	5 mg. T.I.D., a.c. and 10 mg. h.s. orally
propantheline	Pro-Banthine	same as methantheline	same as diphemanil	15 mg. T.I.D., 30 mg. h.s., up to 60 mg. Q.I.D. orally; 30 mg. I.M., I.V. q6h
scopolamine		preoperative preparation for anesthesia, motion sickness, eye diseases and disorders	disorientation, delirium, tachycardia, dryness of mouth, mydriasis	300 mcg.-1 mg. T.I.D., Q.I.D. orally; 0.3-0.6 mg. S.C., I.M., I.V.

The Narcotic Analgesics

Narcotics are probably one of the oldest group of drugs known to man, their use being recorded in ancient writings dating back several thousand years. The opiate narcotics, such as morphine, codeine, and heroin are obtained from the unripe pod of a certain species of the poppy plant—Papaver somniferum. Turkey and the countries of the Far East produce most of the raw opium used in the United States, by pharmaceutical companies for legal medical products, and by criminal factions interested in the illegal buying and selling of narcotics.

Pain is a sensation, just as heat and cold are sensations. The sudden occurrence of pain that lasts for short periods of time is different from pain that has persisted for a long period of time. The type of pain experienced will sometimes determine the type of **analgesic** prescribed by the physician.

Types of Narcotic Analgesics

There are two types of narcotic analgesics: (1) the **opiates** such as morphine and codeine and (2) the **synthetic** narcotics such as meperidine (Demerol). Morphine is considered the prototype or "model" narcotic,

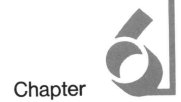

Chapter **35**

The Narcotic Analgesics and the Narcotic Antagonists

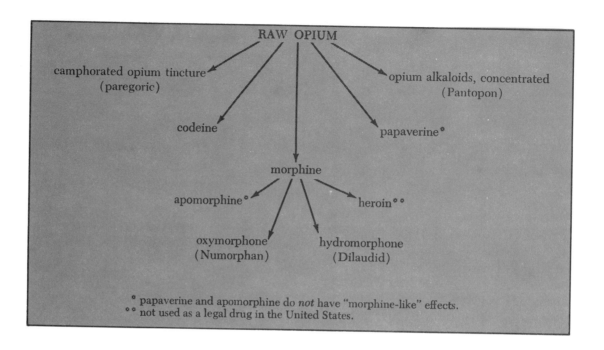

RAW OPIUM

camphorated opium tincture (paregoric)

opium alkaloids, concentrated (Pantopon)

codeine

papaverine°

morphine

apomorphine°

heroin°°

oxymorphone (Numorphan)

hydromorphone (Dilaudid)

° papaverine and apomorphine do *not* have "morphine-like" effects.
°° not used as a legal drug in the United States.

and the actions and uses of other narcotic analgesics are usually compared to the actions and uses of morphine.

The white poppy is the source of the *opiate* narcotics. The unripe seed pods are cut and the dried juice or resin is collected. This sticky brown mass is *raw opium,* from which the natural narcotics are obtained.

Raw opium contains about twenty alkaloids, many of which have no value in medicine. Above is a chart showing the preparations obtained from raw opium that are used in medicine.

The first *synthetic* narcotic analgesic was meperidine (Demerol). Although this drug does not chemically resemble morphine, its action is very similar to that of morphine. Other synthetic narcotics soon followed, but like morphine, they all have addiction potential.

General Drug Action

Morphine, as well as other narcotic analgesics, relieves pain, but exactly *how* is not fully understood. Morphine may dull the ability of the patient to perceive pain, perhaps by depressing the thalamus and sensory cortex of the central nervous system. Morphine may also act on areas of the brain that are responsible for fear, anxiety, and pain, thereby allowing the patient to tolerate pain. Morphine is an extremely effective analgesic for many types of moderate to severe pain.

Morphine affects many areas of the body:

CONSCIOUSNESS—drowsiness, euphoria, sleep, and mental clouding usually occur. Codeine is less likely to depress the consciousness; however, some patients will experience these effects to a lesser degree. The synthetic narcotics also vary in their effect on the consciousness, but most synthetics, such as meperidine (Demerol), appear to have a somewhat less depressing effect.

EYE—morphine and the other opiates cause constriction (miosis) of the pupil. Codeine has little or no effect on the pupil in lower doses. The synthetic narcotics appear to have minimal effect on the pupil, although some patients may experience slight mydriasis (dilatation of the pupil).

RESPIRATORY—the respiratory rate and depth is depressed by morphine and to a varying degree by the other opiates. Synthetic narcotics also depress the respiratory center.

COUGH REFLEX—morphine and other opiates have **antitussive** (depression of the cough reflex) action because of their ability to depress the cough reflex center of the medulla. Codeine is used as an antitussive agent.

MEDULLA—the chemoreceptor trigger zone (CTZ) may be stimulated, resulting in nausea and vomiting. But the narcotic analgesics also depresss the vomiting center. Therefore nausea and vomiting may or may not occur. Apomorphine, an opiate with no narcotic-like activity, acts only on the CTZ, producing immediate emptying of stomach contents.

PITUITARY—the opiates and synthetic narcotics stimulate the release of antidiuretic hormone (ADH) resulting in a decrease in urinary output. This decrease may or may not be significant.

GASTROINTESTINAL TRACT—morphine slows peristalsis in the stomach, duodenum, and small and large intestines. The emptying time of the stomach is delayed and the digestive process slowed. Gastric, pancreatic, and biliary secretions are decreased. This results in constipation and anorexia. Other opiates and the synthetic narcotics appear to be constipating, especially when taken for a few days or more.

GALLBLADDER AND COMMON BILE DUCT—spasms of the biliary tract may occur in some patients during the administration of morphine. Other opiates and the synthetic narcotics have a lesser effect on the biliary tract.

GENITOURINARY TRACT—narcotic analgesics induce spasms of the ureter. Urinary urgency may also result due to the action of these drugs on the detrusor muscle of the bladder. Some patients may experience difficulty in voiding due to contraction of the bladder sphincter.

The ability of the narcotic analgesics to relieve pain depends on several factors—the drug, the dose, the patient, and the type of pain. For mild pain, the physician will usually prescribe a non-narcotic analgesic. In some cases of mild pain a narcotic analgesic such as codeine may be necessary. Moderate to severe pain usually requires drugs such as morphine, meperidine (Demerol), alphaprodine (Nisentil), anileridine (Leritine), or any of the other narcotic analgesics.

Uses of the Narcotic Analgesics

The chief use of the narcotic analgesics is to relieve pain; however, they also have other uses. Papaverine is an alkaloid of opium but does *not* have morphine-like action. Papaverine does not have analgesic properties or addiction potential. This drug exerts its chief effect on smooth muscles of blood vessels, resulting in vasodilatation. Papaverine is classified as a vasodilator and not as a narcotic analgesic.

Paregoric (camphorated opium tincture) and opium, powdered, U.S.P., are used as antidiarrheal agents. The chief constituent of raw opium is morphine. It is

the effect of morphine on the gastrointestinal tract—the slowing of peristalsis—that makes paregoric and opium, powdered, U.S.P., effective antidiarrheal agents. The opium, powdered, U.S.P., is added to other drugs to soothe as well as slow the small and large intestines. Examples of these combinations are Donnagel-PG (kaolin, pectin, hyoscyamine, atropine, hyoscine, and opium, powdered, U.S.P.) and Pecto-Kaolin (kaolin, pectin, and opium, powdered, U.S.P.). Paregoric and opium, powdered, U.S.P., have addiction potential.

Apomorphine is a semisynthetic derivative of morphine. This drug has *very little* analgesic activity but does have a strong stimulating effect on the vomiting center. Apomorphine is classed as an **emetic**—a drug that causes or has the ability to cause a patient to vomit. This drug has limited use in medicine but may be employed in the emergency treatment of poison ingestion. Apomorphine or any emetic is contraindicated in the following: ingestion of petroleum products (gasoline, kerosene, cleaning fluids), corrosive acids or alkali, and caustic substances; and in comatose or semicomatose patients who may aspirate vomitus.

Alphaprodine (Nisentil) is a congener (a drug that chemically resembles another drug) of meperidine (Demerol). This drug is a short-acting narcotic analgesic that may be used for minor orthopedic procedures, urological procedures, minor surgical procedures, and as part of the preoperative medication for major surgery.

Other synthetic analgesics are anileridine (Leritine), levorphanol (Levo-Dromoran), fentanyl (Sublimaze), and methadone (Dolophine). Fentanyl is a potent drug that may be combined with droperidol (Inapsine) to produce anesthesia. This type of anesthesia is called **neuroleptanalgesia.** Fentanyl may also be used preoperatively as well as during the immediate postoperative period. Methadone (Dolophine) is used in the detoxification and maintenance treatment of heroin and opiate addiction. It may also be used as an analgesic for the relief of severe pain.

Codeine, hydromorphone (Dilaudid), oxymorphone (Numorphan), oxycodone, and opium alkaloids, concentrated (Pantopon) are opium derivatives used for their analgesic activity. Codeine is a mild analgesic, when compared to morphine and other opiates, and is of little value in the relief of severe pain. Codeine may be combined with other analgesics, for example Codasa (aspirin and codeine) and Empirin Compound with codeine phosphate (aspirin, caffeine, phenacetin, and codeine). Oxycodone may be combined with aspirin, phenacetin, and caffeine (Percodan) and like codeine is an analgesic for mild to moderate pain. Hydromorphone (Dilaudid), oxymorphone (Numorphan), and opium alkaloids, concentrated (Pantopon) are similar to morphine in analgesic activity, and are used in the relief of moderate to severe pain.

Some narcotics, such as codeine, are utilized for their antitussive effect. These drugs may be used alone or more commonly as components in tablets or syrups.

Side Effects of Narcotic Analgesics

The side effects that may occur with the administration of narcotic analgesics depend on several factors: (1) the patient, (2) the dose administered, (3) the route of administration, (4) the length of time the narcotic has been given (that is, one dose versus administration over a period of days), and (5) at times the disease or general condition of the patient.

Narcotic analgesics are capable of causing drowsiness, euphoria, and sleep, the degree of which will vary. Many times sleep or drowsiness is desirable, for example in the patient who has had major surgery. At times, this side effect may well be undesirable, as in the patient with a head injury being observed for neurological changes, especially the level of consciousness.

Morphine and morphine derivatives cause miosis (pinpoint pupils). Occasionally miosis or mydriasis (dilatation of the pupil) may be seen with the use of meperidine (Demerol), alphaprodine (Nisentil), and anileridine (Leritine).

Suppression of the cough reflex may be undesirable in some patients, for example those who have had chest surgery. In order to avoid this, the physician orders a narcotic analgesic in lower than normal doses.

Respiratory depression, the degree of which will vary, occurs during the administration of all narcotic analgesics.

Nausea and vomiting may occur; the physician should be notified. On occasion, a patient may experience nausea and/or vomiting with one narcotic but not with another.

Hypotension and tachycardia have been known to occur after the administration of meperidine (Demerol) and its congeners. This is more likely to happen if the patient suddenly changes position, especially from a supine to a sitting position. Also, bradycardia can occur during the administration of morphine.

Constipation is relatively common with the long-term administration of the opiates and synthetic narcotics. Anorexia may accompany constipation due to the delaying of the digestive process.

Biliary spasms may be seen in some patients. Usually the patient complains of pain and/or discomfort in the right upper quadrant. Urinary urgency, difficulty in voiding, and a decrease in urinary output may be seen during administration of narcotic analgesics. The decrease in urinary output may be insignificant and pose no problem, except in patients with chronic renal disease. Ureteral spasms may be noted, especially in those with ureteral calculi.

All narcotic analgesics have *addiction potential.* Addiction can occur at varying times and each patient receiving a narcotic should be observed for signs of addiction, especially those patients taking a narcotic for more than 7-10 days.

Clinical Considerations

Narcotics are dangerous drugs, not only because of their addiction potential but also because of their widespread effects on many organs and structures. A narcotic is *never* given without a physician's order. However, the patient in pain should *never* be denied a narcotic because it has addiction potential. Administration of narcotics for several days will not cause addiction! A patient may need a potent analgesic, especially after major surgery. If a patient requests or appears to need a more potent analgesic, the physician should be informed of this problem.

All narcotics are to be kept under lock and key at all times. Narcotics should not be removed from the locked drawer until they are to be administered. Narcotics and the instruments used to administer them (needle and syringe) in parenteral form are not to be left unattended on a counter or table. After use, the needle and syringe must be removed from the patient's environment and destroyed immediately, if disposable. Glass syringes and reusable needles should be returned to the medicine room and stored as per hospital policy. These precautionary measures are taken to prevent illicit acquisition of these materials and/or drugs by addicts. Unfortunately, it is possible to assume a false sense of security in a hospital situation. It must be remembered that *anyone* is capable of taking drugs and/or the instruments used to administer them. This includes physicians, nurses, nurse's aides, orderlies, cleaning personnel, patients, and visitors. When a nurse or physician takes the responsibility of administering a narcotic he or she also assumes the responsibility of following the correct procedures of administration and disposal of the materials used.

The respiratory rate is to be counted *before* a narcotic is administered, due to the depressing effect of these drugs. If the respiratory rate is 10 or below, the drug should be withheld and the physician notified. Twenty to 30 minutes *after* parenteral administration the nurse should check:

1. respiratory rate and depth and pulse
2. general appearance of the patient
3. blood pressure. If the patient appears pale, the pulse is rapid and/or thready, and mild

to moderate diaphoresis is noted, the physician should be notified

4. patient's response to the analgesic effect

If the drug was given intravenously, the patient should be observed during and 10 minutes after administration.

Any occurrence of a decreased respiratory rate requires close nursing supervision until the rate returns to normal. It is necessary to notify the physician, since for some patients this can be a precarious situation. A narcotic antagonist may be needed to reverse the effect of the narcotic. Other medical measures may also be necessary to prevent further complications of a decrease in the respiratory rate and depth.

Since narcotics are administered for pain, they should be given as soon as possible after the patient asks for, or appears to need, an analgesic. The time limit ordered by the physician (that is, q4h, q6h, etc.) must be observed. If the patient requests an analgesic more often than is ordered, the physician should be informed of this problem. The dose of the medication may have to be increased, a different drug may be necessary, a more serious disease process may be present, or addiction may be occurring.

A patient should be told that the medication is for pain. On some occasions, a patient may believe the injection or tablet is for something else besides pain. Anxiety and discomfort may follow, while the patient "waits" for an analgesic. This problem is more likely to occur in patients also receiving tablets or injections for reasons other than pain several times a day.

Anxiety, regardless of the reason, can also *lessen* the effect of a narcotic.

Other Potent Analgesics

There is a newer group of drugs, not classified as narcotics, yet more potent than the non-narcotic analgesics (aspirin and related drugs). This group evolved during a search for drugs that would have analgesic properties similar to morphine and the other opiates, yet *not* have addiction potential.

Pentazocine (Talwin) and methotrimeprazine (Levoprome) are examples of potent analgesics used in the relief of mild to moderate pain.

Pentazocine (Talwin) has (1) a mild depressing effect on the respiration, (2) the ability to reduce gastric secretions, and (3) some sedation qualities. The usual side effects seen are anorexia, nausea, vomiting, and sedation. Hypotension and hypertension, weakness, and visual disturbances may also be seen. The oral form of pentazocine appears to cause fewer side effects than parenteral administration. The latter appears to have more analgesic ability.

Methotrimeprazine (Levoprome) is a phenothiazine derivative (see Chapter 28). Not only an analgesic, as a phenothiazine it will also relieve the anxiety and tension that often accompany pain. Since phenothiazines have antiemetic and tranquilizing properties, this drug may be used in obstetrics, as a preoperative medication, and as a postoperative analgesic and antiemetic.

Hypotension, weakness, dizziness, and euphoria

may be encountered during the use of methotrimeprazine (Levoprome). This drug is given only by the intramuscular route.

Clinical Considerations

Observe the patient for the appearance of side effects. Since hypotension can occur during use of either drug, the blood pressure should be taken *before* parenteral administration. The patient should be checked 20-30 minutes *after* administration, to determine the analgesic effect of the drug as well as the occurrence of hypotension (tachycardia; cold, clammy skin; drop in blood pressure) and other side effects.

In some instances, pain may not be relieved and a narcotic may be necessary.

The Narcotic Antagonists

The word antagonist means "one that goes against." A narcotic *antagonist* abolishes the effects of opiate and opiate-like narcotics.

Types of Narcotic Antagonists

There are two types of narcotic antagonists:

Total antagonists which abolish the effects of an opiate and have *no* other effect on the body. An example of this type is naloxone (Narcan).

Partial antagonists which abolish the effects of an opiate but also have varying degrees of opiate-like activity. Examples of this type are levallorphan (Lorfan) and nalorphine (Nalline).

Table 6-1.
USES OF NARCOTIC ANTAGONISTS

Use	LEVAL-LORPHAN (LORFAN)	NALORPHINE (NALLINE)	NALOXONE (NARCAN)
treatment of *severe* respiratory depression caused by morphine or drugs with morphine-like effects (hydromorphone, meperidine, heroin, methadone, *et al.*)	√	√	√
treatment of *severe* respiratory depression caused by pentazocine (Talwin) or propoxyphene (Darvon)			√
narcotic maintenance programs			√
prophylactically in conjunction *with* narcotics to prevent respiratory depression	√		
treatment of asphyxia of the newborn resulting from the mother receiving a narcotic	√	√	
treatment of respiratory depression when the type of depressant drug is not known			√
diagnosis of narcotic addiction*		√	√

* Use of this method of determining addiction is recommended only when it is important to recognize addiction and other methods of detection are not available.

General Drug Action

Exactly *how* the narcotic antagonists abolish the effect of the opiates is not clearly understood, but it is thought that these drugs compete with the opiates and synthetic narcotics at receptor sites of the respiratory center. A narcotic antagonist displaces the narcotic molecule, thus reversing the effect of the narcotic, namely respiratory depression.

Side Effects of Narcotic Antagonists

Naloxone (Narcan), a total antagonist, has no apparent pharmacological activity in the absence of narcotics. Side effects are rare.

Nalorphine (Nalline), in the absence of narcotics, produces effects similar to morphine, namely, respiratory depression, slight decrease in the pulse, and constriction of the pupils. There may also be signs of anxiety, vivid dreams, hallucinations, nausea, and sweating. When nalorphine is given to patients who have received a narcotic and are experiencing narcotic side effects, the effects of the narcotic will be abolished.

Levallorphan (Lorfan), in the absence of narcotics, may produce respiratory depression. When it is given to patients who have received a narcotic the results are the same as nalorphine (Nalline).

Clinical Considerations

The dose of the narcotic antagonists is usually based on the amount or dose of the narcotic, if known. In some cases this may not be known and the physician may order a repeat dose of the antagonist.

The following points are to be considered when a patient is given a narcotic antagonist:

1. closely observe the patient for the abolishment of the effects of the narcotic. This includes counting the respirations, taking the pulse and blood pressure, observing for mental changes, checking the pupil size.
2. if the drugs are administered intravenously, the antagonistic effect will be noticeable in 2-5 minutes. When they are administered subcutaneously or intramuscularly the effect should occur in 5-20 minutes.
3. observe the patient for the appearance of narcotic withdrawal symptoms if addiction is suspected. These symptoms include: profuse perspiration, tearing, nausea, vomiting, gooseflesh, yawning, dilated pupils. The intensity of withdrawal signs may vary.
4. if narcotic overdose or idiosyncrasy is the *suspected* cause of respiratory depression, a narcotic antagonist is administered. Accurate observations must be made as to the patient's response to the drug, as a narcotic may *not* be the cause of respiratory depression and other disease processes may be present. If this is the case, side effects of the antagonist (unless naloxone is used), particularly increased respiratory depression, will appear.
5. the effects of narcotic antagonists usually last 1-4 hours; therefore the effect of the antagonist may wear off *before* the effect of the narcotic. Observation for 4 or more hours is necessary.

Table 6-2.
POTENT ANALGESICS AND NARCOTIC ANTAGONISTS

Generic Name	Trade Name	Uses	Side Effects	Dose Ranges
Narcotic Analgesics				
alphaprodine	Nisentil	analgesia, preoperative preparation, analgesia during labor and prior to urological and minor surgical procedures	same as morphine	10-30 mg. I.V.; 10-60 mg. S.C.
anileridine	Leritine	analgesia, preoperative preparation, analgesia during labor	same as morphine	25-50 mg. orally, S.C., I.M.; 5-10 mg. I.V.
codeine		analgesia, antitussive	same as morphine but less pronounced	15-60 mg. orally, S.C.
fentanyl	Sublimaze	preoperative preparation, neuroleptanalgesia, immediate postoperative analgesia	skeletal and thoracic rigidity, apnea, plus the side effects of morphine	PREOPERATIVE: 50-100 mcg. I.M. 30-60 minutes prior to surgery. DURING SURGERY: 25-100 mcg. I.V.; POSTOPERATIVE: 50-100 mcg. I.M.
hydromorphone	Dilaudid	same as codeine	same as morphine	1-4 mg. S.C., I.M., I.V., orally
levorphanol	Levo-Dromoran	analgesia, preoperative preparation	same as morphine	2-3 mg. S.C., orally
meperidine	Demerol	same as anileridine	same as morphine plus cardiac arrhythmias	50-150 mg. orally, I.M., S.C. As an anesthesia supplement may be given I.V.
methadone	Dolophine	analgesia, treatment of narcotic addiction	same as morphine when used as an analgesic	2.5-10 mg. orally, I.M., S.C. In treatment of addiction doses are appreciably higher

Generic Name	Trade Name	Uses	Side Effects	Dose Ranges
morphine sulfate		analgesia, preoperative preparation	miosis, constipation, nausea, vomiting, respiratory depression, euphoria, hypotension, sweating, decrease in body temperature, urinary retention and frequency, ureteral and/or biliary spasms, physical dependence	2-20 mg. S.C., I.M.; 2.5-15 mg. I.V.
opium alkaloids, concentrated	Pantopon	analgesia	same as morphine	5-20 mg. S.C., I.M.
oxycodone (with aspirin, phenacetin, caffeine)	Percodan	analgesia	same as morphine plus side effects of aspirin, phenacetin, caffeine	1 tablet
oxymorphone	Numorphan	same as anileridine	same as morphine	1-1.5 mg. S.C., I.M.; 500 mcg. I.V.; 2-5 mg. suppository
paregoric (camphorated opium tincture)		diarrhea	same as morphine but less pronounced	ADULT: 5-10 ml. CHILD: 2-4 ml. per square meter of body surface

Potent Non-Narcotic Analgesics

Generic Name	Trade Name	Uses	Side Effects	Dose Ranges
methotrimeprazine	Levoprome	analgesia, sedation	postural hypotension, sedation, euphoria, headache, nausea, vomiting, pain at site of injection	2-30 mg. I.M. (patient should be kept supine for 6-12 hours after administration)
pentazocine	Talwin	analgesia, preoperative preparation	sedation, nausea, vomiting, anorexia, diarrhea, constipation, hypotension, weakness, euphoria, dry mouth	50-100 mg. orally; 30-60 mg. I.M., S.C.; 20 mg. I.V.

Table 6-2. (*Continued*)

GENERIC NAME	TRADE NAME	USES	SIDE EFFECTS	DOSE RANGES
OTHER OPIATE DERIVATIVES (DO NOT HAVE OPIATE-LIKE EFFECTS)				
apomorphine		emetic	central nervous system depression	5-10 mg. S.C. INFANT: 1 mg. S.C.
papaverine		treatment of cardiovascular diseases	flushing, hypotension, dizziness, nausea, abdominal distress	100 mg. orally several times daily; 30-120 mg. S.C., I.M., I.V.
NARCOTIC ANTAGONISTS				
levallorphan	Lorfan	narcotic overdose or idiosyncrasy	respiratory depression	1-3 mg. S.C., I.M., I.V.
nalorphine	Nalline	same as levallorphan plus diagnosis of narcotic addiction	miosis, drowsiness, sweating, nausea, vomiting; in large doses vivid dreams, hallucinations, nightmares	5-10 mg. I.V.; 1-3 mg. S.C. (for diagnosis of addiction). INFANT: 200 mcg. I.M., S.C. or through the umbilical cord
naloxone	Narcan	same as levallorphan and nalorphine plus treatment of opiate addiction	drug has no apparent pharmacological activity in the absence of opiates	400 mcg. I.V., I.M., S.C. Treatment of opiate addiction: doses are appreciably higher and given orally

The salicylates, in the form of methyl salicylate (oil of wintergreen), were known to the ancients during the time of Hippocrates. In the mid-nineteenth century sodium salicylate was first used as an internal medicine in the treatment of fever and rheumatic fever. Aspirin (acetylsalicylic acid), the most commonly used salicylate, was not synthesized until the turn of the century.

Types of Non-Narcotic Analgesics

There are two types of non-narcotic analgesics:

the **salicylates**
the **nonsalicylates**: coal-tar derivatives and other analgesics not related to the salicylates

General Drug Action

THE SALICYLATES

The precise mechanism of action of the analgesic effect of the salicylates is unknown. It is thought that the drugs may work on structures deep within the brain, probably on the thalamus. Salicylates may also act on peripheral structures, such as blood vessels.

The **antipyretic** (fever-reducing) effect of salicylates is also not well understood. They

Non-Narcotic Analgesics

may directly affect the *hypothalamus,* the heat regulating center of the body. Nerve impulses from the hypothalamus are sent to superficial blood vessels and sweat glands. Dilatation of blood vessels and increased activity of sweat glands aid in lowering the body temperature. With the dilatation of peripheral blood vessels, more blood—which is *warm*—comes in contact with *cooler* surrounding tissues. This in turn lowers the temperature of the blood by the process of radiation and conduction. Increased sweat gland activity cools the skin, and body heat is lost. Salicylates do *not* lower the body temperature of individuals who do *not* have a fever.

Salicylates have an **anti-inflammatory** effect. How they reduce inflammation is not well understood. Salicylates also reduce swelling, heat, and redness in patients with acute and chronic inflammatory disorders such as rheumatic fever and rheumatoid arthritis. Salicylates do *not* prevent damage to joints and connective tissue but may delay the progressive disability resulting from these diseases.

Salicylates have a **uricosuric** effect, increasing the secretion of **urates** (uric acid salts) in the urine. This is of value in the treatment of gout, a metabolic disease characterized by acute inflammation of the joints. Patients with gout tend to have elevated uric acid levels and the salts of uric acid (urates) are deposited in and around joints.

THE NONSALICYLATES

Coal-tar derivatives (para-aminophenol derivatives) are **analgesics** and **antipyretics** but do *not* have anti-inflammatory or uricosuric activity. Acetaminophen (Tylenol) may be used alone whereas phenacetin is usually included in products that contain other analgesics, for example Empirin Compound. The precise mechanism of action of these drugs is unknown; the action of the salicylates most probably applies to the coal-tar derivatives.

Other **non-narcotic analgesics** include propoxyphene hydrochloride (Darvon) and propoxyphene napsylate (Darvon-N). The analgesic effect of these drugs appears to be through action on the central nervous system. They have little antipyretic or anti-inflammatory activity.

Uses of Non-Narcotic Analgesics

The most common use of the salicylates is to relieve mild to moderate pain. Salicylates are also effective antipyretic (fever-reducing) drugs, and are used in the home and hospital.

The anti-inflammatory effect of these drugs makes them useful in the treatment of inflammatory disorders. On occasion, they may be combined with other drugs as part of the medical management of these diseases.

Acetaminophen (Tylenol), a coal-tar derivative, is an analgesic used in mild to moderate pain. It also has antipyretic activity. Patients who are not able to tolerate aspirin and other salicylates often can tolerate acetaminophen.

As stated above, phenacetin is usually included in combination-type analgesic compounds such as Empirin Compound (aspirin, phenacetin, caffeine).

Phenacetin is a mild analgesic and antipyretic but like acetaminophen has no anti-inflammatory activity.

Aspirin (acetylsalicylic acid) is available as a plain or enteric-coated (also written as E.C.) tablet. The enteric coating prevents absorption and/or disintegration of the tablet in the stomach. Once the tablet has left the stomach, alkaline secretions of the duodenum dissolve the coating, and the drug is absorbed into the bloodstream. The enteric coating may prevent gastric distress, a common side effect of aspirin.

Some aspirin products are available with buffering agents—usually magnesium carbonate or aluminum hydroxide—which are added to reduce gastric distress caused by the irritating effect of aspirin on the stomach lining.

Combination-type analgesics such as those containing aspirin, phenacetin, and caffeine have not definitely proved to be any more effective than aspirin. Although advertising claims may state otherwise, aspirin products are very much alike. Unfortunately, a great amount of money is spent on products that are supposed to fizz or be faster. All these products produce one effect—the relief of pain—the same effect produced by plain aspirin U.S.P.

Side Effects of Non-Narcotic Analgesics

THE SALICYLATES

In normal doses, salicylates produce few side effects.

Gastrointestinal disturbances including nausea, vomiting, and epigastric burning or distress appear to be the most common side effects. These may involve drug idiosyncrasy, drug allergy, or concentration of aspirin particles in the mucosa (lining) of the stomach. These symptoms are more likely to occur in patients receiving large doses of aspirin for treatment of arthritic-type diseases.

Gastrointestinal bleeding has also been observed in patients taking even small amounts of aspirin. In some patients blood loss may result in anemia, hematemesis (vomiting of blood), and blood in the feces.

Aggravation of bleeding disorders may occur during salicylate administration; therefore these drugs are contraindicated in patients

1. with vitamin K deficiencies
2. who are scheduled for surgery
3. who are receiving anticoagulant drugs
4. with bleeding disorders
5. with an active ulcer or a history of ulcer
6. who bruise easily (unless use has been approved by the physician)

This caution includes products that contain aspirin, such as Darvon Compound (propoxyphene, aspirin, phenacetin, caffeine) and Empirin Compound.

Hypersensitivity reactions, though rare, have been known to occur. The patient will experience swelling of the throat, mouth, and lips and have difficulty in breathing. Hypotension may accompany these symptoms. Death can occur in hypersensitive individuals.

Salicylism (see Table 7-1) may be noted in patients taking larger than normal doses of salicylates or in patients who repeat a normal dose in less than the 3-4 hours recommended.

Table 7-1.
SIGNS OF SALICYLISM AND SALICYLATE INTOXICATION

SALICYLISM	SALICYLATE INTOXICATION
tinnitus (ringing or roaring sound in the ears)	effects of salicylism, more pronounced
headache	PLUS
mental confusion, drowsiness	restlessness
fever	excitement
nausea, vomiting	incoherent speech
increased respiratory rate	tremors
increased pulse rate	delirium
	euphoria
	hallucinations
	convulsions

Salicylate intoxication (see Table 7-1) may be seen during prolonged high dosage therapy or after a single toxic dose. The latter is usually seen in small children who have ingested a large number of tablets at one time. Apparently some children do not mind the bitter taste of adult aspirin. Baby aspirin, which is flavored, may also be found and ingested by a child.

The higher the dose, the more pronounced are the symptoms of salicylate intoxication.

Enteric-coated tablets, taken routinely, may produce signs of salicylism since it has been reported that the absorption time of the tablet is variable and may be delayed.

THE NONSALICYLATES

ACETAMINOPHEN AND PHENACETIN

Acetaminophen (Tylenol) and phenacetin appear to be relatively nontoxic when used in normal doses. When these drugs are taken consistently over a long period of time, side effects may occur.

Kidney damage has been reported with the prolonged use of both these drugs, although phenacetin has been reported to be more likely to cause damage. This fact is clearly stated on the labels of analgesic compounds containing phenacetin; however, some individuals do not heed warnings on drug labels, especially those purchased without a prescription.

Hemolytic anemia and methemoglobinemia may be seen in some patients who have taken these drugs for long periods of time. Methemoglobinemia is the development of an abnormal blood pigment (methemoglobin) which is incapable of carrying oxygen to body cells. The patient then experiences symptoms of anemia. Hemolytic anemia is the destruction of red blood cells. This condition may lead to kidney failure and death.

Hypersensitivity reactions, the same as those seen with the salicylates, as well as rashes, urticaria (hives), and gastrointestinal disturbances may occasionally occur.

PROPOXYPHENE

Propoxyphene hydrochloride (Darvon) and propoxyphene napsylate (Darvon-N) administration may result in dizziness, headache, rash, gastrointestinal disturbances, and sedation. Occasionally, physical and psychological dependence has been known to occur with long-term use. Acute toxicity, due to overdose, may produce symptoms of narcotic intoxication, namely: respiratory depression, coma, and hypotension. Convulsions have been reported.

Clinical Considerations

It is important to know the contraindications and precautions of salicylate therapy. These drugs are given with caution to patients with gastritis, ulcers, or history of ulcers, and are not to be given to patients receiving anticoagulants. These warnings are also to be included in discharge teaching plans. The physician may tell a cardiac patient who is being discharged on anticoagulant therapy "not to take *any* drugs without first checking with me." This admonition should be reinforced, and perhaps reexplained to the patient. The word "drugs" may have various connotations, and the patient may believe that it refers only to prescription drugs. It should be emphasized that "all drugs" also refers to those which can be obtained without a prescription, including aspirin.

Patient histories should be obtained at the time of admission to the hospital. This procedure should include asking about prescription *and* nonprescription medications that are used on both a regular and occasional basis.

When salicylates or acetaminophen are used as antipyretics, they may be given orally or rectally in suppository form. The following points should be considered during and after administration of these drugs:

1. if drugs are given rectally, check to see if the suppository is being retained. This should be done two or three times during the first hour after administration. If expelled the suppository must be reinserted
2. drug effect may be seen in approximately one-half hour, but this time may vary
3. length of action is 2-4 hours. Since salicylates act on the fever and not on underlying disease processes, the temperature may begin to rise after this time. In some instances it may be necessary to monitor the temperature hourly or more often, until it stabilizes in the normal range
4. use of a rectal suppository may give inaccurate readings if a rectal probe or rectal thermometer is used to obtain the temperature, since the probe may be adjacent to the suppository instead of to the rectal wall. In order to insure accurate readings, check the rectum by digital examination, and if necessary move the suppository away from the tip of the probe
5. if profuse sweating occurs, bedding and gown changes will be necessary. A bath towel placed over the pillow will help absorb perspiration

When these drugs are used as anti-inflammatory/analgesic agents for arthritic conditions note whether pain, redness, swelling, and tenderness remain the same, increase, or decrease. Abatement of these symptoms is gradual and would be noted over a period of days. The patient may be helpful in evaluating these changes. Intensification of symptoms should be brought to the physician's attention, as an increase in dose or a change in medication may be necessary.

Large doses of salicylates—6 or more Grams per day—will affect the clotting mechanism of the blood. Easy bruising and bleeding tendencies may be noted. In some patients this occurs even when lower doses are prescribed.

In the hospital setting these drugs require a physician's order. If a patient requests an aspirin, it is necessary to refuse. Explain that even though anyone can purchase aspirin, nonprescription drugs can affect laboratory tests, mask symptoms of disease, or interfere with other drugs. This is why nonprescription drugs cannot be dispensed or administered unless they are ordered by the physician.

Acute salicylate toxicity is serious and requires prompt emergency intervention, namely gastric lavage, support of respiration, administration of intravenous fluids, and close patient observation.

Discharge Teaching

Discharge teaching for the patient on long-term salicylate therapy should include the following points:

1. these medications should be kept in a locked drawer if there are children in the home
2. if the patient is referred to another physician or has a dental appointment, the physician or dentist should be informed of the type and dose of salicylates
3. patients should have the signs of salicylism explained. The physician must be contacted if salicylism is noted

Table 7-2.
NON-NARCOTIC ANALGESICS

Generic Name	Trade Name	Uses	Side Effects	Dose Ranges
acetaminophen	Tylenol, Nebs	analgesic, antipyretic	nausea, vomiting, rash, urticaria, gastrointestinal disturbances, hemolytic anemia, methemoglobinemia, kidney damage	300-600 mg. orally
acetylsalicylic acid (aspirin)	many trade names	analgesic, antipyretic, anti-inflammatory	nausea, vomiting, rash, epigastric distress, G.I. bleeding, aggravation of bleeding disorders, hypersensitivity reactions, salicylism in overdoses	300 mg.-1.0 Gram orally or by rectal suppository
propoxyphene hydrochloride	Darvon	analgesic	dizziness, headache, rash, gastrointestinal disturbances, sedation, euphoria, physical and psychological dependence	65 mg. orally
propoxyphene napsylate	Darvon-N	analgesic	same as propoxyphene hydrochloride	100 mg. orally

NOTE: There are many products containing aspirin plus other drugs or ingredients such as caffeine, phenacetin, buffering agents, propoxyphene, codeine. Use of combination-type drugs requires observation for side effects that may occur with *each* ingredient.

A **sedative** is a drug that produces a relaxed, calming effect. Sedatives are usually given during the day; while they may make a patient drowsy, they usually do not produce sleep.

A **hypnotic** is a drug that induces sleep; that is, it allows the patient to fall asleep and stay asleep. This type of drug is administered at night or h.s. (at bedtime).

Types of Sedatives and Hypnotics

There are two types of sedative/hypnotic drugs, the **barbiturates** and the **nonbarbiturates**. Both types are capable of producing central nervous system depression resulting in sedation and/or sleep. Small doses of these drugs have sedative or antianxiety effects; higher doses result in hypnotic effects.

General Drug Action

All the **barbiturates** basically have the same action described above. The only difference among them involves the *onset of action* and the *duration of action*. A comparison of barbiturate preparations is given in Table 8-1.

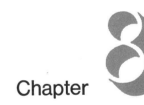

Chapter 8

55

Sedatives and Hypnotics

Table 8-1.
RELATIVE DURATION OF ACTION OF SEDATIVE/HYPNOTICS

ULTRA-SHORT-ACTING	SHORT- TO INTERMEDIATE-ACTING	LONG-ACTING
methohexital (Brevital)	amobarbital (Amytal)	phenobarbital (Luminal)
thiamylal (Surital)	aprobarbital (Alurate)	
thiopental (Pentothal)	butabarbital (Butisol)	
	talbutal (Lotusate)	
	pentobarbital (Nembutal)	
	secobarbital (Seconal)	

Individual patients may react differently to a barbiturate, and the duration of action may vary. The ultra-short-acting barbiturates are used as anesthetic agents.

All barbiturates are **general depressants,** that is, they depress many organs and structures of the body. Their major action, in normal doses, is on the central nervous system, respiratory system, and gastrointestinal tract.

The effect produced by a barbiturate **depends on** the drug, the dose, the route, and the patient.

The central nervous system depression produced by the barbiturates is not completely understood. It is thought that they act principally at the level of the thalamus, preventing transmission of impulses to the cerebral cortex. They also depress the sensory cortex.

In *normal* doses, most barbiturates exert a minimal effect on the respiration of the average patient. The ultra-short-acting barbiturates have a more pronounced effect on respiration.

Barbiturates decrease intestinal peristalsis, but this effect is less pronounced than the effect on the central nervous system.

Barbiturates are detoxified by the liver. All drugs that enter the body ultimately leave the body. Some leave virtually unchanged whereas others are transformed into other chemicals or compounds. The liver is the organ that changes the barbiturates into other compounds that are excreted by the kidney.

The **nonbarbiturates** also depress the central nervous system. Ethchlorvynol (Placidyl) and flurazepam (Dalmane) have muscle relaxant and anticonvulsant properties as well.

Uses of Sedatives and Hypnotics

Sedatives, which are almost always administered during daytime hours, have a variety of uses, generally in the treatment of anxiety and apprehension. Patients with chronic diseases may require sedatives, not only to reduce anxiety but also as adjuncts in the treatment of the disease. Patients with hypertension, for example, may have some apprehension about their illness. Apprehension can raise the blood pressure. Administration of a sedative with or without other antihypertensive agents may lower the blood pressure. Patients with coronary artery disease and gastrointestinal disorders also may benefit from the use of a barbiturate or nonbarbiturate sedative.

These drugs are also used to reduce preoperative apprehension and are given immediately prior to office dental procedures, minor surgical procedures, or for several days prior to major surgery. The patient who faces radical major surgery usually has varying degrees of apprehension, and use of a sedative may alleviate some of this preoperative anxiety.

Paraldehyde is used as a sedative or hypnotic in the treatment of delirium tremens (D.T.'s) in alcohol withdrawal.

When barbiturates or nonbarbiturates are used as hypnotics, larger doses are usually required to produce sleep. The elderly patient may require smaller doses. Drugs with a wider margin of safety, such as chloral hydrate, may be prescribed for the elderly patient who may experience excitement and confusion when barbiturates or other nonbarbiturates are administered.

Side Effects of Sedatives and Hypnotics

All sedatives and hypnotics have the ability to cause *psychological dependence*; that is, after a period of time the patient has difficulty sleeping without the use of a hypnotic. This is not seen in all patients. Use of barbiturates and some nonbarbiturates can also lead to *physical dependence*.

The side effects of the barbiturates are: rash, vertigo, euphoria, dizziness, nausea, vomiting, headache, drug "hangover." Some patients may exhibit excitement and confusion.

The nonbarbiturates also have various side effects. Ethinamate (Valmid) has few reported side effects when given in normal doses. Chloral hydrate usually has few side effects, but nausea, vomiting, and epigastric distress may occur in some individuals, apparently caused by the drug's irritating effect on the stomach lining.

Paraldehyde has a wide margin of safety. Taken orally it may produce gastric distress, especially when given in liquid rather than capsule form. This drug causes pain on injection. Although not a side effect, the disagreeable odor and taste of the liquid preparation may be a deterrent for some patients, whereas others do not appear to be disturbed by the drug's pungent odor and taste. Added to orange juice or tomato juice, the liquid oral form may be more palatable for some patients. The odor permeates the patient's surroundings and is noticeable on the breath.

Side effects most commonly seen in the nonbarbiturates are nausea, vomiting, sedation, dizziness, and euphoria. Side effects specific to particular drugs are given at the end of the chapter.

Clinical Considerations

Barbiturates and nonbarbiturates have very little analgesic action; therefore they should not be administered to the patient who has pain and cannot sleep.

Sedative/hypnotics should *not* be administered together with narcotic analgesics, nor should both types be administered within a short period of time, unless specifically ordered by a physician. Both types are central nervous system depressants, and in some instances the combined drug response could be profound, with depresssed respiration, bradycardia, and unresponsiveness. If there is any doubt regarding the administration times of either type of drug, the physician should be contacted and the situation explained.

Before giving a hypnotic, determine the patient's needs:

1. is the patient uncomfortable? If the reason for discomfort is pain, an analgesic may be needed
2. is it too early for the patient to receive the drug? Is a later hour preferred?
3. on previous nights has the drug helped the patient sleep? If not, a different drug or dose may be needed
4. does the patient receive narcotic analgesics every 4-6 hours? A hypnotic may not be necessary, or the physician may have to be contacted regarding the advisability of the use of the hypnotic
5. are there disturbances that may keep the patient awake and decrease the effectiveness of the drug?

Hypnotics are *never* left at the patient's bedside, to be taken at a later hour. This rule applies to *all* drugs, with the exception of drugs that are specifically ordered to be left at the patient's bedside, such as:

> 6/6
> nitroglycerin tablets at bedside to be taken for angina.
> p r. n
> Dr. Greene

> 2/17
> Maalox 15ml. q2h. leave bottle at bedside
> Dr. James

Hypnotics should not be left unattended in the medicine room, nurses' station, in the hall on a cart, or in other areas to which patients, visitors, or hospital personnel have direct access. If these drugs are prepared in advance, they should be placed in a *locked* drawer until time of administration.

Excessive drowsiness and/or headache in the morning (drug "hangover") may occur in some patients. A smaller dose or different drug may be necessary.

When drugs are used as daytime sedatives, excessive drowsiness and intermittent sleep may prevent the patient from sleeping at night, even when a hypnotic is administered. A decrease in the sedative dose may be necessary. In some instances daytime sedation may be an integral part of treatment and the dose and/or drug cannot be changed. Drowsiness may disappear after a period of time.

Side rails should be raised and a call light placed within easy reach for all patients receiving hypnotics or sedatives, since some patients may experience confusion if they awake during the night and try to get out of bed without assistance. Elderly patients may show excitement, restlessness, and confusion after the administration of barbiturates and should be checked frequently during the night. As noted above, many physicians prefer the use of the nonbarbiturates, such as chloral hydrate, in elderly patients.

Many hospitalized patients have difficulty sleeping at night. Environmental disturbances should be minimized as much as possible. If half side rails instead of full side rails are used, patients may still get out of bed. In a darkened room, chairs, footstools, slippers, and hospital equipment are difficult to see, leading to accidents and falls. These should be placed well away from the bed and any area where the patient may walk. If full side rails are used a call light should be within *easy* reach.

Some nonbarbiturates, such as ethchlorvynol (Placidyl), are short-acting, and help patients who need a drug only to get to sleep. Others may not benefit from a short-acting type hypnotic; this should be brought to the physician's attention. For many hospitalized patients, a good night's rest is an integral part of recovery.

Paraldehyde is very painful when injected, and assistance may be needed when the drug is administered. If more than 5 ml. is ordered, the dose is best given in divided, DEEP I.M. doses in both buttocks. If the parenteral form is discolored it should not be used. Given as an oral liquid, it can be mixed with cold orange juice or tomato juice. In capsule form, for example, Paral, additional fluids or juices are usually not needed unless the patient develops mild epigastric distress.

Discharge Teaching

Patients discharged from the hospital should be warned that other drugs can potentiate the action of barbiturates and nonbarbiturates. Discharge teaching should include the following points:

1. *only* the number of tablets prescribed by the physician should be taken. If the medication does not help, the physician should be contacted. The dose must *never* be increased without approval
2. alcohol and barbiturates *do not mix*. Alcohol should not be taken *before* or *after* drugs used for sleep. This warning also includes the nonbarbiturates. THIS POINT SHOULD BE STRESSED
3. keep these medications out of the reach of children as well as other members of the family
4. varying degrees of drowsiness may be experienced with the use of daytime sedatives. Driving a car, operating machinery, or performing any task that constitutes a potential danger may be hazardous. Most patients develop some degree of tolerance after taking these drugs over a period of time. Although the sedative effect may have disappeared, reflexes may still be slowed and there remains some degree of danger even though the patient feels alert

Table 8-2.
SEDATIVES AND HYPNOTICS

Generic Name	Trade Name	Uses	Side Effects	Dose Ranges
BARBITURATES				
amobarbital	Amytal	sedative, hypnotic	skin eruptions, dizziness, nausea, headache, drug hangover, excitement, euphoria, judgment may be impaired, physical and psychological dependence	SEDATIVE: 20-60 mg. 2-3 times/day orally; HYPNOTIC: 100-200 mg. orally, I.M.
aprobarbital	Alurate	sedative, hypnotic	same as amobarbital	SEDATIVE: 20-40 mg. T.I.D. orally; HYPNOTIC: 80-160 mg. orally
butabarbital	Butisol	sedative, hypnotic	same as amobarbital	SEDATIVE: 8-60 mg. 3-4 times/day orally, I.M.; HYPNOTIC: 100-200 mg. orally, I.M.
methohexital	Brevital	short-acting anesthetic	hiccups, laryngospasm, muscular twitching, respiratory depression	varies
pentobarbital	Nembutal	sedative, hypnotic	same as amobarbital	SEDATIVE: 15-40 mg. 3-4 times/day orally; HYPNOTIC: 60-120 mg. orally, I.M.; 30-200 mg. rectal suppository
phenobarbital	Luminal	sedative, hypnotic	same as amobarbital	SEDATIVE: 15-30 mg. 2-4 times/day orally, S.C., I.M.; HYPNOTIC: 100-300 mg. orally, S.C., I.M., I.V.
secobarbital	Seconal	sedative, hypnotic	same as amobarbital	SEDATIVE: 15-50 mg. 3-4 times/day orally; HYPNOTIC: 100-200 mg. orally, I.M.
talbutal	Lotusate	sedative, hypnotic	same as amobarbital	SEDATIVE: 30-50 mg. 2-3 times/day orally; HYPNOTIC: 120 mg. orally

Generic Name	Trade Name	Uses	Side Effects	Dose Ranges
thiamylal	Surital	short-acting anesthetic	respiratory depression, laryngospasm, hypotension	varies
thiopental	Pentothal	short-acting anesthetic	same as thiamylal	varies
NONBARITURATES chloral hydrate		sedative, hypnotic	nausea, vomiting, rash, epigastric distress	SEDATIVE: 250 mg. orally T.I.D.; HYPNOTIC: 500 mg.-1.0 Gram orally, rectally
ethchlorvynol	Placidyl	sedative, hypnotic	vertigo, headache, nausea, vomiting, drug hangover, ataxia	SEDATIVE: 200-600 mg. per day orally, in divided doses; HYPNOTIC: 500 mg.-1.0 Gram orally
ethinamate	Valmid	hypnotic	rare	500 mg.-1.0 Gram orally
flurazepam	Dalmane	hypnotic	dizziness, ataxia, confusion, lightheadedness, nausea, vomiting, anorexia, diarrhea	15-30 mg. orally
glutethimide	Doriden	sedative, hypnotic	nausea, vomiting, anorexia, confusion, rash, headache, drowsiness	SEDATIVE: 125-250 mg. orally T.I.D.; HYPNOTIC: 500 mg.-1.0 Gram orally
methaqualone	Quaalude, Parest, Sopor	sedative, hypnotic	headache, dizziness, nausea, vomiting, dry mouth, tachycardia, epigastric distress	SEDATIVE: 75 mg. orally Q.I.D.; HYPNOTIC: 150-300 mg. orally
methyprylon	Noludar	sedative, hypnotic	nausea, vomiting, constipation, drowsiness, headache, rash	SEDATIVE: 50-100 mg. orally T.I.D.; HYPNOTIC: 200-400 mg. orally
paraldehyde		sedative, hypnotic	nausea, vomiting, gastric distress	4-15 ml. in juice; 5 ml. or more I.M.; 10-20 ml. per rectum (NOTE: use glass syringes)

NOTE: *All* barbiturates have addiction potential. Some nonbarbiturates may cause psychological and/or physical dependence.

Opium was used by ancient civilizations and it is quite probable that some were addicted to the drug. The seriousness of opium addiction was not realized until the middle of the nineteenth century. Today we are faced with problems not only of drug addiction, but also of the abuse of drugs that are not addicting, but just as deadly.

Drug abuse may be defined as the use of a drug to produce a change in mood or behavior in a way that departs from approved medical or social patterns.

Compulsive drug abuse is the *need* to use any drug or chemical repeatedly to produce desired effects. The need to use a drug may be *physical, psychological,* or *both.*

Physical need, or **physical dependence,** is the *body's* dependence on *repeated* administration of a drug. **Psychological need** or **psychological dependence** is the *mind's* dependence on repeated use of a drug.

When an individual is physically and psychologically dependent on a drug he has a craving to take the drug repeatedly. If and when the drug is stopped, symptoms of *drug withdrawal,* also called the abstinence syndrome, occur. The abstinence syndrome can range from very mild to very severe, depending on the drug(s) involved, the dose used, the frequency of use, the length of time the drug has been taken, and the individual.

Chapter

Drug Abuse

Drug addiction may be defined to include the following:

1. a compulsive desire or craving to use a drug or chemical
2. an involvement with the drug to the exclusion of all other activities such as work, recreation, family, school
3. a *strong* tendency to return to the drug after withdrawal
4. a tendency to increase the dose
5. physical dependence
6. the absence of the drug—or abstinence syndrome—produces a moderate to severe physical reaction
7. detriments to society can exist in the drug and its use, as well as in the user.

Drug habituation may be defined to include the following:

1. a desire to use a drug continually for the effects produced
2. little or no tendency to increase the dose
3. no *physical* dependence; rather, psychological dependence
4. when the drug is withdrawn there is no true *physical* abstinence syndrome
5. the detrimental effect, if any exists, is on the individual rather than on society.

Heroin

Heroin (sometimes called "Horse," "H," "Smack," "Harry") is obtained from morphine, the principal alkaloid of raw opium. It is the strongest and most addicting of all opium derivatives. Thus heroin poses a serious socioeconomic problem for several reasons:

1. it is physically addicting
2. the resale value is very high, making it a very profitable venture for the sellers
3. continued use may result in other physical problems such as hepatitis, physical neglect, malnutrition, septicemia.

Heroin may be inhaled ("sniffed") or taken subcutaneously ("skin popping") or intravenously ("mainlining"). A dose of the drug is called a "fix." The desired effects on the user are euphoria and drowsiness. Other effects are anorexia, fixed pinpoint pupils, constipation, and decreased pulse and respiratory rate. Continued intravenous use results in scarring of the veins with skin markings often referred to as "tracks."

Signs of heroin withdrawal (abstinence syndrome) are: yawning, perspiration, tearing of the eyes, increased nasal discharge, gooseflesh, abdominal cramps, bone and muscle pain, nausea, vomiting, diarrhea, dilatation of the pupils, restlessness, increase in body temperature, increase in pulse and respiratory rate, marked mental depression or despair, an intense desire (craving) for the drug.

The symptoms will usually begin when the next dose of the drug is due, reach a peak in 36-72 hours, and gradually diminish in 4-5 days.

Some addicts take or are given overdoses. Signs and symptoms of overdose are: stupor, pinpoint pupils, nausea, vomiting, decreased pulse and respiratory rate, signs of shock. Coma may be present.

Heroin crosses the placental barrier; therefore a child

born of an addicted mother will also be addicted to the drug. The infant will need immediate treatment, but despite this, many of these infants die.

Other Opiates

Other opiate derivatives are used less frequently than heroin, except as substitutes when heroin is unavailable. Addiction to opiate derivatives may occur in people who receive them while under the care of a physician, as in the case of a terminally ill cancer patient. These patients, though addicts, are not denied a narcotic (nor should they be) because of their illness.

Others may procure opiates by falsifying prescriptions or obtaining the drugs in various ways—for example by feigning illness. Members of the medical profession—physicians, pharmacists, nurses—have ready access to drugs, and for varied reasons many use and are addicted to drugs such as morphine and meperidine (Demerol).

Heroin addicts unable to purchase a daily supply may steal from drugstores or warehouses, purchase cough medicines or analgesics that contain small amounts of codeine, or feign illness in an emergency room or outpatient department in an effort to receive a narcotic analgesic.

Nurses, physicians, and pharmacists administer, prescribe, and dispense many different types of medications. A few may be tempted to experience the effects of a narcotic, after which use of the drug might continue, although it does not in all cases.

Those addicted to opiates and other narcotics have a similar abstinence syndrome and incur many of the same dangers of heroin addiction.

Cocaine

Cocaine is an alkaloid obtained from coca leaves. In the late nineteenth century it was used (most unsuccessfully) in the treatment of morphine addiction and as a local anesthetic. It still has limited use as a local anesthetic. Slang terms for cocaine include "Dust," "Coke," "C," "Snow."

The heroin addict does not use cocaine *instead of* heroin, but may mix it with heroin to obtain a greater effect. This combination is called a "speedball."

Cocaine *stimulates* the central nervous system, producing marked euphoria and excitement when sniffed or inhaled. Overdose produces marked anxiety, hallucinations, and convulsions. Cocaine is not addicting but psychological dependence often occurs.

Cocaine's danger lies in its ability to cause psychological dependence and permanent damage to nasal mucosa; it can probably cause mental impairment. Weight loss and malnutrition usually occur with continued use. On some occasions the user may injure himself or others while in a state of excitement, which often accompanies cocaine use.

The chronic cocaine user may be identified by aggressive behavior, rapid pulse and respiratory rate, and dilated pupils. Abrupt withdrawal does not produce a physical abstinence syndrome, but the chronic user may require psychiatric treatment once the drug is stopped. Psychological dependence can produce an intense craving to return to the drug.

The Hallucinogens

MARIJUANA

A hallucinogen is a drug capable of producing a state of delirium characterized by visual and sensory disturbances that are bizarre and distorted. **Marijuana** ("Grass," "Mary Jane," "Tea," "Pot") belongs to the family of plants called Cannabis and is a hallucinogen. The substance that gives the hallucinogenic effect is a resin in the dried plants—THC or tetrahydrocannabinol.

Hashish is a more potent cannabis product that comes from plants grown in the Middle East. It is eight to ten times more potent than the American-grown variety.

The user may experience a variety of effects: euphoria, drowsiness, dizziness, lightheadedness, visual distortions, sensory distortions, hunger (especially for sweets), giddiness, and hallucinations. Sometimes other effects occur, such as panic, depression, nausea, vomiting, diarrhea, dryness of the mouth, and burning of the eyes.

The effects usually last 2-4 hours, but this is highly variable.

The signs of the user include inflammation of the eyes, dilatation of the pupils, increase in pulse, drop in blood pressure, and the odor of marijuana on the clothes.

The chronic user *may* show a change in personality and living habits, such as:

1. a lack of interest in school, work, other people
2. carelessness in personal hygiene, clothes
3. a preoccupied appearance
4. lack of motivation
5. memory difficulty
6. passiveness, apathy

Marijuana use may result in psychological dependence.

It is not known for sure whether marijuana is harmful, but there is some evidence that chronic use can lead to brain changes and possibly brain deterioration.

LSD

LSD—lysergic acid diethylamide—is a potent hallucinogen. Along with visual and sensory disturbances it causes changes in mood, affect, time/space perceptions, and body image.

Taking the drug, sometimes called "Acid," is usually referred to as a "trip," which may be a good or bad trip. The "good trip" is a pleasurable experience whereas the "bad trip" is one of panic, despair, frightening visual and/or sensory experiences, and a fear of insanity. The user never knows whether a trip will be good or bad, and there appears to be no way to avoid a bad trip.

Another potentially dangerous aspect of LSD use is the occurrence of a repeat trip—without taking the drug again. It is not clear why a repeat trip, which may occur as long as two years later, happens; it is not experienced by all who use the drug. Another risk is permanent psychosis; that is, the user does not "return" from the "trip." Whether this effect is temporary or permanent is not known; only time will tell whether a particular victim will recover.

Death, which has occurred during the use of LSD or during a repeat trip, is not due to the drug but to a false sense of ability or strength which may induce feats that cause death. The user may attempt to fly, walk on water, stop moving cars, etc., ending his or her life trying to accomplish such distorted ideas. Physical dependence does not occur and psychological dependence is rare.

Peyote cactus grows in the southwest United States and in Mexico. The small round growths (called buttons) are chopped off and chewed or brewed as tea. Peyote contains an alkaloid—mescaline—a white, crystalline substance used in capsule, liquid, or tablet form.

Use of peyote and mescaline produces euphoria and a state similar to that experienced with LSD.

DMT (dimethyltryptamine), **DET** (diethyltryptamine), and **STP**, also known as **DOM** (dimethoxymethylamphetamine), are also hallucinogens which produce effects similar to those of LSD.

Other substances enjoy fleeting popularity—nutmeg, meat tenderizer, smoking crushed aspirin, etc. These substances are not true hallucinogens but may produce a euphoric state, often with serious if not deadly results.

The greatest dangers in the use of hallucinogens are permanent psychosis, suicide, injury to self and others, and possible chromosome damage.

Stimulants and Depressants

Although stimulants and depressants may be used alone, drug users often take them along with or between the use of other drugs.

AMPHETAMINES AND METHAMPHETAMINES

The **amphetamines** and **methamphetamines** are adrenergic drugs originally used as central nervous system stimulants and anorexiants (drugs that control the appetite). Due to drug abuse potential, physicians are using other drugs or regimens in the treatment of obesity and in those diseases or conditions requiring central nervous system stimulation. If use of these drugs is necessary, therapy should be under the strict control of the physician.

The amphetamines/methamphetamines produce euphoria, alertness, and a sense of excitation. The user will appear talkative, restless, and excitable, and may perspire freely. The pupils may be dilated. Some take the drug orally; it is also used intravenously to produce an instant euphoric effect, which is greater in intensity. The user is called a "speed freak" and may increase the dose once tolerance develops. Large doses can produce convulsions, coma, and death.

These stimulants may be used for several days, during which time the individual is in a constant state of euphoria (called a "high") with minimal food intake and sleep. The drug is discontinued because of exhaustion, confusion, or disorientation. A period of mental depression follows. Tranquilizers and barbiturates may be taken to come off of a "high," to avoid the period of nervousness and restlessness that sometimes prevents sleep. Under the influence of these drugs physical harm may result to the user and others. Users may be belligerent, develop severe psychosis, and become depressed and suicidal. There is strong evidence that these drugs have addiction potential.

THE BARBITURATES AND NONBARBITURATES

As we have seen, these drugs have their proper use in medicine, but like other drugs they do have abuse potential. Drug tolerance can develop in the chronic barbiturate user and in some cases physical addiction and psychological dependence occur. The abstinence syndrome includes abdominal cramps, nausea, vomiting, weakness, and tremors. Overdose, which is not uncommon, can cause convulsions, delirium, and coma, as well as permanent brain damage and death. In some cases withdrawal from barbiturates may be more harmful, physically, than withdrawal from heroin.

The nonbarbiturate sedative/hypnotics are also subject to abuse. Methaqualone (Quaalude) and glutethimide (Doriden) are two examples of this group. Use of these drugs can result in psychological and physical dependence.

Withdrawal from the barbiturates and nonbarbiturates should be accomplished gradually, with the dose tapered off over a period of time. *Abrupt* withdrawal can result in serious consequences and even death.

TRANQUILIZERS

Use of tranquilizers can result in drug tolerance and physical and psychological addiction. (See Chapter 28.) This group of drugs is misused and abused—not only by those involved with illegal drugs but also by segments of the population who do not consider themselves "drug users."

Withdrawal, when it does occur, resembles barbiturate withdrawal, with the intensity depending on the severity of drug dependence and the length of time the drug has been taken. Psychological withdrawal will result in anxiety, nervousness, and a desire to return to the drug.

Unfortunately, some may be led to believe that tranquilizers are "safe" drugs, thus using them indiscriminately. Children growing up in an atmosphere of tranquilizer-popping parents can hardly be blamed for turning to drugs.

The Volatile Hydrocarbons

The volatile hydrocarbons are used by adults as well as children, although their greatest use appears to be in the younger segment of the population. Glue-sniffing produces euphoria and exhilaration which may be followed by stupor, dizziness, hallucinations, slurred speech, nausea, and vomiting. These effects usually begin after a few deep inhalations of the vapor. Intoxicating effects may last 30-60 minutes. Glue and other volatile hydrocarbons (gasoline, kerosene, cleaning fluids) may permanently damage the brain, heart, kidneys, liver, and bone marrow. When a plastic bag is placed over the head to contain the vapors and produce a more rapid drug effect, asphyxia and death can occur.

Conclusion

Drug abuse is dangerous, regardless of the drug(s) used. Members of the medical profession may be tempted to abuse drugs since they work with many different types of medications. To take a couple of antibiotic capsules because of a cold, or a barbiturate to get some sleep, or a marijuana cigarette because it makes things a little easier—all may be invitations to trouble, even discounting legal implications (which are still positive deterrents). Use of an antibiotic *could* result in anaphylactic shock and death. The barbiturate may be the start of a cycle in which it becomes necessary to use barbiturates to sleep, amphetamines to stay awake, and more barbiturates to sleep.

Table 9-1.

DRUGS OF ABUSE

Drug	Symptoms of Use / Symptoms of Overdose	Physical Dependence	Psychological Dependence	Methods of Treatment
heroin	USE: stupor, drowsiness, bradycardia, decrease in respiratory rate, euphoria, constipation, anorexia, weight loss, pinpoint pupils, needle marks OVERDOSE: stupor to coma, increase in pulse, slow shallow respirations, pinpoint pupils, nausea, vomiting, pale to cyanotic color	Yes	Yes	rehabilitation programs, psychiatric treatment, drug substitution programs oxygen, artificial ventilation if necessary, narcotic antagonist, treat shock, monitor vital signs, antibiotics if infection present
opiate-like narcotics	USE: same as heroin (needle marks not present if taken orally)	Yes	Yes	same as heroin
marijuana	USE: euphoria, drowsiness, odor on clothes, nausea, vomiting, dilated pupils, dry mouth, panic, depression, burning of eyes	No	Yes (?)	usually none needed; may need psychiatric care
other hallucinogens	USE: dilated pupils, rambling conversation, laughing, crying, incoordination, mild hypertension, may "see" sounds and "hear" colors, time and body image distorted, panic, psychotic episodes, may try to harm others OVERDOSE: "bad trip"?	No	Yes	emotional support, diazepam (Valium) may terminate trip; may need psychiatric care

Table 9-1. (Continued)

DRUG	SYMPTOMS OF USE SYMPTOMS OF OVERDOSE	PHYSICAL DEPENDENCE	PSYCHOLOGICAL DEPENDENCE	METHODS OF TREATMENT
amphetamine, methamphetamine	USE: hypertension, tachycardia, increased respirations, excitability, restlessness, dilated pupils, perspiration, hallucinations OVERDOSE: heart failure, severe tachycardia, extreme hypertension, coma, shock	Yes (?)	Yes	gastric lavage if taken orally; sedation may be necessary oxygen, artificial ventilation, I.V. fluids, vasopressors for shock, monitor vital signs
barbiturates, nonbarbiturates	USE: drowsiness, stupor, confusion, ataxia, pulse weak and rapid OVERDOSE: stupor to coma, hypotension, respirations shallow, pulse weak and rapid, pale to cyanotic color	Yes	Yes	monitor vital signs, treat hypotension, gastric lavage artificial ventilation, gastric lavage, I.V. fluids, treat shock, maintain airway
tranquilizers	resemble barbiturate intoxication	Rare	Yes	monitor vital signs; treatment depends on severity of overdose
volatile hydrocarbons	USE: euphoria, stupor, dizziness, hallucinations, slurred speech, mental confusion, nausea, vomiting, tinnitus, irritation of mucous membrane, tachycardia, characteristic odor OVERDOSE: coma, hypotension, signs of anoxia, respiratory difficulty; may be dead on arrival	No	Yes	emotional support; hypotension may occur oxygen, artificial ventilation, I.V. fluids; if heart, liver, kidney, brain, bone marrow damage occur, treat as symptoms are presented

NOTE: Methods of treatment may vary. Use of a combination of these drugs may also require a different approach to treatment. Physician preference for drugs and/or other methods of treatment may differ from the information noted above.

Although many drugs indirectly affect the heart, a special group of drugs is employed for direct action on cardiac tissue. There are two types of cardiac drugs: the **cardiotonics**, also called cardiac stimulants, and the **cardiac depressants**, also called antiarrhythmic drugs.

The Cardiotonics

These drugs, in crude form, were known to the ancient Egyptians and Romans, but their specific use and action were not completely understood until William Withering, in 1785, published his observations on the use of digitalis in the treatment of "dropsy" (edema). In the last fifty years the action and use of digitalis and related glycosides have been defined, and they are still among the chief medications used in the treatment of heart disease.

General Drug Action of Cardiotonic Drugs

The heart, weakened by disease, age, or both, is often in need of drug therapy. The cardiotonics—digitalis and the related glycosides—exert their chief action on the myocardium (heart muscle). A **glycoside** is obtained from plant sources and consists of a chemical and sugar.

Chapter 10

The Cardiotonics and the Cardiac Depressants

Table 10-1.
COMPARATIVE ACTIONS OF
DIGITALIS PREPARATIONS

DIGITALIS PREPARATION	ONSET	DURATION
digitalis, whole leaf	slow	long
digitoxin	slow	long
digoxin	short	short
lanatoside C	variable	short

Digitalis preparations basically have the same drug action, the only difference being in:

the *speed* of action
the *duration* of action.

These variations allow for choosing a preparation that will best suit the needs of the patient.

The main pharmacological action of digitalis and related glycosides is the ability to *increase the force of contraction* of cardiac muscle. These drugs probably act directly on muscle fibers of the myocardium. When the force of contraction is increased, cardiac *output* is increased. Cardiac output is the amount of blood, in milliliters (ml.) leaving the left ventricle each time the myocardium contracts. A heart weakened by disease or age cannot pump a sufficient amount of blood; thus there is a decrease in the amount of oxygenated blood leaving the left ventricle during each myocardial contraction. A *marked decrease* in cardiac output deprives the kidneys and other vital organs of an adequate blood supply. The kidneys are unable to remove water, electrolytes, and waste products; excess fluid (edema) in the lungs and/or tissues may result. The body attempts to make up this deficit by increasing the heart rate.

Cardiotonic drugs *slow the heart rate* and *strengthen the force of myocardial contraction.* The *increased* force of contraction improves blood flow to the kidneys and other vital organs. Peripheral and/or pulmonary edema may respond to therapy.

Cardiotonic drugs also slow the pulse by vagal nerve stimulation, but this drug action is thought to be minimal; the greatest drug effect appears to be on the myocardium. The tenth cranial nerve, the vagus nerve, normally slows the heart, and provides a "braking" mechanism when the pulse rate rises. Stimulation of the vagus increases its ability to slow the heart.

The effects of digitalis therapy are indicated in the chart on page 73.

Uses of Cardiotonic Drugs

Cardiotonic drugs are used primarily

1. in the treatment of **congestive heart failure**
2. to correct **cardiac arrhythmias,** namely: atrial fibrillation, heart block (under certain conditions), paroxysmal atrial or nodal tachycardia

Side Effects of Cardiotonic Drugs

There is a narrow margin of error between full *therapeutic effect* and *drug toxicity.* Signs of toxicity may also be seen with normal doses (Table 10-2).

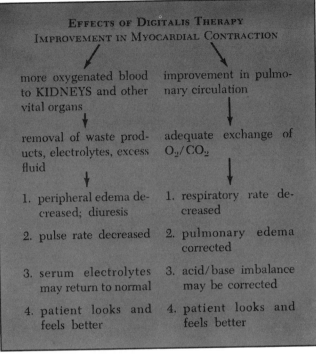

EFFECTS OF DIGITALIS THERAPY
IMPROVEMENT IN MYOCARDIAL CONTRACTION

more oxygenated blood to KIDNEYS and other vital organs

improvement in pulmonary circulation

removal of waste products, electrolytes, excess fluid

adequate exchange of O_2/CO_2

1. peripheral edema decreased; diuresis
2. pulse rate decreased
3. serum electrolytes may return to normal
4. patient looks and feels better

1. respiratory rate decreased
2. pulmonary edema corrected
3. acid/base imbalance may be corrected
4. patient looks and feels better

Table 10-2.
SIGNS OF DIGITALIS TOXICITY

GASTROINTESTINAL	NEUROLOGICAL	CARDIAC
anorexia	blurred vision	change in pulse rate and rhythm (extrasystoles, bigeminal pulse, bradycardia, tachycardia)
nausea	halos around dark objects	
vomiting	disturbance in yellow/green vision	
epigastric discomfort		
diarrhea	headache	
abdominal cramps	muscle weakness	

Clinical Considerations

Digitalis and allied glycosides are *potent* drugs. Signs of drug toxicity can occur, even when normal doses are administered. When a patient receives these drugs, certain measures must be instituted during the entire period of drug therapy.

1. an *apical-radial* pulse should be taken when the patient receives a cardiotonic for the first time. Later, radial rates may be taken unless ordered otherwise.

2. a *radial rate* is taken for a *full minute before* the drug is administered. If the pulse is *60 or below* in adults, or *70 or below* in children, the drug is *not* given and the physician notified. The exception to this rule is a specific written order of a physician changing the minimum pulse rate.

> 7/8
> Digitalis 0.09 Gm. q.d. May be given if pulse is (55) or more.
> Dr. Greene

3. signs of toxicity are to be reported to the physician. Some signs of toxicity may be difficult to detect, for example, anorexia. The bed patient could have a poor appetite for several reasons—restriction of activity, presence of illness, or dislike for hospital food. It becomes difficult to determine if the loss of appetite is due to the drug or to other factors.

When digitalis or one of the allied glycosides is given to the patient for the first time, the patient is being **digitalized,** a term used to describe successive doses of a cardiotonic drug. A **digitalizing dose** is that amount of drug needed to obtain therapeutic effects. Once the therapeutic effects are reached, the patient is placed on a **maintenance dose**—the amount of drug required to maintain therapeutic effects.

The example given here shows a rapid digitalizing dose of digoxin. The physician may elect to digitalize the patient slowly by ordering 0.5 to 1 mg. of digoxin daily. The choice of rapid or slow digitalization usually depends on the patient's condition, his cardiac status, and physician preference. Digoxin may also be given by the intravenous route for rapid digitalization. The drug index at the end of the chapter lists other cardiotonic preparations with digitalizing doses, maintenance doses, and route of administration.

The physician determines whether the patient is fully digitalized by:

1. the pulse rate and quality
2. electrocardiogram (ECG) changes
3. improvement in the patient's condition
4. appearance of side effects (signs of digitalis toxicity)

When a patient is being digitalized, note the patient's general appearance, monitor vital signs, record

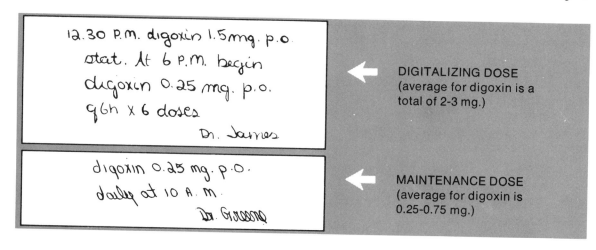

12.30 P.M. digoxin 1.5mg. p.o. stat. At 6 P.M. begin digoxin 0.25 mg. p.o. q6h x 6 doses
Dr. James

DIGITALIZING DOSE (average for digoxin is a total of 2-3 mg.)

digoxin 0.25 mg. p.o. daily at 10 A.M.
Dr. Giacobbe

MAINTENANCE DOSE (average for digoxin is 0.25-0.75 mg.)

the intake and output as well as report any changes in the patient's appearance. Side effects must be reported to the physician. The development of an arrhythmia must be reported immediately, as other modes of medical management may be necessary.

B.P.	
Pulse rate, quality	
Respirations	
Color	
Edema (where?)	
Weight	
Urinary output	
Fluid intake	
Cough?	
Restlessness	
Dyspnea	
Orthopnea	
Other complaints	

Great care must be taken in the administration of cardiotonic drugs. References should be consulted for average digitalizing doses. If in doubt, do *not* give the drug; check with the patient's physician.

Not every patient can be digitalized or maintained on cardiotonic drugs without side effects. As stated above, there is a narrow margin between full therapeutic effect and drug toxicity. Maintenance doses must be individualized and may vary from patient to patient.

Discharge Teaching

Discharge teaching should include:

1. teaching the patient *how* and *when* to take his pulse
2. explaining when the drug is *not* to be taken
3. explaining side effects (the patient might be given a list of the side effects to aid him in remembering the most significant and pertinent ones) and what to do if and when they occur
4. indicating the time of day the medication is to be taken
5. stressing the importance of taking the medication exactly as prescribed (failure to do so will lessen the effectiveness of drug therapy)
6. stressing the importance of keeping office or clinic appointments

Points 1 to 3 of the above should be given to a patient only with the approval of the physician. Information to be presented to patients should be checked by the physician for accuracy.

The signs of digitalis toxicity should be presented to the patient in a positive way, with the explanation that these symptoms are not unusual but must be reported to the physician. A change in medication may be necessary, since each patient's response to cardiotonic drugs is different.

The nurse or a family member, rather than the physician, may be the first to detect signs of toxicity, since patients are likely to discuss what appear to be minor complaints (anorexia, etc.) with the nurse or other health professional.

Cardiac Depressants

We have seen that cardiotonic drugs are used to strengthen the myocardium. Cardiac depressants are used to treat cardiac arrhythmias. Patients with heart disease may have not only a weakened myocardium, but also disturbances in heart rhythm (arrhythmia). Cardiodepressants are also called antiarrhythmic drugs.

Types of Cardiac Depressant Drugs

Quinidine and procainamide (Pronestyl) are cardiac depressants, and while unrelated chemically have similar actions. Both drugs had been in use a relatively long period of time before newer drugs with antiarrhythmic abilities were introduced. Lidocaine (Xylocaine), propranolol (Inderal), and diphenylhydantoin (Dilantin) are examples of newer preparations. Lidocaine is a local anesthetic but also has the ability to abolish cardiac arrhythmias. Propranolol (Inderal) is a beta adrenergic blocking agent; diphenylhydantoin (Dilantin) is used to treat epilepsy and also has the ability to abolish some cardiac arrhythmias.

General Drug Action of Cardiac Depressant Drugs

Quinidine and quinine are alkaloids obtained from the bark of the cinchona tree. Quinidine is a cardiac depressant; quinine is used primarily to treat malaria. Procainamide (Pronestyl) is chemically related to procaine, a local anesthetic.

Quinidine and procainamide (Pronestyl) *depress myocardial excitability* by *increasing* the threshold of cardiac muscle. Cardiac muscle has the attributes of

nerves and *muscle*, and therefore will have the properties of both kinds of structure.

A stimulus (which is a form of energy) must be of a specific intensity before it can be transmitted along a nerve fiber. If it is of less intensity, the stimulus cannot be transmitted. This characteristic of nerve fibers is called the *all or none* response. *Threshold* is a term applied to the stimulus of lowest intensity that will give rise to a response.

Some cardiac arrhythmias are caused by the generation of an abnormal number of (electrical) stimuli of the S.A. (sino-atrial) node or of the myocardium (atrial or ventricular myocardium). The entire cardiac muscle responds to this abnormal number of stimuli, thus creating an arrhythmia. If the threshold of cardiac fibers is *raised*, then *only* those stimuli of greater intensity will be transmitted, with a subsequent response of cardiac muscle—a decrease in the number of contractions of the myocardium. Cardiac depressants *decrease* the excitability of the myocardium by *increasing* the threshold of cardiac muscle fibers, thereby *decreasing* the response (contraction of cardiac muscle) to the increased number of stimuli.

In order to visualize this phenomenon, think of a bowl of gelatin sitting on a table. A slight rap on the table causes the gelatin to quiver. If the gelatin were placed in a freezer until it was almost frozen and then placed on the table, a rap would not produce the same response.

Quinidine and procainamide (Pronestyl) *lengthen the refractory (rest) period*. All nerves have a refractory period, which is the *interval of time* between transmissions of impulses along a nerve fiber. An impulse cannot pass along a nerve fiber until the end of the refractory period.

If the refractory period is lengthened, the number of impulses transmitted over a given period of time is *decreased*. For illustration, a refractory period of 0.25 second is assigned to a nerve fiber. The time required for a nerve impulse to travel along this fiber is 0.5 second. The total time is 0.75 second.

If the refractory period is *lengthened* to 0.5 second, the total time becomes 1 second. Thus the number of impulses that can be transmitted within a given period of time—say for example 60 seconds—*decreases*, because the refractory period is lengthened.

Quinidine and procainamide (Pronestyl) *slow the speed of the conduction of impulses* along cardiac fibers. If an impulse travels at a *decreased* rate of speed, the number of impulses transmitted within a given period of time decreases. For example, if the travel time along the nerve fiber is increased to 0.75 second, the total is now 1.25 seconds. Lengthening the refractory period and slowing the speed of conduction slows the heart rate.

Propranolol (Inderal), a beta adrenergic blocking agent (see also Chapter 3), is capable of blocking the effects of the sympathetic nervous system on cardiac muscle, thus decreasing the heart rate. This drug also has quinidine-like action. Lidocaine (Xylocaine) has an action similar to that of quinidine and procainamide (Pronestyl) and raises the threshold of cardiac muscle. Diphenylhydantoin (Dilantin) appears to stabilize cell membranes of cardiac muscle, thus preventing a response to excessive stimuli.

Uses of Cardiac Depressant Drugs

Cardiac depressants are used to treat a variety of cardiac arrhythmias. Although cardiotonics may also be used to treat cardiac arrhythmias, the greatest use of these agents is in the treatment of congestive heart failure. The drug tables at the end of the chapter list the types of arrhythmias responding to each cardiac depressant.

QUINIDINE is used in the treatment of ventricular and atrial arrhythmias

PROCAINAMIDE (Pronestyl) is used in the treatment of ventricular and some atrial arrhythmias

LIDOCAINE (Xylocaine) is used in the treatment of ventricular arrhythmias occurring during cardiac surgery or following a myocardial infarction. This drug is administered intravenously and rapidly abolishes these arrhythmias. Advantages of lidocaine are its rapid action and brief duration. This permits alteration of treatment —that is, an increase or decrease in the drug dose as the patient responds to therapy

PROPRANOLOL (Inderal) is used in the treatment of supraventricular tachycardias

DIPHENYLHYDANTOIN (Dilantin) is used in the treatment of paroxysmal atrial tachycardia, especially when due to digitalis toxicity, and in atrial and ventricular arrhythmias not responsive to other cardiac depressants.

Side Effects of Cardiac Depressant Drugs

Quinidine is a dangerous drug and like digitalis preparations has side effects, some of which may be serious. The most common side effects involve the gastrointestinal tract: diarrhea, nausea, and vomiting. Other side effects are headache, vertigo, fever, tinnitus (ringing in the ears), rash, urticaria, visual disturbances, and mental confusion. These side effects may occur even when low doses of the drug are used. More serious side effects, hypotension and respiratory difficulty, are more apparent during parenteral administration of the drug.

Procainamide (Pronestyl), like quinidine, is also a dangerous drug with similar side effects: anorexia, nausea, vomiting, and diarrhea. Weakness, a bitter taste in the mouth, mental depression, giddiness, and hallucinations can also occur. Hypotension may occur during intravenous administration. Occurrence of cardiac arrhythmias, more common with intravenous administration, may require emergency measures.

The most serious side effects of propranolol (Inderal) are bradycardia, asystole, and hypotension. The incidence of these side effects is reduced when the patient's response is observed on a cardiac monitor. With oral administration, nausea, vomiting, diarrhea, constipation, mental confusion, insomnia, and headache may occur. This drug is contraindicated in patients with asthma.

Lidocaine (Xylocaine) is administered intravenously. The side effects of this drug can be serious, requiring constant cardiac monitoring and patient observation. Central nervous system and gastrointestinal side effects include vertigo, visual disturbances, nausea, vomiting, and convulsions. Cardiovascular side effects are hypotension and cardiac arrest.

The most common side effects of diphenylhydantoin (Dilantin) seen during the cardiac use of the drug are rash, nausea, and vomiting. When this drug is used for long periods of time, as in the treatment of epilepsy, other side effects may be seen.

Clinical Considerations

Clinical considerations for the administration of cardiac depressant drugs are similar to those of the cardiotonic preparations.

It is usually advisable to take an apical-radial pulse rate during the administration of quinidine, procainamide (Pronestyl), and diphenylhydantoin (Dilantin), especially when drug therapy is first instituted. Taking apical-radial rates or cardiac monitoring is advisable during intravenous administration of any cardiac depressant drug—especially propranolol (Inderal) and lidocaine (Xylocaine). Hypotension can occur during use, especially when drugs are administered intravenously.

All side effects, even those not found in reference sources, should be reported to the physician. Although not all symptoms or complaints are drug-related, a physician's determination of their importance is required.

The bitter taste which sometimes occurs during procainamide (Pronestyl) therapy may be relieved by mouth wash or hard candy (if allowed). If gastrointestinal disturbances occur, the drug should be withheld until the physician is notified. Excessive vomiting and/or diarrhea can result in loss of electrolytes; this condition can precipitate cardiac arrhythmias.

The dose of cardiac drugs must be measured accurately. The physician's order sheet should be carefully checked before preparing the drug for administration.

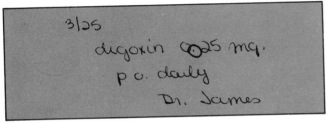

3/25
digoxin 0.25 mg.
p.o. daily
Dr. James

Because lidocaine administration can result in serious side effects, including convulsions and cardiac arrest, an airway should be available at the patient's bedside—in plain sight. If hypotension or cardiac arrhythmias occur during intravenous administration, the infusion should be slowed to the *lowest* possible number of drops per minute until the physician can examine the patient and determine the advisability of continued therapy. It is important to be familiar with resuscitation procedures should cardiac arrest be evident.

Cardiotonics and cardiodepressants can *cause* serious arrhythmias as well as correct them. *Any change* in the pulse rate, rhythm, or quality is of importance.

Patients receiving cardiac drugs may be aware of the fact that they have heart disease. This knowledge, coupled with hospitalization, may provoke anxiety, fear of the unknown, and worry about the future. Some patients need to verbalize their feelings, and you should be prepared to listen to them. Patients who are incapacitated by their illness may need referral to social agencies.

Discharge Teaching

Discharge teaching should include:

1. explaining side effects to the patient and/or family*
2. stressing the importance of drug therapy and the role of drugs in the treatment of disease
3. stressing the importance of taking the medication exactly as prescribed
4. indicating the time of day the medication is to be taken
5. stressing the importance of keeping office or clinic appointments

* The physician should be consulted as to the advisability of explaining side effects.

Table 10-3.
CARDIAC DRUGS

GENERIC NAME	TRADE NAME	USES	SIDE EFFECTS	DOSE RANGES
CARDIOTONICS				
acetyldigitoxin	Acylanid	management of congestive heart failure, control of ventricular rate in patients with atrial fibrillation, prevention of attacks of paroxysmal atrial or nodal tachycardia, tachycardias of anesthesia and surgery of patients with cardiac disease, heart block (under certain conditions)	anorexia, nausea, vomiting, abdominal cramping, epigastric discomfort, headache, fatigue, muscle weakness, blurred vision, diarrhea, halos around dark objects, disturbance in color vision (green/yellow), cardiac arrhythmias, neuralgia-like pain of jaw and lumbar area	DIGITALIZATION: rapid—1.6-2.2 mg. in 3-4 divided doses orally; slow—1.8-3.2 mg. over a 2-6 day period orally MAINTENANCE: 100-200 mcg. daily orally
deslanoside	Cedilanid-D	same as acetyldigitoxin	same as acetyldigitoxin	DIGITALIZATION: 1.6 mg. in divided doses I.M., I.V. MAINTENANCE: 400 mcg. I.M., I.V. daily (oral cardiotonics are preferable for maintenance when possible)
digitalis		same as acetyldigitoxin	same as acetyldigitoxin	DIGITALIZATION: dose varies. Average is 1.5 Gm. in divided doses orally MAINTENANCE: 100 mg. orally
digitalis purpurea glycosides		same as acetyldigitoxin	same as acetyldigitoxin	parenteral form of digitalis. Dose varies with manufacturer

Generic Name	Trade Name	Uses	Side Effects	Dose Ranges
digitoxin	Crystodigin, Purodigin	same as acetyldigitoxin	same as acetyldigitoxin	DIGITALIZATION: 200 mcg. B.I.D. × 4 days orally, followed by maintenance dose. Also given as 30-50% of total digitalizing dose followed by ⅛-¼ the total dose at 3-6 hour intervals. MAINTENANCE: 50-300 mcg. daily
digoxin	Lanoxin	same as acetyldigitoxin	same as acetyldigitoxin	DIGITALIZATION: 2-3 mg. in divided doses orally; 1-1.5 mg. I.V. in divided doses. MAINTENANCE: ¼ of the digitalizing dose daily in single or divided doses orally, I.M., I.V.
gitalin	Gitaligin	same as acetyldigitoxin	same as acetyldigitoxin	DIGITALIZATION: rapid — 2.5 mg. orally, then 750 mcg. q6h until therapeutic results obtained; slow — 1.5 mg. daily × 4-6 days. MAINTENANCE: 250 mcg.-1.25 mg. daily
lanatoside C	Cedilanid	same as acetyldigitoxin	same as acetyldigitoxin	DIGITALIZATION: total dose 8-10 mg. over 3-4 days orally. MAINTENANCE: 500 mcg.-1.5 mg. daily orally

Table 10-3. (*Continued*)

GENERIC NAME	TRADE NAME	USES	SIDE EFFECTS	DOSE RANGES
ouabain	G-Strophanthin	same as acetyldigitoxin	same as acetyldigitoxin	DIGITALIZATION: total dose of 1 mg. I.V. in divided doses

CARDIODEPRESSANTS

diphenylhydantoin	Dilantin	supraventricular and ventricular arrhythmias, digitalis-induced arrhythmias	rash, nausea, vomiting	vary according to reason for use
lidocaine	Xylocaine	acute management of ventricular arrhythmias	vertigo, visual disturbances, nausea, vomiting, convulsions, muscular twitching, bradycardia, hypotension, cardiac arrest	BOLUS INJECTION: 50-100 mg. I.V. Intravenous infusion: 1 Gram added to 1000 ml.
procainamide	Pronestyl	ventricular extrasystoles and tachycardia, atrial fibrillation, paroxysmal atrial tachycardia, cardiac arrhythmias associated with anesthesia and surgery	anorexia, nausea, vomiting, diarrhea, cardiac arrhythmias, mental changes, bitter taste, hypotension	500 mg.-1.25 Grams orally; 500 mg.-1 Gram I.M.; 200 mg.-1 Gram I.V. diluted in intravenous solution

Generic Name	Trade Name	Uses	Side Effects	Dose Ranges
propranolol	Inderal	paroxysmal atrial tachycardia, sinus tachycardia, atrial extrasystoles, atrial flutter and fibrillation, tachyarrhythmias of digitalis intoxication; occasionally used to treat ventricular tachycardias if other drugs or methods fail	hypotension, bradycardia, asystole, nausea, vomiting, diarrhea, constipation, mental confusion, headache, insomnia	10-40 mg. T.I.D., Q.I.D. orally; 1-3 mg. I.V.
quinidine		ventricular and atrial arrhythmias: paroxysmal atrial fibrillation, atrial flutter, paroxysmal supraventricular tachycardias, premature atrial or ventricular systoles, ventricular tachycardia	anorexia, nausea, vomiting, diarrhea, abdominal pain, confusion, headache, fever, vertigo, tinnitus, visual and mental disturbances, cardiac arrhythmias, rash, urticaria, hypotension with I.V. use	330-660 mg. per dose orally, 400-600 mg. per dose I.M., 800 mg. per dose I.V.

Anticoagulant drugs are used to prevent the formation of blood clots. They do *not* "thin" the blood, nor can they dissolve clots that have already formed. Anticoagulants are valuable adjuncts in the treatment of various cardiovascular conditions.

Types of Anticoagulants

There are two types of anticoagulant drugs: (1) **heparin** and (2) the **oral anticoagulants**.

Heparin is manufactured by *mast cells,* which are located around capillaries. For commercial use, heparin is extracted from the lungs of animals.

Oral anticoagulants are drugs of two different chemical types: the **coumarin derivatives** and the **indandione derivatives** (see Table 11-1). Drugs of the coumarin class are the ones most widely used in the United States. Dicumarol is the prototype oral anticoagulant.

General Drug Action

Anticoagulants interfere with the clotting mechanism of blood. This is a complex chemical process that occurs in three stages, shown in the chart on the following page.

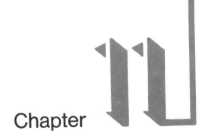

Chapter 11

85

Anticoagulant Drugs

Table 11-1.
ORAL ANTICOAGULANTS

Generic Name	Trade Name	Duration of Action
COUMARIN DERIVATIVES		
acenocoumarol	Sintrom	1½-3 days
dicumarol, U.S.P.		2-6 days
warfarin potassium	Athrombin-K	1-5 days
warfarin sodium	Coumadin; Panwarfin	1-5 days
INDANDIONE DERIVATIVES		
anisindione	Miradon	1½-5 days
diphenadione	Dipaxin	10-21 days
phenindione	Hedulin	1-4 days

Although its exact mechanism of action is not clearly understood, it appears that heparin:

1. inactivates thromboplastin (stage 1)
2. this in turn interferes with the conversion of prothrombin to thrombin (stage 2)
3. and fibrinogen is prevented from forming fibrin (stage 3)

Heparin acts on the blood clotting mechanism; it also appears to keep platelets from clumping together and enhancing the formation of a blood clot.

The **oral** anticoagulants—the coumarin and indandione derivatives—reduce the blood's ability to clot by interfering with the synthesis of prothrombin in the

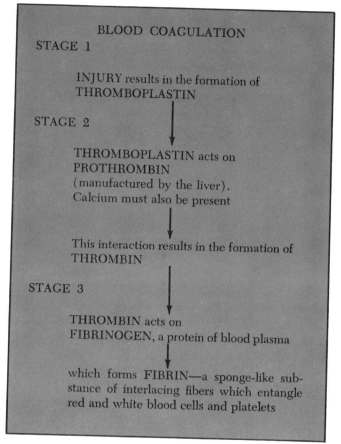

BLOOD COAGULATION

STAGE 1

INJURY results in the formation of THROMBOPLASTIN

STAGE 2

THROMBOPLASTIN acts on PROTHROMBIN (manufactured by the liver). Calcium must also be present

This interaction results in the formation of THROMBIN

STAGE 3

THROMBIN acts on FIBRINOGEN, a protein of blood plasma

which forms FIBRIN—a sponge-like substance of interlacing fibers which entangle red and white blood cells and platelets

liver (stage 2). The liver needs vitamin K to synthesize prothrombin. The oral anticoagulants prevent the use of vitamin K, so that the amount of **prothrombin** circulating in the blood drops. This is called *hypoprothrombinemia* (low prothrombin in the blood).

Uses of Anticoagulant Drugs

Heparin is used as a prophylactic (preventive):

1. to prevent the formation of a blood clot, that is, a thrombus (a clot formed in a blood vessel or cavity) or an embolus (a clot in a vessel or cavity that has traveled to that area from another area)
2. to prevent the extension of thrombi
3. to prevent the clotting of blood that is removed from the body as in extracorporeal circulation—the shunting of blood outside the body. Extracorporeal circulation is utilized in open heart surgery and hemodialysis procedures.

Diseases and conditions that may require the use of heparin are: thrombophlebitis, pulmonary embolus, and prevention of complications of cardiac and vascular surgery, extracorporeal circulation, and hemodialysis. Heparin may also be used in conjunction with oral anticoagulants.

The oral anticoagulants are used in the treatment of:

1. venous thrombosis
2. acute coronary thrombosis
3. prophylaxis and treatment of pulmonary emboli

COMPARISON OF HEPARIN AND ORAL ANTICOAGULANTS

ROUTES OF ADMINISTRATION: Heparin cannot be given orally; it must be administered by the intravenous, intramuscular, or subcutaneous route. The repository (long-acting) form may be administered by deep subcutaneous or intramuscular route. The coumadin and indandione derivatives are only given orally.

ONSET OF ACTION: Heparin has a rapid onset of action, making it particularly useful in emergency situations. The oral anticoagulants require hours or days before producing a therapeutic effect.

DURATION OF ACTION: Heparin, with the exception of the repository form, has a shorter duration of action.

LONG-TERM THERAPY: Heparin must be administered in the hospital and therefore cannot be used for long-term therapy.

TOXICITY: Heparin is relatively nontoxic. Bleeding tendencies appear to be less common than with the oral anticoagulants.

Side Effects of Anticoagulant Drugs

HEPARIN

Side effects of heparin are somewhat rare. The only serious side effect is hemorrhage, which may be minor, as in local ecchymosis (extravasation of blood into the skin and mucous membranes), or major. The action of heparin can be immediately reversed by the administration of intravenous protamine sulfate.

ORAL ANTICOAGULANTS

As with heparin, the most common side effect of the oral anticoagulants is hemorrhage, which can be major or minor. The action of oral anticoagulants can be reversed by the administration of vitamin K preparations such as menadione (Hykinone) or phytonadione (Mephyton). Several hours are usually required for the reversal of anticoagulant action.

Other side effects are:

COUMARIN DERIVATIVES—nausea, vomiting, anorexia, diarrhea, dermatitis

INDANDIONE DERIVATIVES—dermatitis, blood dyscrasias, diarrhea, nausea

Clinical Considerations

HEPARIN

Heparin is measured in *units* and is available as 1000 U, 5000 U, 7500 U, 10,000 U, 15,000 U, 20,000 U, 40,000 U per milliliter (ml.). The vial must be checked to be sure the dose administered corresponds to the strength used. If the dose ordered does *not* compare to the heparin strength available, the dose must be computed. The nurse should use the strength ordered whenever possible. If the strength ordered is not available on the hospital unit, it should be obtained from the pharmacy, unless an emergency situation exists.

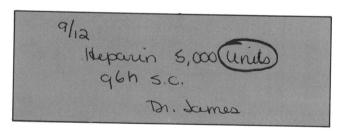

The dose of heparin is usually ordered according to the patient's response to the drug. This is determined by venous clotting time determinations, such as the Lee-White time or the partial thromboplastin time (PTT). The optimum drug effect is reached when the clotting time is 2½ to 3 times the control or the PTT is 1½ to 2 times normal.

The following are to be done according to hospital policies:

1. Notify the laboratory for venous clotting time determinations according to the physician's order. Heparin therapy will be regulated according to laboratory results, since these tests are done immediately prior to the time the heparin dose is due.
2. Notify the physician of the venous clotting times and obtain the order for the next dose of heparin. After a few days the physician may discontinue the laboratory tests and order the amount of heparin that maintains the venous clotting time at the desired level.

As stated above, heparin is administered by the intravenous, subcutaneous, and intramuscular routes, the subcutaneous route being the most common. The injection site should *not* be massaged *before* or *after* injection of the drug.

Protamine sulfate should be readily available in case it becomes necessary to reverse the effects of heparin.

Throughout the period of heparin therapy the possibility of the occurrence of side effects should be considered. In formulating a plan of care, all personnel must plan to check the patient for signs of bleeding. This includes:

1. notations on the Kardex, preferably in *red*: "PATIENT RECEIVING HEPARIN"
2. notation on the Kardex regarding points of observation: "check for easy bruising, check urine and stool for the appearance of blood, check the mouth for bleeding"

ORAL ANTICOAGULANTS

Patients receiving oral anticoagulants for the first time require a daily adjustment of the drug dose, which is determined by blood prothrombin levels. Prior to the first dose, a base line—the patient's normal prothrombin level—should be obtained. The nurse should check with the physician regarding initial prothrombin levels *before the drug is administered*. In most cases the physician writes a specific order requesting a prothrombin time before the initial dose of an oral anticoagulant is administered.

Optimum therapeutic results are achieved when prothrombin levels are 1½ to 3 times the control value. Prothrombin values depend on the procedure and materials used and therefore vary slightly from hospital to hospital.

Although hospital patient records vary, most include an anticoagulant chart for recording prothrombin levels, the control value, and the dose of anticoagulant given.

The patient's response to oral anticoagulant therapy is sometimes unpredictable. Since laboratory values vary, appropriate personnel or hospital policy books should be consulted to find the safe maximum limit of prothrombin levels. Whenever a laboratory report exceeds this limit, the physician must be contacted.

Bleeding can occur at any time, even when prothrombin levels appear to be within a safe limit. Bleeding is an indication that the prothrombin level is too high for the particular patient. Any bleeding, *no matter how slight*, is a warning and necessitates notifying the physician as soon as possible. If bleeding is detected prior to the administration of the oral anticoagulant, the drug is *not* to be given. This also applies to prothrombin levels that are higher than the accepted maximum limit; the drug is *not* to be given until the physican has been notified.

All nursing personnel should be informed of patients receiving anticoagulants, including nurses and assistants. A notation on the Kardex along with a review of drug therapy in a team conference will help alert nursing personnel, especially those working part-time who may not readily know the drug therapy of all patients. Notations should be made in red, along with specific nursing observations:

CHECK THE FOLLOWING AREAS
FOR BLEEDING AND REPORT

urinal (or catheter drainage unit), bedpan, emesis basin, nasogastric suction EACH TIME EMPTIED

toothbrush, emesis basin during oral care

easy bruising, nosebleeds, excessive bleeding from minor cuts or scratches

---

The antidotes for oral anticoagulants—the vitamin K preparations menadione (Hykinone) or phytonadione

Table 11-2.
DRUGS AND CONDITIONS AFFECTING
THE RESPONSE TO ANTICOAGULANTS*

Increased Effectiveness (patient can bleed)	Decreased Effectiveness (effectiveness of drug is lost)
ANTIBIOTICS—may destroy intestinal bacteria that manufacture vitamin K	DIARRHEA—hinders the absorption of oral anticoagulants
ASPIRIN and other salicylates —may affect prothrombin synthesis	MINERAL OIL—same reason as diarrhea
OTHER DRUGS—phenylbutazone (Butazolidin), thyroid preparations, quinidine, ethacrynic acid (Edecrin)	OTHER DRUGS—barbiturates, glutethimide (Doriden), ethchlorvynol (Placidyl)

* This is only a partial list. Appropriate references should be consulted for a complete list of agents that increase or decrease the effectiveness of oral anticoagulants.

(Mephyton)—should be readily available and stocked in the medicine room.

Certain drugs and conditions can alter the effectiveness of oral anticoagulants by either increasing or decreasing prothrombin levels. If these levels are *decreased*, the effectiveness of the anticoagulant may be lost, if *increased*, bleeding can occur (Table 11-2).

Discharge Teaching

Discharge teaching should include the following points:

1. the drug is to be taken as directed
2. importance of visits to the physician's office
3. if another physician or dentist is seen, he should be made aware of anticoagulant drug therapy
4. other nonprescription drugs should not be taken without first consulting the physician. This includes aspirin, all other analgesics, laxatives, cold and hay fever medications, etc.
5. identification, such as MEDIC-ALERT, should be carried. In case of an accident or sudden illness this will alert hospital personnel
6. any signs of bleeding as well as other side effects must be reported to the physician *at once*. The drug should *not* be taken until the physician has been contacted
7. the physician should be called without delay if a problem occurs.

Long-term anticoagulant therapy requires cooperation on the part of the patient and the family. Caution should be exercised in teaching, so that the patient is not unduly alarmed. Teaching should progress at the patient's pace and level of understanding. It may help if important points are written down for the patient's future reference.

Table 11-3.
ANTICOAGULANT DRUGS

Generic Name	Trade Name	Uses	Side Effects	Dose Ranges
acenocoumarol	Sintrom	prophylaxis and treatment of: intravascular clotting, postoperative thrombophlebitis, pulmonary embolus, emboli and thrombi of peripheral arteries, myocardial infarction	nausea, vomiting, anorexia, abdominal cramping, diarrhea; overdose may produce bleeding tendency	INITIAL DOSE: 8-28 mg. daily orally MAINTENANCE: 2-10 mg. daily orally
anisindione	Miradon	same as acenocoumarol	same as acenocoumarol	INITIAL DOSE: 100-300 mg. daily orally MAINTENANCE: 25-200 mg. daily orally
dicumarol		same as acenocoumarol	same as acenocoumarol	INITIAL DOSE: 200-300 mg. daily orally MAINTENANCE: 25-200 mg. daily orally
heparin sodium	Panheprin	prophylaxis and treatment of thromboembolitic disorders, used during extracorporeal circulation procedures	local irritation, hematoma at injection site, bleeding tendency	dose based on venous clotting time
phenindione	Hedulin	same as acenocoumarol	same as acenocoumarol	INITIAL DOSE: 100-300 mg. in divided doses orally MAINTENANCE: 50-150 mg. daily orally
warfarin potassium	Athrombin-K	same as acenocoumarol	same as acenocoumarol	same as warfarin sodium; given only by oral route
warfarin sodium	Coumadin, Panwarfin	same as acenocoumarol	same as acenocoumarol	INITIAL DOSE: 10-60 mg. daily orally, I.M., I.V. MAINTENANCE: 2-10 mg. daily orally, I.M., I.V.

Table 11-3. (*Continued*)

Generic Name	Trade Name	Uses	Side Effects	Dose Ranges
HEPARIN ANTAGONIST				
protamine sulfate		heparin antagonist	hypotension, bradycardia, flushing	up to 50 mg. by *slow* intravenous injection
ORAL ANTICOAGULANT ANTAGONISTS				
menadiol sodium diphosphate	Synkayvite	antagonist: oral anticoagulants; treatment of prothrombin deficient states		5-10 mg. orally, I.M.
menadione sodium bisulfate	Hykinone	same as menadiol sodium diphosphate		50-100 mg. by *slow* I.V. injection; other deficiency states: 500 mcg.-2 mg. S.C., I.M., I.V.
phytonadione	Mephyton, Konakion	same as menadiol sodium diphosphate		2.5-25 mg. I.M., S.C., I.V., orally

Diseases of the arteries can cause three serious problems: heart disease, cerebral vascular disease, and peripheral vascular disease. Vasodilating drugs sometimes relieve the symptoms of these diseases, but in some cases drug therapy affords only minimal relief.

Types of Vasodilating Agents

There are several types of vasodilating agents that bear no chemical relationship to one another. The most commonly used are **papaverine; the nitrites; miscellaneous agents** such as cyclandelate (Cyclospasmol), isoxsuprine (Vasodilan), and dipyridamole (Persantine); and **alpha adrenergic blocking agents** (see Chapter 3).

General Drug Action

Vasodilating agents principally affect the smooth muscle of blood vessels. The exact action of some of these drugs is not known, whereas others possess alpha adrenergic blocking activity. Relaxation of the smooth muscle layer of blood vessels results in vasodilation, which increases the amount of blood available to the area. Some vasodilating drugs, such as the nitrites, are effective in the treatment of specific vascular diseases, whereas

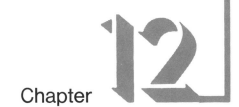

Chapter

Vasodilating Agents

others with more generalized action may prove only moderately effective. In some instances, drug therapy brings about only partial, short-lived improvement.

Uses of Vasodilating Agents

Papaverine, a derivative of opium that possesses *no* narcotic-like effects, is sometimes used in the treatment of peripheral vascular diseases. Some physicians feel that the effectiveness of the drug is limited.

The nitrites are used chiefly in the treatment of angina pectoris. Amyl nitrite has a pungent odor and is used only as an inhalant. It is packaged in crushable glass ampuls; the ampul is crushed in a handkerchief and the vapors inhaled. Other nitrites, which are easier to use and work equally well, have largely replaced amyl nitrite.

Glyceryl trinitrate (nitroglycerin), erythrityl tetranitrate (Cardilate), and isosorbide dinitrate (Isordil) belong to the nitrite group and are used in the treatment of coronary insufficiency and angina pectoris. Dipyridamole (Persantine), although not related to the nitrites, is also used in the treatment of angina.

Cyclandelate (Cyclospasmol) and isoxsuprine (Vasodilan) are used in the treatment of peripheral vascular diseases.

Side Effects of Vasodilating Agents

Side effects of these drugs are usually results of their action, that is, vasodilatation. Headache, flushing of the skin, dizziness, lightheadedness, weakness, gastrointestinal distress, sweating, and rash may be seen. In some patients these side effects may be minimal; in others they are more pronounced.

Clinical Considerations

Nitroglycerin is given in the form of *sublingual* tablets placed *under* the tongue and allowed to dissolve. A patient may have to be shown *how* to use the drug for the first time. The drug is *not* to be swallowed, since this destroys its effectiveness and may cause gastric distress. One form of nitroglycerin—Nitroglyn—is a sustained-action preparation that is swallowed.

Nitroglycerin is usually ordered p.r.n.—that is, it is taken whenever the patient requires relief from the pain of angina. Since angina attacks often come without warning, the physician may order the drug to be kept at the patient's bedside, where it is available for immediate relief.

If nitroglycerin is left at the bedside, it is important to keep an accurate account of the number of tablets used each day. The patient can be given a pad and pencil to record the times the medication was needed and whether the drug relieved the pain. Not all patients are able or willing to keep this record; to those who are, it may be of value in the assessment of their disease. The physician, knowing the exact number of tablets used and the relief afforded will be able to determine whether or not different therapy should be instituted in the future. Further studies, such as X-ray, may be needed and surgery may be planned if angina is not relieved by drug therapy.

In the event that the patient cannot keep a record of nitroglycerin use, the nurse should record this information. It may be necessary to check several times a day, since patients have a tendency to forget how many tablets were taken and at what time the tablets were necessary. In the event dizziness, headache, or weakness occurs during or after taking the drug, the patient should be instructed to remain quiet, breathe deeply, and move the legs. This may relieve the symptoms.

Occasionally the patient may ask if the drug nitroglycerin will explode. The patient should be assured that this form of nitroglycerin will *not* explode and that there is no need to fear handling the drug.

Usually six to ten nitroglycerin tablets are left at the patient's bedside unless ordered otherwise by the physician. The supply can be replenished as needed; however, excessive use of the drug may require contacting the physician, as a more serious situation may be developing.

When a vasodilator is used to treat peripheral vascular diseases such as Raynaud's disease or Buerger's disease, the patient's response to drug therapy should be assessed. Usually response is slow; it may be several days before there are noticeable changes in the patient's condition. The patient may be of assistance in comparing overt changes before and during drug therapy.

In assessing the patient's response to drug therapy in peripheral vascular disease, skin color (pale, mottled, or cyanotic) and temperature (cool or warm) and the presence or absence of pain (increased or diminished) should be noted and recorded in the patient's chart. *Abrupt* changes should be reported immediately. Intense white or dark areas may indicate the development of a more serious problem, and the physician should be contacted immediately.

Table 12-1.
VASODILATING AGENTS

Generic Name	Trade Name	Uses	Side Effects	Dose Ranges
amyl nitrite		angina	marked flushing, headache, throbbing of head	1 ampul, crushed in handkerchief, vapors inhaled
cyclandelate	Cyclospasmol	management of occlusive vascular disease, nocturnal leg cramps, leg ulcers, cerebral edema	flushing, tingling of extremities, dizziness, headache, sweating, tachycardia, gastrointestinal disturbances	200-400 mg. Q.I.D., a.c., h.s. orally
dipyridamole	Persantine	coronary insufficiency	same as cyclandelate	25-50 mg. T.I.D. a.c. orally
erythrityl tetranitrate	Cardilate	angina	headache, nausea	5-10 mg. T.I.D. sublingual, oral
glyceryl trinitrate (nitroglycerin)		angina	flushing, headache	400-600 mcg. sublingual q2-3h p.r.n.
isosorbide dinitrate	Isordil	same as dipyridamole	same as cyclandelate	5-10 mg. sublingual; 5-30 mg. Q.I.D. a.c. and h.s. orally
isoxsuprine	Vasodilan	arteriosclerosis, Raynaud's disease	dizziness, lightheadedness	10-20 mg. T.I.D., Q.I.D. orally; 5-10 mg. I.M.
pentaerythritol tetranitrate	Peritrate	angina	headache, nausea, visual disturbances	20 mg. Q.I.D. a.c. and h.s. orally

The composition of body fluids remains fairly constant despite the many demands placed on the body each day. On occasion, these demands cannot be met and drugs and fluids must be given in an attempt to restore equilibrium.

Types and Uses of Solutions Used in the Management of Body Fluids

Blood plasma, dextran, serum albumin, protein hydrolysate, and **glucose** are used in an attempt to correct fluid deficiencies or treat certain diseases or conditions.

Blood plasma is the liquid part of blood, containing in solution, water, sugar, electrolytes, fats, gases, proteins, bile pigment, and clotting factors. Human plasma, also called *human pooled plasma,* is obtained from the liquid portion of donated blood. While whole blood must be typed and cross-matched because it contains red blood cells carrying blood type and Rh factors, human plasma does not require this procedure. Because of this, plasma can be given in acute emergencies. Plasma is used to increase the blood volume when:

1. hemorrhage has occurred and fluid must be administered immediately
2. plasma alone has been lost, for example in severe extensive burns.

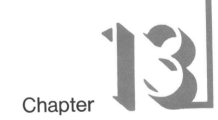

Chapter 13   97

Management of Body Fluids

Plasma is also used to provide lost proteins in kidney and liver disease. Plasma is given intravenously.

Dextran is a polysaccharide manufactured as 6% dextran in sodium chloride. Like plasma, dextran is used to increase blood volume when hemorrhage has occurred, until whole blood is available.

Serum albumin is a sterile solution of albumin obtained from healthy human donors. One hundred milliliters of serum albumin is equivalent to approximately 500 ml. of whole blood since it increases plasma volume by 400 to 500 ml.

Serum albumin is used (1) as a plasma expander, (2) in the treatment of edema of nephrosis, and (3) to treat severe cirrhosis. The therapeutic value of serum albumin in the latter two conditions has been questionable and use may be reserved for those who do not respond to other forms of therapy.

Protein hydrolysates are mixtures of amino acids administered intravenously for the treatment of protein deficiency, a condition seen in those who cannot ingest, digest, or assimilate protein.

Glucose (dextrose) is available in concentrations of 2.5% to 50%. The lower concentrations are used to supply calories and water when food and/or liquids cannot be taken orally. Fifty percent glucose is an osmotic diuretic used to *remove* excess fluid from the body.

Types and Uses of Electrolytes and Salts Used in the Management of Body Fluids

A **cation-exchange resin,** sodium polystyrene (Kayexalate), is used in the treatment of HYPERkalemia (*high* blood potassium) in patients with kidney disease or damage to the kidney resulting from crushing injury. Routes of administration are oral or rectal, in the form of a retention enema. The mode of action is exchange of ions across a membrane—the intestine. Most of the exchange action takes place in the large intestine, regardless of whether the resin is given orally or rectally.

Potassium (K^+) preparations such as potassium chloride, potassium bicarbonate (K-Lyte), and potassium gluconate (Kaon) are given for HYPOkalemia (*low* blood potassium). Extensive burns, uncontrolled diabetes, loss of fluid due to excessive diuresis, and loss of fluid from the gastrointestinal tract due to vomiting, diarrhea, nasogastric suction, or intestinal fistulas result in hypokalemia. Potassium may be administered orally or intravenously, depending on the type used and the reason for use. When the intravenous route is used the drug *must be diluted* in 500 or 1000 ml. of intravenous solution and administered *slowly.*

Potassium is a major cation (an ion with a positive charge) of the body fluid and is necessary for the transmission of nerve impulses, the contraction of muscles (including cardiac muscle), and other physiological processes.

Calcium (Ca^{++}), for example, calcium chloride and calcium gluconate, is given for HYPOcalcemia (*low* blood calcium). Disease, accidental removal of the parathyroid glands, pregnancy, and malnutrition may result in hypocalcemia. Calcium is necessary for the functioning of nerves and muscles, the clotting of blood, the building of bones and teeth, and other physiological processes.

Sodium bicarbonate ($NaHCO_3$) is a salt used as

an antacid (see Chapter 30) and to treat acidosis. Some causes of acidosis are severe renal disease, uncontrollable diabetes, cardiac arrest, and severe dehydration. It is bicarbonate, not sodium, that is effective. This drug may be given orally or intravenously.

Sodium (Na^+), as sodium chloride, is administered for HYPOnatremia (*low* blood sodium). It may be given orally or intravenously. Excessive diaphoresis, severe vomiting and/or diarrhea, and intestinal fistulas are some causes of hyponatremia. Sodium is essential in the maintenance of normal heart action and in the regulation of osmotic pressure in body cells.

Side Effects of Solutions Used in the Management of Body Fluids

BLOOD PLASMA: There is a risk of transmitting serum hepatitis through blood plasma administration. In laboratories where donors are carefully screened, this risk is greatly minimized. Circulatory overload, due to rapid infusion, can lead to cardiac failure and pulmonary edema.

DEXTRAN: There are no side effects to dextran administration except circulatory overload due to rapid infusion of the intravenous solution. Rarely urticaria and anaphylactoid reactions may be seen.

SERUM ALBUMIN: Though rare, risk of transmitting serum hepatitis is possible. Circulatory overload may also occur.

PROTEIN HYDROLYSATES: Should be infused slowly, especially when first started, since nausea, vomiting, and a feeling of warmth may occur. Slowing the infusion to 2-5 drops per minute may eliminate these effects, but if they continue it may be necessary to discontinue the infusion.

GLUCOSE: There are no side effects to glucose administration except circulatory overload due to rapid infusion of the intravenous solution.

Side Effects of Electrolytes and Salts Used in the Management of Body Fluids

CATION-EXCHANGE RESINS: Potassium deficiency (hypokalemia) can occur if doses are too high. The amount of resin to be given is calculated according to serum potassium levels.

POTASSIUM: Abdominal discomfort, diarrhea, nausea, and vomiting may be noted with the oral or intravenous administration of potassium salts. Overdose or rapid intravenous administration can result in HYPERkalemia, with signs of mental confusion, listlessness, weakness, numbness of the extremities, paralysis, hypotension, and cardiac arrhythmias. Death due to cardiac arrhythmias can occur if the situation is not recognized.

CALCIUM: There are no side effects to calcium chloride administration except signs of overdose (HYPERcalcemia), including weakness, anorexia, constipation, and weight loss. Cardiac arrhythmias may result from intravenous administration.

SODIUM BICARBONATE: The only danger involved in the use of sodium bicarbonate is overdose, resulting in *alkalosis*—a state of alkali excess. In emergency situations, such as cardiac arrest, it may be difficult to avoid some degree of alkalosis since the drug is administered rapidly, with no time available to await the results of laboratory studies regarding the degree of acidosis present or the patient's response.

Baking soda is sodium bicarbonate. Excessive use as a remedy for gastric distress could also result in alkalosis.

SODIUM: Excessive amounts of sodium chloride can result in edema. In some patients this places an added strain on the heart.

Clinical Considerations

Patients receiving intravenous dextrose, serum albumin, and plasma should be observed for signs of circulatory overload, namely a weak and rapid pulse, dyspnea, and hypotension. Given when the circulatory volume is *decreased*, these solutions are capable of increasing the volume. If solutions are administered too rapidly, the fluid deficit may be more than met, and overload results. At the first sign of circulatory overload the infusion should be slowed to 1-3 drops, or at least as slow as possible, until the physician examines the patient.

As with any intravenous administration, the needle site should be inspected frequently for signs of tissue infiltration. The patient should be made as comfortable as possible, although under some circumstances this may be difficult. A large needle, which may also cause discomfort, is required for the administration of serum albumin.

When cation-exchange resins are administered rectally, a cleansing enema is usually given first. Then the powdered resin is mixed with water and administered with a large rectal catheter. The viscous fluid flows in by gravity and must be stirred frequently. The solution should remain in place for 4 hours; however, this often proves difficult for most patients. Elevating the hips may help in retaining fluid. The bed should be protected with absorbent pads or by plastic sheeting beneath the draw sheet. The patient may experience abdominal cramping due to the pressure of the fluid in the colon. A saline enema is given to remove the resin.

When potassium is given intravenously, it *must* be diluted in 500-1000 ml. of intravenous solution and given in *not less than 4 hours*, unless specifically ordered otherwise by the physician. In order to administer the mixture in 4 or more hours, correct calculation is necessary:

1. Determine the number of drops per ml. delivered by the brand of intravenous administration set used. This is stated on the container. (The number of drops per ml. administered by each product varies with the manufacturer.)

2. Several approaches can be used in making calculations; one example is given here. These computations can be expressed as:

(a) $\dfrac{\text{TOTAL AMOUNT OF SOLUTION}}{\text{NUMBER OF HOURS}} =$
number of ml./hr.

(b) $\dfrac{\text{ML./HR.}}{60} =$ number of ml./minute

(c) ML./MIN. $\times$ NUMBER OF DROPS/ML.
$=$ number of drops/minute

1000 ml. (amount of I.V. solution)

8 hours (the time the solution is to infuse—this time is selected by the physician or nurse)

number of ml. per hour: $1000 \div 8 = 125$ ml.

number of ml. per minute: $125 \div 60 = 2.08$ ml./m. (round off to 2 ml. per minute)

If there are 14 drops per ml. delivered by the brand of intravenous infusion set being used, there are 28 drops in 2 ml. Since the desired amount to be infused per minute is 2 ml., the infusion should be timed at 28 drops per minute.

When sodium bicarbonate is given by the intravenous route, the solution must be checked frequently to assure that infusion is at the rate ordered by the physician. When used during cardiopulmonary resuscitation procedures, the 50 ml. ampul size may be administered intravenously every 10 minutes, although this time span can vary.

Excessive doses of sodium can result in edema, with additional strain on the cardiovascular system. Intravenous solutions containing sodium as sodium chloride ("normal saline") are contraindicated in patients with cardiac disease. If use of intravenous solutions containing sodium is necessary, these patients should be observed for circulatory overload and pulmonary edema.

All intravenous solutions, for example 5% dextrose in water, should be administered with great care. *At no time* should *any* intravenous solution be run at a rapid rate unless there is a specific written order for rapid infusion. The *average* length of time for the infusion of 1000 ml. of solution is 4-8 hours.

Whenever an electrolyte, salt, or intravenous solution is given to a patient great care must be exercised. Use of these drugs and solutions is commonplace, but complacency should never replace the vigilance necessary for safe drug administration.

Discharge Teaching

The frequent use of sodium bicarbonate (baking soda) should be discouraged since excessive use can lead to alkalosis. In addition, use of this common household product may disguise a more serious problem.

Discharge teaching for patients taking oral potassium should include mention of the importance of measuring the medication accurately and possible side effects. The patient should be encouraged to call his physician if side effects occur and to discontinue taking the medication until the physician has been made aware of the problem.

Table 13-1.
DRUGS USED IN THE MANAGEMENT OF BODY FLUIDS

Generic Name	Trade Name	Uses	Side Effects	Dose Ranges
calcium lactate		treatment of hypocalcemia	overdose: hypercalcemia	4 Grams T.I.D. 1 hour p.c. orally
calcium gluconate		same as calcium acetate	same as calcium acetate	1-15 Grams daily in divided doses, given 1 hour p.c. orally; 5-20 ml. of 10% solution slowly I.V.
potassium bicarbonate	K-Lyte	treatment of hypokalemia	listlessness, mental confusion, tingling of extremities, gastrointestinal disturbances, nausea, vomiting, diarrhea; hypotension, cardiac arrhythmias with overdose	1 tablet or 1 dose COMPLETELY DISSOLVED in water B.I.D., Q.I.D. orally
potassium gluconate	Kaon	same as potassium bicarbonate	same as potassium bicarbonate	15 ml. in 1 or more ounces of water B.I.D., Q.I.D. orally
sodium bicarbonate		treatment of metabolic acidosis	overdose: alkalosis	varies with severity of acidosis
sodium chloride		treatment of hyponatremia	overdose: edema, electrolyte disturbance	adjusted to patient's need
sodium polystyrene	Kayexalate	treatment of hyperkalemia	hypokalemia, hypocalcemia, constipation, anorexia, nausea, vomiting	15-60 Grams daily orally, rectally

Diuretics

Many conditions or diseases can cause retention of excess fluid (edema), such as heart failure, endocrine disturbances, and kidney and liver diseases. Diuretic therapy may be instituted to rid the tissues of the body of excess fluid.

Types of Diuretic Agents

There are various types of diuretic agents. Some have specific uses; the diuretic mannitol, for example, is used in the treatment of oliguria (decreased urine secretion). Other diuretics are used in the treatment of edema regardless of the cause.

The types of diuretics are: **osmotic diuretics, mercurial diuretics, thiazide diuretics, carbonic anhydrase inhibitors, aldosterone antagonists,** the xanthines, and **miscellaneous agents.**

General Drug Action of Diuretic Agents

Most diuretics act on the tubules of the kidney nephron. There are approximately one million nephrons in each kidney filtering the bloodstream to remove waste products and impurities. During this process electrolytes and water are also filtered.

Chapter **14**

Diuretics and Antihypertensive Agents

The filtrate, which normally contains ions (potassium, sodium, chloride), waste products (ammonia, urea), and water passes through the proximal and distal convoluted tubules and the loop of Henle. At these points selective *reabsorption* of amino acids, glucose, some electrolytes, and water takes place. Thus ions and water required by the body are returned to the bloodstream by minute capillaries that surround the tubules.

An osmotic diuretic increases the density of the glomerular filtrate. This prevents selective reabsorption, and water is excreted.

The mercurial and thiazide diuretics depress tubular reabsorption of sodium and chloride ions. Sodium and chloride are then excreted in the urine. Since excess sodium causes edema, loss of sodium will reduce the amount of edema.

Furosemide (Lasix) acts on both the distal and proximal tubules and loop of Henle. The mode of action is similar to that of mercurial diuretics. Ethacrynic acid (Edecrin) is similar to furosemide (Lasix) in mode of action.

Carbonic anhydrase, an enzyme found in the body, produces free hydrogen ions which are then exchanged for sodium ions in the kidney tubules. Carbonic anhydrase inhibitors prevent the exchange of sodium and hydrogen ions, and sodium and bicarbonate ions are excreted. Water loss subsequently follows the sodium loss.

Aldosterone, a hormone secreted by the adrenal cortex, enhances the *reabsorption* of sodium in the distal convoluted tubule. An aldosterone antagonist blocks the effect of this hormone on the kidney tubule and sodium and water are excreted.

Caffeine, theophylline and theobromine are xanthines with relatively weak diuretic activity. Aminophylline U.S.P. (theophylline ethylenediamine) is the most effective xanthine-type diuretic. The precise mode of action is unknown, but it is generally believed that xanthines act on the kidney tubule. These drugs have been replaced by newer and more potent diuretics.

Uses of Diuretic Agents

Diuretics are mainly used to treat edema—the retention of excess fluid in body tissues. A variety of diseases or conditions may give rise to edema—liver disease, hypertension, kidney disease, congestive heart failure, and pregnancy, as well as some drugs, such as corticosteroids.

The diuretic that will best suit the patient is selected. Mild forms of edema usually respond to use of the less potent diuretics, usually as oral preparations. Moderate to severe forms usually require a more potent diuretic, the route depending on the speed of action desired and the patient's general condition.

Some nonedematous states are treated with diuretics. Glaucoma and epilepsy may be treated with carbonic anhydrase inhibitors such as acetazolamide (Diamox). Osmotic diuretics, such as mannitol (Osmitrol), may be used to increase the secretion of urine in cases of severe oliguria and anuria. Uses of the different types of diuretic agents are indicated as follows.

OSMOTIC DIURETICS: prevention of acute renal failure during and after prolonged surgery, treatment of mercury poisoning, treatment of anuria and oliguria due to shock, hemorrhage, and dehydration

MERCURIAL DIURETICS: edema due to congestive heart failure and nephrosis, ascites due to cirrhosis

THIAZIDE DIURETICS: congestive heart failure when other diuretics are ineffective, edema due to nephrotic syndrome, edema of pregnancy, premenstrual syndrome, edema due to drugs, hypertension

CARBONIC ANHYDRASE INHIBITORS: glaucoma, selected cases of petit mal and grand mal epilepsy, premenstrual syndrome

ALDOSTERONE ANTAGONISTS: treatment of edema when other diuretics are ineffective; may also be used alone or more effectively with other diuretics

XANTHINES: pulmonary edema, edema associated with congestive heart failure

MISCELLANEOUS AGENTS: ethacrynic acid (Edecrin) and furosemide (Lasix) are used in edema associated with congestive heart failure, acute pulmonary edema, when other diuretics are ineffective, edema due to the nephrotic syndrome, hepatic cirrhosis, lymphedema

Side Effects of Diuretic Agents

OSMOTIC DIURETICS: *Mannitol*—headache, nausea, circulatory overload; *Urea*—nausea, vomiting, headache, hypotension, mental confusion

MERCURIAL DIURETICS: stomatitis, gastric disturbances, vertigo, electrolyte disturbances; cardiac arrhythmias can occur with I.V. use

THIAZIDE DIURETICS: electrolyte disturbances, gastrointestinal disturbances, rash

CARBONIC ANHYDRASE INHIBITORS: mild acidosis, drowsiness

ALDOSTERONE ANTAGONISTS: headache, mental confusion, rash; larger doses: drowsiness, ataxia, abdominal discomfort

XANTHINES: *oral*—gastrointestinal disturbances, headache, rash, electrolyte disturbances; *intramuscular*—pain at site of injection, electrolyte disturbances; *intravenous*—headache, flushing, hypotension, cardiac arrhythmias

MISCELLANEOUS AGENTS: *ethacrynic acid* (Edecrin)—electrolyte disturbances, anorexia, nausea, vomiting, abdominal discomfort, diarrhea, rash, headache; *furosemide* (Lasix)—rash, electrolyte disturbances, nausea, vomiting, diarrhea

Clinical Considerations

The chief side effect of diuretic therapy in edema is the loss of electrolytes and water. In some patients the diuretic effect of these drugs is moderate, whereas in others a large volume of urine is secreted. Regardless of the amount of fluid lost, there is always the possibility of excessive electrolyte loss, which in some cases can be serious.

Table 14-1.

FOR PATIENTS ON DIURETIC MEDICATIONS

SIGNS OF HYPOKALEMIA	SIGNS OF HYPONATREMIA
muscle cramps	oliguria, anuria
muscle weakness	decreased skin turgor
cardiac arrhythmias	dry mucous membranes
postural hypotension	hypotension
apathy, malaise	tachycardia
anorexia	apprehension
vomiting	
abdominal distension, paralytic ileus	
thirst	
shallow respirations	

On occasion, concurrent replacement drug therapy will be ordered, that is, additional use of salt (*sodium chloride*) and the administration of potassium. While this is not necessary in all cases, it may be of importance to those losing excessive amounts of sodium and potassium.

In order to recognize early signs of electrolyte loss, the signs of hyponatremia and hypokalemia should be known by all members of the nursing team. A list of these signs, posted in the medicine room, will aid as a reminder (Table 14-1).

Patients receiving any diuretic for the first time should be placed on intake and output. This, plus daily weight measurement—which should be done at approximately the same time each day—will aid in determining the effectiveness of drug therapy. Anuric and oliguric patients receiving osmotic diuretics must be placed on *accurate* intake and output. The amount of fluid intake and urinary output may be measured every 15-30 minutes. In some instances it may be necessary to use a Urimeter or other device to insure absolute accuracy.

Patients should be told that the injections or tablets will cause frequent voiding. Failure to relate this information may precipitate undue worry and anxiety.

A call light should also be nearby if the patient requires assistance in getting out of bed or using the urinal or bedpan. Patients who are experiencing postural hypotension should be warned to get out of bed slowly or ask for assistance.

Diuretics administered by the intravenous route must be given *slowly* and with *great care*. Although rare, there have been fatal reactions, usually from ventricular fibrillation.

The patient receiving diuretics for the first time requires observation during the first few days of therapy. Complaints that indicate electrolyte loss may necessitate withholding the next dose of the drug until the physician is contacted. Indwelling catheter drainage bags may also require emptying *before* the end of each shift and should be checked periodically during the day.

Some patients experience interruption of sleep during the first few days of therapy. Since many patients stabilize after a few days, this problem sometimes corrects itself.

Discharge Teaching

Discharge teaching should include the following points:

1. the signs and symptoms of electrolyte loss
2. the importance of taking the medication as scheduled by the physician. The medication may be taken daily or only several days per week, such as every second or third day. A calendar, with the proper dates circled, will aid in remembering which day the drug is to be taken
3. the patient should be encouraged to contact the physician if signs of weakness, marked thirst, or any unusual problems occur.

Antihypertensive Agents

Drug therapy for hypertension is directed toward various body systems, namely: blood vessels, the central nervous system, and the extracellular fluid compartment.

Types of Antihypertensive Agents

Most cases of hypertension have an unknown cause, and as in many other diseases and conditions there is no one "best" drug for appropriate treatment. There is a variety of antihypertensive agents, enabling the physician to select the drug he believes will best suit a particular patient.

Adrenergic blocking agents, ganglionic blocking agents, diuretics, veratrum alkaloids, MAO inhibitors, and **sedatives** and **tranquilizers** are used in the treatment of hypertension.

General Drug Action of Antihypertensive Agents

The exact mechanism of action of the adrenergic blocking agents is not well understood. Even though the actions of some of these drugs are slightly different, the results are the same.

Ganglionic blocking agents block the transmission of impulses at the ganglia (plural of ganglion) of the sympathetic and parasympathetic nervous systems. A ganglion is a mass of nerve cell tissue that lies outside the central nervous system. A preganglionic fiber comes before the ganglion, and a postganglionic fiber comes after the ganglion. Preganglionic fibers of the sympathetic and parasympathetic nervous systems secrete acetylcholine.

Ganglionic blocking agents act on sympathetic *and* parasympathetic nerve fibers; therefore the effect of these drugs resembles the effects of adrenergic blocking and cholinergic blocking agents.

The diuretics, especially the thiazides, remove excess water and sodium from the body, thus reducing blood volume and lowering the blood pressure. This appears to be the *immediate* action of diuretics; however, on a long-term basis, these drugs appear to act in a different manner, which is not clearly understood.

The veratrum alkaloids reflexly stimulate the vasomotor center and impulses are then sent to the heart and blood vessels. Heart action is slowed and blood vessels dilated. This in turn results in a drop in blood pressure.

The MAO (*monoamine oxidase*) inhibitors are antidepressant drugs, but one—pargyline (Eutonyl)—is used expressly in the treatment of hypertension. The precise mechanism of action is not fully understood.

Sedatives and tranquilizers may be used to treat hypertension but in themselves do not have true antihypertensive action. These drugs are usually used in conjunction with other antihypertensive agents. Their ability to relieve apprehension and anxiety is of value in the treatment of this disease.

Uses of Antihypertensive Agents

After the severity and, if possible, the etiology of hypertension in the patient have been determined, an agent must be selected for treatment. Some antihypertensive agents, such as the rauwolfia alkaloids, are used to treat mild to moderate forms of hypertension. The veratrum alkaloids are almost always used in moderate to severe forms. The patient's response to drug therapy must also be considered; since response can be quite variable, the therapy may have to be altered until the optimum drug/dose response is attained.

Side Effects of Antihypertensive Agents

ADRENERGIC BLOCKING AGENTS: bradycardia, nausea, fatigue, diarrhea, and nasal stuffiness. Episodes of hypotension may also occur, especially during the use of methyldopa (Aldomet) and guanethidine (Ismelin).

GANGLIONIC BLOCKING AGENTS: produce a wide variety of side effects arising from their ability to block both sympathetic and parasympathetic ganglia. The side effects most commonly seen are dryness of the mouth, blurred vision, nausea, vomiting, diarrhea or constipation, urinary retention, and postural hypotension.

DIURETICS: when used as antihypertensive agents have the same side effects as those seen when they are used in treatment of edema. Electrolyte disturbance is the chief side effect, but gastrointestinal effects may also be seen.

VERATRUM ALKALOIDS: potent antihypertensive agents with a narrow margin of safety. Hypotension and bradycardia are the most common side effects, but nausea, vomiting, perspiration, salivation, flushing, and dizziness are also seen. Adjustment of dosage may relieve some of these side effects.

MAO INHIBITOR, pargyline (Eutonyl): may cause nausea, vomiting, dryness of the mouth, insomnia, peripheral edema, constipation, headache, and postural hypotension. Drugs such as barbiturates, alcohol, narcotic analgesics, and antihistamines must be used with caution when patient is receiving an MAO inhibitor. Certain foods such as aged cheeses, beer, coffee, and cola beverages can produce *hypertensive crisis*. Liver damage and anemia have also been reported, requiring periodic liver function tests and blood counts.

The chief side effect encountered during the use of sedatives and tranquilizers is excessive drowsiness. Psychological and physical dependence can occur with the use of barbiturates, and psychological dependence must be considered with the use of tranquilizers.

Clinical Considerations

The blood pressure, pulse, and patient's general appearance are general indications of the success or failure of drug therapy. If there is no specific written order for blood pressure and pulse determinations, judgment must be used regarding frequency. Patients who have received these drugs for a period of time and appear to be well stabilized probably require these readings two or three times per day. During the the initial phase of drug therapy, the blood pressure and pulse should be taken every 1-4 hours. This is especially important in cases of severe hypertension and in the use of potent antihypertensive agents.

Postural hypotension may cause dizziness and lightheadedness. The patient should be instructed to assume a sitting or standing position *slowly*. The nurse should take time to explain the hazards of this problem, since it may persist for some time and must be tolerated. The following points are to be explained:

1. the side effect is not unusual
2. the side effect may persist
3. sitting on the edge of the bed for a few minutes or rising from a chair slowly may minimize the symptoms
4. if dizziness persists, return to bed
5. do not attempt to walk unassisted if dizziness and lightheadedness persist for more than 1-2 minutes

The above points can also be included in discharge teaching, if the problem remains. Some patients may require assistance in getting out of bed or a chair. A call light should be nearby within easy reach of the bed or chair.

Blood pressure readings may also be ordered when the patient is in a supine as well as a sitting and standing position. If not so ordered, they should be taken whenever the patient experiences postural hypotension.

Awareness of the side effects that may occur will help in observing the patient's response to drug therapy. If the patient complains of dryness of the mouth, the use of mouth wash or frequent sips of water may alleviate this problem. Appearance of nausea, vomiting, or bradycardia, on the other hand, requires contacting the physician at once.

Discharge Teaching

Discharge teaching may include teaching the patient or a member of the family how to take a blood pressure reading. The physician should be consulted first since not all patients need constant surveillance of vital signs. If the patient inquires as to where a stethoscope and sphygmomanometer may be purchased, it is best to advise a purchase from a reputable medical/surgical supply company rather than from mail order companies that are not medical supply specialists.

Antihypertensive agents must be administered *at the time intervals ordered*. Taking the drug late may interfere with drug action, resulting in drug ineffectiveness and/or an exaggeration of side effects.

Discharge teaching should also include this point, and the patient should be advised to adhere to the dose schedule. It is often of help if the patient is told that the drug works best when taken *exactly* as directed on the prescription container.

Table 14-2.
DIURETICS AND ANTIHYPERTENSIVE AGENTS

Generic Name	Trade Name	Uses	Side Effects	Dose Ranges
Diuretic Agents				
ALDOSTERONE ANTAGONIST				
spironolactone	Aldactone A	treatment of edema resistive to other drugs	headache, mental confusion, rash; abdominal discomfort, drowsiness, ataxia in larger doses	100 mg. daily in divided doses orally
CARBONIC ANHYDRASE INHIBITORS				
acetazolamide	Diamox	glaucoma, petit and grand mal epilepsy, premenstrual syndrome	drowsiness, mild acidosis	250-375 mg. in A.M. daily orally
ethoxyzolamide	Cardrase, Ethamide	same as acetazolamide	nausea, dizziness, numbness of extremities	62.5-750 mg. daily in divided doses orally
MERCURIAL DIURETICS				
chlormerodrin	Neohydrin	ascites, cardiac and nephrotic edema	stomatitis, gastric disturbances, vertigo, electrolyte disturbances	55-110 mg. daily orally
mercaptomerin	Thiomerin	same as chlormerodrin	same as chlormerodrin	0.5-2 ml. S.C.

Generic Name	Trade Name	Uses	Side Effects	Dose Ranges
OSMOTIC DIURETICS				
mannitol	Osmitrol	prevention of acute renal failure during and after prolonged surgery, treatment of mercury poisoning, treatment of anuria and oliguria due to hemorrhage, shock, dehydration	headache, circulatory overload, hyponatremia	50-200 Grams over 24-hour period I.V.
urea	Urevert	reduce or prevent increased intracranial pressure, treatment of cerebral edema, prevention of acute renal failure during and after prolonged surgery	nausea, vomiting, headache, hypotension, mental confusion, tachycardia	up to 120 Grams in 24 hours I.V.; 40-100 Grams daily orally
THIAZIDE DIURETICS				
bendroflume-thiazide	Naturetin	congestive heart failure, when other diuretics are ineffective, edema of nephrotic syndrome, edema of pregnancy, premenstrual syndrome, edema due to drugs, hypertension	electrolyte disturbances, gastrointestinal disturbances, rash	5-20 mg. daily orally
benzthiazide	Exna	same as bendroflumethiazide	same as bendroflumethiazide	50-200 mg. daily orally
chlorothiazide	Diuril	same as bendroflumethiazide	same as bendroflumethiazide	500 mg.-1 Gram daily or B.I.D. orally, as diuretic; 250 mg. B.I.D.-500 mg. T.I.D. orally as antihypertensive; 500 mg. (as sodium salt) I.V.
hydrochloro-thiazide	HydroDIURIL, Esidrix	same as bendroflumethiazide	same as bendroflumethiazide	25-100 mg. daily or B.I.D. orally

Table 14-2. (*Continued*)

GENERIC NAME	TRADE NAME	USES	SIDE EFFECTS	DOSE RANGES
methyclothiazide	Enduron	same as bendroflumethiazide	same as bendroflumethiazide	2.5-20 mg. daily orally
polythiazide	Renese	same as bendroflumethiazide	same as bendroflumethiazide	1-4 mg. daily orally
trichlor-methiazide	Naqua	same as bendroflumethiazide	same as bendroflumethiazide	2-16 mg. daily orally
XANTHINE				
aminophylline U.S.P.		pulmonary edema, edema of congestive heart failure	oral: gastrointestinal disturbances, headache, rash; I.M.: pain at site of injection; I.V.: headache, flushing, hypotension, cardiac arrhythmias	100-200 mg. T.I.D., Q.I.D. orally; 250-500 mg. I.V.
MISCELLANEOUS AGENTS				
ethacrynic acid	Edecrin	edema of congestive heart failure, pulmonary edema, when other diuretics are ineffective, edema due to nephrotic syndrome, hepatic cirrhosis, lymph-edema	electrolyte disturbances, anorexia, gastrointestinal disturbances, rash, headache	50-400 mg. daily orally; 50 mg. I.V. (as sodium ethacrynate)
furosemide	Lasix	same as ethacrynic acid	rash, electrolyte disturbances, nausea, vomiting, diarrhea	40-600 mg. daily orally; 20-40 mg. I.M., I.V.

Generic Name	Trade Name	Uses	Side Effects	Dose Ranges
ANTIHYPERTENSIVE AGENTS				
ADRENERGIC BLOCKING AGENTS				
alseroxylon	Rauwiloid	treatment of mild, labile hypertension	nasal congestion, nausea, fatigue, diarrhea, bradycardia	2-4 mg. daily orally
guanethidine	Ismelin	moderate to severe hypertension	dizziness, weakness, exertional hypotension, bradycardia, diarrhea, nasal congestion	10-50 mg. daily orally
methyldopa	Aldomet	same as guanethidine	headache, dizziness, hypotension, bradycardia, diarrhea, nasal stuffiness	500 mg.-2 Grams daily orally; 250-500 mg. q6h I.V.
GANGLIONIC BLOCKING AGENTS				
mecamylamine	Inversine	moderate to severe hypertension	dryness of mouth, blurred vision, constipation, urinary retention, nausea, vomiting, postural hypotension	2.5-25 mg. daily in divided doses orally
pentolinium	Ansolysen	essential hypertension	same as mecamylamine	20-100 mg. T.I.D., Q.I.D. (may be higher as tolerance develops); 1-10 mg. S.C., I.M.
trimethaphan	Arfonad	used during neurosurgery and vascular surgery to create controlled hypotension	hypotension	administered by anesthesiologist

Table 14-2. (Continued)

Generic Name	Trade Name	Uses	Side Effects	Dose Ranges
MAO INHIBITOR				
pargyline	Eutonyl	moderate to severe hypotension	nausea, vomiting, dryness of mouth, insomnia, nightmares, constipation, headache, hypotension, peripheral edema	25-75 mg. daily orally
VERATRUM ALKALOID				
alkavervir	Veriloid	essential, renal, and malignant hypertension	hypotension, bradycardia, nausea, vomiting, perspiration, salivation, flushing, dizziness	3-5 mg. T.I.D. p.c. orally

NOTE: The dosages for sedatives and tranquilizers when used in conjunction with antihypertensive agents may vary and are usually adjusted according to the patient's response to therapy. The dose for diuretics is also adjusted according to patient response, and may be the same as or less than the dose required for diuresis.

Caffeine, one of the oldest stimulant drugs, is found in coffee and tea. Some central nervous system stimulants such as picrotoxin are rarely used today, whereas others are used to treat specific medical disorders.

Types of Central Nervous System Stimulants

The **xanthine group** of drugs includes three related alkaloids: caffeine, theophylline, and theobromine. Other central nervous system stimulants are **miscellaneous agents** with various clinical applications.

General Drug Action

These drugs act on the cerebrum, brain stem, or spinal cord. Drugs that act principally on the cerebrum are generally referred to as *psychomotor stimulants*. Those with principal action on the brain stem are referred to as *analeptic agents*. Stimulants capable of inducing a convulsion—that is, *convulsants*—act on the brain stem and spinal cord. The xanthine drugs are central nervous system stimulants with additional peripheral activity.

The xanthines—caffeine, theophylline, and theobromine—stimulate the central nervous

Chapter 15

Central Nervous System Stimulants

system (cerebrum and spinal cord) and act on the following peripheral structures:

HEART—stimulation of the myocardium resulting in an increase in rate, contraction, and cardiac output

BLOOD VESSELS—dilatation of peripheral blood vessels, constriction of cerebral blood vessels

SMOOTH MUSCLES—relaxation, especially smooth muscles of the bronchi

KIDNEY—increase in urinary output

Uses of Central Nervous System Stimulants

Strychnine is rarely used in medicine because of the danger of toxicity. Picrotoxin is occasionally used in the treatment of respiratory depression due to barbiturate overdose, but usually other methods of treatment are tried first. Pentylenetetrazol (Metrazol) has been used to produce convulsions as a treatment for certain types of mental illness, a form of treatment rarely used today. This drug is presently used as a diagnostic agent for epilepsy. Doses smaller than one necessary to produce a grand mal seizure are administered while EEG (electroencephalogram) recordings are taken. Changes in brain wave patterns may indicate the area of the brain that is the focus of the epileptic seizure.

Nikethamide (Coramine) is a brain stem stimulant whose chief effect is on the respiratory center. It is used as a respiratory stimulant in cases of barbiturate overdose and anesthesia idiosyncrasy. Ethamivan (Emivan) and doxapram (Dopram) are used as respiratory stimulants to combat the respiratory depressant effects of anesthesia and to hasten awakening from anesthesia when the patient has an idiosyncrasy to anesthetic agents. These two agents are *not* used when the anesthetized patient is going through a normal postoperative recovery period.

Methylphenidate (Ritalin) is a mild central nervous system stimulant used in the treatment of (1) mild depression (2) narcolepsy (overwhelming attacks of sleep), and (3) hyperkinetic children. Such children are overactive with limited attention spans, easily distracted, and generally difficult to manage. Although a central nervous system *stimulant* is prescribed, the response to drug therapy is one of mild sedation and manageability. Deanol (Deaner), like methylphenidate (Ritalin), is used to treat mild cases of apathy and depression and hyperkinetic behavior disorders.

Caffeine, a xanthine, is used medically in the form of caffeine and sodium benzoate, as a respiratory stimulant in barbiturate intoxication and alcoholic stupor. Other drugs, such as ethamivan (Emivan) have largely replaced the medical use of caffeine. Coffee and tea, which contain caffeine, are used nonmedically as stimulants. Both beverages can increase mental alertness and relieve weariness, but the stimulating effect of caffeine in these beverages is mild. Caffeine is also included in some analgesic preparations such as Anacin (aspirin and caffeine) and Empirin Compound (aspirin, phenacetin, and caffeine). The addition of caffeine is for analgesic purposes, rather than central nervous system stimulation, as caffeine has a *mild* constricting effect on pulsating cerebral blood vessels, which may help relieve pain. Caffeine is also available in OTC, nonprescription preparations promoted for their ability to relieve weariness. Unless coffee or tea produces gastric upset or is disliked, the advantage of products such as No-Doz over the liquid beverage appears to be negligible.

Aminophylline, a xanthine, is a salt of theophylline mainly used for its effects on the bronchi and kidneys. It has central nervous system stimulating ability similar to that of caffeine. The bronchodilating effect of aminophylline makes it particularly useful in treating bronchial asthma, pulmonary edema, and congestive heart failure. Intravenous use in the asthmatic patient usually results in increased ease in breathing. Less severe attacks may be treated with the rectal suppository form. Oral aminophylline and theophylline may be used as a prophylactic method of treatment.

Acute pulmonary edema may be treated with intravenous administration of aminophylline, as well as other drugs such as morphine, vasopressors, and cardiotonics. The bronchodilating effect of aminophylline allows more air to move into the lung.

The diuretic effect of aminophylline and theophylline is mild; these drugs are rarely used solely for this purpose. The mild diuretic effect is of value in the treatment of acute pulmonary edema and congestive heart failure. Theobromine has little medical use today, as it is being replaced by other preparations that are more effective.

Side Effects of Central Nervous System Stimulants

Strychnine and picrotoxin are highly toxic drugs, capable of causing convulsions and death. Due to their toxicity, they are rarely used today.

Pentylenetetrazol (Metrazol) is capable of creating convulsive seizures and technically has no side effects except convulsions. Nikethamide (Coramine) is also capable of causing convulsions with overdose.

The side effects of ethamivan (Emivan) involve excessive stimulation of the central nervous system. The patient recovering from anesthesia may thrash about and unless protected may incur injury. Laryngospasm, muscular twitching, and flushing may also be seen.

The administration of doxapram (Dopram) can result in nausea, vomiting, cardiac arrhythmias, broncho- and laryngospasm, hypertension, and hyperactivity. As with ethamivan (Emivan), injury can result if the patient is not protected.

The side effects that may be seen with the administration of methylphenidate (Ritalin) are insomnia, nervousness, anorexia, and nausea. These side effects may disappear with lower doses. This drug should be given with caution to patients who are emotionally unstable—especially those who have a history of drug dependence and/or alcoholism—since tolerance and psychological dependence have been reported.

Use of beverages and tablet preparations containing caffeine may produce nervousness, nausea, tachycardia, and insomnia. Medical use of caffeine and sodium benzoate can cause tachycardia, nervousness, tremors, and insomnia when doses are exceeded.

Theophylline and aminophylline are more toxic than caffeine. Intravenous use of aminophylline can result in headache, dizziness, tachycardia, and hypotension. This drug must be given *slowly*, since fatal cardiac arrhythmias and hypotension have been known to occur. The occurrence of serious side effects is minimal if care is exercised in administration. Intramuscular injection is painful. Oral use may cause gastrointestinal disturbances such as nausea, vomiting, and diarrhea. Rectal administration may irritate the rectal mucosa (lining) and stimulate the defecation reflex with expelling of the suppository. Uneven and slow absorption of the drug when used rectally may or may not be a problem, since drug response is sometimes noted even with partial absorption.

Clinical Considerations

Pentylenetetrazol (Metrazol) may be used to diagnose epilepsy. An oral airway should be readily available in case a grand mal seizure occurs. The patient must be protected from injuring himself, and all objects capable of causing injury should be removed from the patient's area. This includes pillows, tables or stands over or near the cart or bed, and restraining devices.

When central nervous system stimulants are used in depression, narcolepsy, or behavior disorders, the response to the drug should be documented. The patient should be observed for increased alertness and interest in surroundings, increased energy, and—in the case of hyperkinetic children—an improvement in attention span and manageability.

Parents of a hyperkinetic child should be encouraged to keep a record of the child's response to medication and to bring this record with them each time the child sees the physician.

Use of respiratory stimulants requires close patient observation. If they are given to counteract the respiratory depressant effect of drugs or anesthesia, the response should be carefully noted, as failure of the drug to stimulate respiration may require other emergency measures. If the patient does respond, excitement may occur. *Manual* restraining may be necessary until the patient is fully responsive. The patient must *not* be left alone when these drugs are administered for this purpose. Additional personnel may be needed until the patient is fully responsive. Restraining devices should be avoided if possible, as these may cause more excitement as the patient begins to regain consciousness.

When aminophylline is administered for bronchial asthma, pulmonary edema, or congestive heart failure, the patient should be observed for relief of symptoms, namely, improvement in breathing and color. The rectal suppository may be expelled due to stimulation of the defecation reflex. The patient should be checked 15-30 minutes after insertion and the suppository reinserted if necessary.

When administered intravenously in dilute form, aminophylline is added to an intravenous solution—usually dextrose and water. The physician may order a specific number of milliliters per hour to insure adequate drug response. This will require timing the rate of infusion every 15-30 minutes. When administered in undiluted form the drug must be given *slowly*. Vital signs should be taken before and after administration.

If the patient fails to respond to treatment or appears to become suddenly worse, the physician should be notified. Prolongation of an asthmatic attack is physically and emotionally taxing. Other medical measures may be necessary.

Table 15-1.
CENTRAL NERVOUS SYSTEM STIMULANTS

Generic Name	Trade Name	Uses	Side Effects	Dose Ranges
aminophylline U.S.P.		treatment of asthma, congestive heart failure, pulmonary edema	I.V.: hypotension, cardiac arrhythmias; oral: nausea, vomiting, diarrhea; I.M.: pain at site of injection; rectal: irritation of rectal mucosa	100-200 mg. T.I.D., Q.I.D. orally, 500 mg. rectally; 250-500 mg. I.V., I.M. Child: 3.5 mg./Kg. I.M., I.V.; 5 mg./Kg. orally; up to 7 mg./Kg. rectally
caffeine and sodium benzoate U.S.P.		respiratory and cerebral stimulant	insomnia, nervousness, nausea, tremors	500 mg.-1 Gram I.M.
deanol	Deaner	treatment of behavior disorders	headache, restlessness, insomnia, constipation	Child: 100-300 mg. daily orally
doxapram	Dopram	treatment of postanesthetic respiratory depression	broncho- and laryngospasm, nausea, vomiting, cardiac arrhythmias, hypertension, hyperactivity, confusion	administered intravenously by anesthetist
ethamivan	Emivan	same as doxapram	laryngospasm, muscular twitching, flushing	administered intravenously by anesthetist
methylphenidate	Ritalin	treatment of mild depression, narcolepsy, hyperkinetic children	insomnia, nervousness, anorexia, nausea, dizziness, headache	10-60 mg. daily in divided doses, orally; child: up to 60 mg. daily orally
nikethamide	Coramine	treatment of respiratory depression	convulsions with overdose	250 mg.-1.25 Grams I.V., I.M., S.C.
pentylenetetrazol	Metrazol	diagnosis of epilepsy	convulsions	dose varies

Diabetes mellitus has been described in the Ebers papyrus and in the writings of Hippocrates, Galen, and Celsus. In 1889, two scientists, von Mering and Minkowski, were able to produce diabetes artificially by removing the pancreas of animals. About 1922, two Toronto scientists isolated insulin from animal pancreas, which upon injection controlled diabetes. In 1955 the oral hypoglycemic agents were introduced.

Types and Uses of Insulin and Oral Hypoglycemic Agents

INSULIN

Insulin for medical use is obtained from animals. There are three types of insulin: (1) rapid-acting insulin, (2) intermediate-acting insulin, and (3) long-acting insulin. The type and amount of insulin selected for a particular patient depends on many factors: age, severity of the disease, eating patterns and habits, physical activity, and the presence of disease, if any.

The following list describes the three properties of insulin—onset, peak, and duration—that are of clinical importance. For a comparison of these properties in various preparations of insulin, see Table 16-1.

Chapter 16

Insulin and Oral Hypoglycemic Agents

1. *Onset*—or *when* the insulin first begins to act in the body
2. *Peak*—the time when the insulin is exerting maximum action
3. *Duration*—the length of time the insulin remains in effect

Table 16-1.
COMPARISON OF INSULIN PREPARATIONS*

INSULIN	ONSET	PEAK	DURATION
RAPID-ACTING INSULINS			
Insulin Injection U.S.P. (regular insulin, regular Iletin)	½-1 hour	2-6 hours	5-8 hours
Prompt Insulin Zinc Suspension (Semilente Iletin, Semilente Insulin)	½-1 hour	3-9 hours	12-16 hours
INTERMEDIATE-ACTING INSULINS			
Globin Zinc Insulin	1-4 hours	6-16 hours	16-24 hours
Insulin Zinc Suspension (Lente Insulin, Lente Iletin)	1-4 hours	7-12 hours	24-30 hours
Isophane Insulin Suspension (NPH Insulin, NPH Iletin)	1-2 hours	7-12 hours	24-30 hours
LONG-ACTING INSULINS			
Extended Insulin Zinc Suspension (Ultralente Iletin, Ultralente Insulin)	4-8 hours	10-30 hours	34-46 hours
Protamine Zinc Insulin Suspension (Protamine, Zinc and Iletin)	1-8 hours	12-24 hours	30-36 hours

* References may vary slightly on these figures.

Insulin is used to treat juvenile-onset diabetes, since this form of diabetes responds poorly to dietary management and oral hypoglycemic therapy. Maturity-onset diabetes is also treated with insulin, but may also be treated by diet and/or hypoglycemic agents. *Brittle diabetes* is a term used to describe the patient who is sensitive to insulin and whose insulin requirements fluctuate widely despite careful medical management and patient cooperation. This form of diabetes may be treated with insulin—usually several injections of regular insulin per day plus the use of semilente insulin at night.

ORAL HYPOGLYCEMIC AGENTS
There are two types of oral hypoglycemic agents: (1) the sulfonylureas and (2) the biguanides.

Table 16-2.
COMPARISON OF ORAL HYPOGLYCEMIC AGENTS*

DRUG	DURATION OF ACTION
SULFONYLUREAS	
acetohexamide (Dymelor)	12-24 hours
chlorpropamide (Diabinese)	up to 60 hours
tolazamide (Tolinase)	12-24 hours
tolbutamide (Orinase)	6-12 hours
BIGUANIDES	
phenformin (DBI)	4-6 hours
phenformin long-acting (DBI-TD)	8-12 hours

* References may vary slightly on these figures.

Oral hypoglycemic agents are used in mild forms of diabetes mellitus. These drugs are *not* used in juvenile-onset type diabetes. The patient who responds most favorably to therapy with these agents is over 40 years of age and not excessively overweight—the maturity-onset type diabetic. Not all maturity-onset type diabetics are candidates for oral hypoglycemic therapy, and whether these agents can be used to treat any one diabetic depends on many factors. Usually, the diabetic who can be controlled on 40 or fewer units of insulin per day responds to oral hypoglycemic therapy.

General Drug Action of Insulin and Oral Hypoglycemic Agents

INSULIN

Insulin stimulates the metabolism of carbohydrates. Although the exact role of insulin in carbohydrate metabolism is not fully understood, it is thought that insulin makes the cell wall more permeable, thus allowing entrance of glucose into the cell.

ORAL HYPOGLYCEMIC AGENTS

The sulfonylureas stimulate the beta cells of the pancreas to increase insulin secretion. Because of this action, these drugs are of value only in those patients whose pancreatic beta cells have some secretory ability.

The exact mechanism of phenformin (DBI), a biguanide, is not known. The drug requires the presence of some insulin—either exogenous insulin (insulin given to the patient) or endogenous insulin (insulin secreted by the patient).

Side Effects of Insulin and Oral Hypoglycemic Agents

INSULIN

HYPERinsulinism (an excess of insulin) with resultant HYPOglycemia may occur in the following instances:

1. the patient receives too much exogenous insulin
2. the patient is a brittle diabetic
3. too little food was eaten after receiving insulin
4. vomiting soon after a meal
5. too much exercise in relation to the insulin dose

Signs of hypoglycemia:

EARLY—behavior changes (may be moody, giddy, belligerent, apprehensive, drowsy), tachycardia, diaphoresis, blurred vision, headache, hunger, fatigue, fine tremors of hands, paleness, numbness of extremities, yawning, incoordination

LATE—loss of consciousness, coma, convulsions

Prolonged, severe hypoglycemia can result in permanent brain damage.

Swelling, redness, warmth, itching may occur at the site of injection—this indicates a localized allergic reaction. These symptoms usually disappear after a few weeks of therapy. Patients may also be allergic to the type of insulin used—that is, pork (porcine) or beef (bovine)—or to the proteins in protamine zinc and globin zinc insulin.

Atrophy and hypertrophy of subcutaneous tissue may occur when sites of injection are not rotated. This can be largely prevented with proper rotation of injection sites.

ORAL HYPOGLYCEMIC AGENTS

Hypoglycemia can occur with the use of sulfonylureas. While the onset of hypoglycemia can often be predicted with insulin use on the basis of insulin's onset and peak of action, it cannot be predicted with use of the sulfonylureas. Hypoglycemia can occur anytime from 30-60 minutes to many hours later. Skin reactions, nausea, vomiting, and diarrhea also may be seen.

The side effects of phenformin (DBI) are anorexia, nausea, vomiting, diarrhea, and a metallic taste in the mouth. Hypoglycemia rarely occurs, but when seen it usually is found in elderly, debilitated patients, alcoholics, or those with impaired kidney or liver function.

Clinical Considerations

In the treatment of patients with diabetes mellitus, patient education is an integral part of the plan for patient care. The newly diagnosed diabetic will need a full, detailed explanation of the diet to be followed, the insulin and/or oral hypoglycemic agent to be taken, the signs of hypo- and hyperglycemia, and the techniques of insulin administration and urine testing. In some hospitals a nurse and dietitian do most or all of the diabetic teaching.

INSULIN

All insulins are given by the subcutaneous route. (The intramuscular route is rarely used since the drug is poorly absorbed from muscle tissue. The nurse must *not* use this route unless specifically ordered by the physician. When the intravenous route is necessary *only* regular insulin may be used.)

The dose of insulin is measured in *units*. The physician writes the dose in units and the bottle is labeled in units.

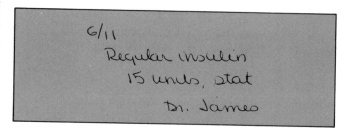

6/11
Regular insulin
15 units, stat
Dr. James

Insulin is available in various strengths—U40, U80, U100. U40 means there are 40 units of insulin per milliliter of solution.

Insulin should be administered in a syringe calibrated to measure units of insulin. Types of insulin syringes include: (1) a syringe with 1 scale used *only* for a specific strength of insulin, such as a U40 syringe; (2) a syringe with 2 scales measuring 2 strengths of insulin, such as a U40/U80 syringe.

In insulin administration, the insulin (strength) and the syringe (scale) must be the same whenever possible.

If a syringe with 2 scales—such as the U40/U80 syringe—is used, care in selecting the correct corresponding scale must be exercised. Occasionally the correct type of syringe may not be available, and an emergency situation may necessitate use of a syringe that does not correspond to the type of insulin. In this case special calculations must be made *before* drawing insulin into the syringe.

A simple method of computing the amount of insulin drawn into a syringe when syringe and insulin do not correspond is as follows:

$$\frac{SYRINGE}{INSULIN} \times DOSE\ ORDERED =$$

AMOUNT MEASURED in the syringe

For example: the physician's order reads "Regular Insulin, 26 units stat." Regular Insulin U40 and a U80 syringe are available. Using the formula above,

$$\frac{80}{40} \times 26 = 52$$

Using the U40 insulin and the U80 syringe, draw insulin up to the 52-unit mark. This equals 26 units of U40 regular insulin.

For convenience in remembering this method, the formula may be abbreviated to $\frac{S}{I} \times D = A$. The practice of using a syringe and insulin that are different is *not* recommended unless it is impossible to obtain the correct syringe and the insulin must be given immediately.

Prior to administration of insulin of the suspension type, which on standing shows a settling of particles, the bottle must be *gently* rotated to insure adequate dispersion of the suspended particles.

As with any medication, the measurement of insulin *must be accurate*. Patients may be very sensitive to minute dose changes, making accurate measurement an absolute necessity.

Patients can have a hypoglycemic reaction even though their insulin needs appear to be regulated. Familiarity with the onset, peak, and duration of *all* insulins is important. Placement of this information, as shown in Table 16-1, in the medicine room where it can easily be seen helps keep all personnel informed.

All patients receiving insulin should be checked at the expected onset *and* peak of action, since it is at these times that hypoglycemic reactions are most likely to occur.

Hypoglycemia is a serious matter and must be terminated as soon as possible. If the patient is conscious and able to swallow with *safety*, oral glucose in the form of fruit juice, cola beverages, or ginger ale is given every 5-10 minutes until there appear to be no further signs of hypoglycemia. As an alternative, 0.5-1 mg. of *glucagon* can be administered by the intramuscular, subcutaneous, or intravenous route. Glucagon is normally produced by the alpha cells of the pancreas and when injected causes a breakdown of glycogen, which is stored in the liver. Glycogen is then converted to glucose. Glucagon is of no value in treating hypoglycemia if liver stores of glycogen are low.

If the patient is unconscious, is uncooperative, or has difficulty in swallowing, oral fluids must *not* be given, as the patient may aspirate. Intravenous 50% dextrose or glucagon are to be given. Hospital policy

Table 16-3.
TYPES OF INSULIN MIXTURES

TYPE OF INSULIN	MAY BE MIXED WITH
Extended Insulin Zinc Suspension (Ultralente Insulin)	Regular Insulin, Insulin Zinc Suspension (Lente Insulin), Prompt Insulin Zinc Suspension (Semilente Insulin)
Insulin Zinc Suspension (Lente Insulin)	Regular Insulin, Extended Insulin Zinc Suspension (Ultralente Insulin), Prompt Insulin Suspension (Semilente Insulin)
Isophane Insulin Suspension (NPH Insulin)	Regular Insulin
Prompt Insulin Zinc Suspension (Semilente Insulin)	Regular Insulin, Insulin Zinc Suspension (Lente Insulin), Extended Insulin Zinc Suspension (Ultralente Insulin)
Protamine Zinc Insulin Suspension (Protamine, Zinc and Iletin)	Regular Insulin
Regular Insulin	All other insulins

and physicians' preferences vary as to the steps taken for immediate treatment of hypoglycemia, and all personnel should be familiar with the procedure to be followed.

Always administer the type of insulin ordered by the physician. One type of insulin must *never* be substituted for another.

When mixing regular insulin with another insulin, be very careful that the correct dose for *each* insulin is taken from the appropriate bottle and measured in the syringe. This point should also be stressed in teaching patients who require two types of insulins to be given at the same time. Patients should also be told to check the labels of insulin bottles before they leave the drugstore to be sure they are given the correct type. Although mistakes rarely happen this remains a good policy.

Various types of insulin mixtures are shown in Table 16-3.

Patients should be instructed not to leave insulin on windowsills or near other sources of heat. Insulin may be stored at room temperature but should be refrigerated if there is any danger of excessive heat. Since patients may forget to keep insulin in a cool place, many physicians prefer to tell their patients to refrigerate insulin. At *no time* must the insulin be placed in the freezer compartment of a refrigerator.

Insulin has an expiration date which is stated on the bottle and on the outside of the carton. The patient should be told to check the expiration date as well as the label *before* leaving the drugstore. In the hospital, if insulin is not used regularly but is stored in the medicine room of the unit, all preparations should be checked periodically and outdated insulin returned to the hospital pharmacy.

All patients receiving insulin must have their urine checked for glucose and ketone bodies (acetone). Although hospital policies vary, urine is normally collected and tested 4 times per day—½ hour before each meal and h.s. The patient should be instructed to void ½ hour *before* the urine sample is collected for testing; otherwise false results may be obtained. Methods used to test urine also vary. Tes-Tape, Clinistix, and Combistix are examples of testing materials.

Some patients require regulation of their insulin; the physician may order regular insulin according to the amount of glucose and acetone present in the urine. This is sometimes referred to as a "rainbow curve" or "sliding scale." The urine is collected and tested ½ hour before each meal and h.s. According to the amount of glucose and acetone present, the corresponding amount of insulin ordered by the physician is then given.

Insulin injection sites are to be *rotated*. After conferring with the physician, the nurse and the patient should work together to plan an orderly pattern for rotation sites. Any progressive order is acceptable. To aid the patient in remembering the order of rotation, a chart can be supplied. Mounting the sheet of paper between pieces of plastic will preserve the drawing.

Patient Education and Discharge Teaching

INSULIN

Each step in the teaching program must be presented clearly, giving the patient ample time to assimilate the material.

Teaching should include the following points:

1. instruction on when to test the urine
2. methods of testing the urine (the physician may have a preference on the type of testing material)
3. the type(s) of insulin to be used
4. how to buy insulin: checking labels as to correct type, expiration dates
5. how to store insulin
6. how to measure insulin in the type of syringe ordered by the physician; reading the syringe
7. principles of aseptic technique
8. how to withdraw insulin from the insulin bottle
9. how to administer insulin; rotation sites
10. signs of hypoglycemia
11. what to do if hypoglycemia occurs
12. the importance of exact measurement of insulin
13. where to buy insulin when traveling; physicians as well as pharmacists usually can supply the patient with information regarding insulin purchase in foreign countries; pharmaceutical companies manufacturing insulin also will supply this information upon written request
14. wearing of tags or bracelets, such as Medic-Alert, identifying the wearer as a diabetic; if the patient is found unconscious—regardless of cause—the identification tags provide medical personnel with information that is essential in treatment

Throughout the teaching program be alert for any difficulty experienced by the patient or family members. Some patients may be unable to read syringe scales and may require special magnifying devices. Other patients may give the impression that they understand the material presented but may be afraid to admit that they really do *not* understand. Having patients *prac-*

tice and *demonstrate* urine testing, using a syringe, and giving their own insulin in the presence of nursing personnel helps insure comprehension of the teaching program.

The physician should be consulted before a teaching program is begun. Some physicians may prefer to do some of the teaching and ask the nurse and dietitian to complete the program.

Recently U100 insulin was introduced in an effort to standardize insulin use and avoid the confusion of using various strengths of insulin. Use of U100 insulin also reduces the injection volume. For example, 50 U of U100 (100 units per ml.) requires the injection of 0.5 ml. of solution whereas 50 U of U40 would require more than 0.5 ml. of solution.

ORAL HYPOGLYCEMIC AGENTS

The diabetic patient who is receiving oral hypoglycemic agents requires the same supervision as the patient receiving insulin. Unfortunately, many patients feel that since they are not taking insulin, strict adherence to medication, dietary restrictions, urine testing, etc. are unnecessary. These patients should be taught *early* about the necessity of strict adherence to the schedule of diet and drug therapy as outlined by their physician.

The patient receiving oral hypoglycemic agents requires the same supervision and teaching discussed above regarding insulin, omitting of course points related to the measurement, administration, and storage of insulin.

Table 16-4.
INSULINS

GENERIC NAME	TRADE NAME OR SYNONYM
Extended Insulin Zinc Suspension U.S.P.	Ultralente Iletin, Ultralente Insulin
Globin Zinc Insulin U.S.P.	
Insulin Injection U.S.P.	regular insulin, regular Iletin, unmodified insulin
Insulin Zinc Suspension U.S.P.	Lente Insulin, Lente Iletin
Isophane Insulin Suspension U.S.P.	NPH Insulin, NPH Iletin, Neutral Protamine Hagedorn Insulin
Prompt Insulin Zinc Suspension U.S.P.	Semilente Iletin, Semilente Insulin
Protamine Zinc Insulin Suspension U.S.P.	PZI; Protamine, Zinc and Iletin

Table 16-5.
ORAL HYPOGLYCEMIC AGENTS

GENERIC NAME	TRADE NAME	SIDE EFFECTS	DOSE RANGES
acetohexamide	Dymelor	hypoglycemia, nausea, vomiting, skin eruptions, diarrhea	250 mg.-1.5 Grams daily orally; dose adjusted to need
chlorpropamide	Diabinese	same as acetohexamide	100-500 mg. daily orally; dose adjusted to need
phenformin	DBI	metallic taste, nausea, anorexia, vomiting, diarrhea, hypoglycemia (rare)	25-300 mg. daily orally; dose adjusted to need
tolazamide	Tolinase	same as acetohexamide	100 mg.-1 Gram daily orally; dose adjusted to need
tolbutamide	Orinase	same as acetohexamide	500 mg.-3.0 Grams daily orally; dose adjusted to need

The sulfonamides or "sulfa" drugs were the first effective chemotherapeutic agents used in the treatment of infections. These drugs were widely used during World War II, because penicillin, though known, was not available in sufficient quantities for general medical use.

Types of Sulfonamide Agents

Sulfonamides are generally classed according to their rate of absorption and excretion. Basically, there are three types of sulfonamide preparations:

1. those which are *rapidly absorbed* into the bloodstream and are *rapidly excreted* from the body. An example of this type is sulfisoxazole (Gantrisin)
2. those which are *rapidly absorbed* into the bloodstream and are *slowly excreted* from the body. An example of this type is sulfameter (Sulla)
3. those which are used for special purposes. These preparations are the topical forms of sulfonamides such as sulfacetamide (Sultrin). Mafenide (Sulfamylon) is another topical agent chemically related to the sulfona-

Chapter 17

The Sulfonamides

mides. There are also sulfonamides that are absorbed into the bloodstream but pass through the body relatively unchanged to be excreted in the urine. An example of this is sulfamethizole (Thiosulfil), used to treat urinary tract infections. Relatively high concentrations of the drug in the urine thereby exert bacteriostatic/bactericidal effects.

General Drug Action

Sulfonamides are *antibacterial* agents, meaning they are active against bacteria. Sulfonamides may be either *bacteriostatic* or *bactericidal*. A bacteriostatic agent retards bacterial growth. A bactericidal agent destroys bacteria.

Whether a drug is bacteriostatic or bactericidal depends on a number of factors: (1) type and dose of the drug (2) concentration of the drug in the bloodstream, body tissues, body fluids, and (3) the bacteria. Sulfonamides are *usually* bacteriostatic.

Therapeutic blood levels are of special importance in the administration of drugs used in the control or eradication of infection. A therapeutic blood level is the minimal level of drug concentration in the body required to produce a desired effect. The desired effect, in the case of sulfonamides and other antibacterial agents, is the bacteriostatic or bactericidal effect.

If a drug is bacteriostatic, bacterial growth is inhibited, thereby allowing the body's own defense mechanisms (white blood cells) to rid the body of invading organisms.

Uses of Sulfonamide Agents

The chief use of sulfonamide preparations is in the treatment or prevention of urinary tract infections. Topical application of mafenide (Sulfamylon) is used in the treatment of severe burns. Sulfacetamide, sulfathiazole, and sulfabenzamide (Sultrin Triple Sulfa) is used topically in some vaginal infections.

Meningococcal meningitis may be treated with sulfonamides such as sulfisoxazole (Gantrisin) and sulfamethoxazole (Gantanol), which are also used prophylactically in those in contact with patients who have meningococcal meningitis.

Side Effects of Sulfonamide Agents

Although not a side effect in the strict sense, one problem encountered with the use of any drug that affects bacterial growth is the development of mutant strains of bacteria that are *resistant* to the drug. If a certain strain of bacteria is resistant to a drug, that particular drug will be of little if any value in the treatment of an infection caused by this strain. If a certain strain of bacteria is *sensitive* to a drug, that particular drug *will* be of value. Development of mutant strains has limited the use of some antibacterials.

The side effects of sulfonamide agents are:

GASTROINTESTINAL: nausea, vomiting, diarrhea
CENTRAL NERVOUS SYSTEM: headache, tinnitus, fatigue, weakness
BLOOD DYSCRASIAS
ALLERGIC REACTIONS: rash, itching, joint pain, Stevens-Johnson syndrome

The Stevens-Johnson syndrome is manifested by fever, cough, muscular aches and pains, and the development of lesions, which appear as red wheals or blisters of the skin, mucous membrane, respiratory tract, eyes, and other organs. Fatalities have occurred with the development of the syndrome.

Crystalluria (crystals in the urine) may also occur during sulfonamide therapy, although infrequently with the newer preparations. Crystalluria occurs, in most instances, when an insufficient amount of fluid is taken by mouth and the urine is highly acid.

Clinical Considerations

Sulfonamides are given with caution to patients with impaired renal function. Such patients should be closely observed for a *decrease in urinary output*, hematuria, pain over the kidney area and diffuse or generalized abdominal pain. Intake and output measurement is an absolute necessity in these patients.

Fluids should be forced and patients should be encouraged to drink two to four extra glasses of fluids (or more!) per day. Drinking additional fluids will have a twofold effect: (1) prevent crystalluria, even though this does not appear to be a major problem with the newer preparations and (2) mechanically wash out the bacteria infecting the urinary tract.

The Stevens-Johnson syndrome, though uncommon, has occurred in some patients. Any occurrence of skin lesions, wheals, or rashes necessitates discontinuing the drug and notifying the physician.

Some patients are placed on a sulfonamide as a prophylactic measure following urological instrumentation or examination. Also, patients may receive lower doses *after* initial treatment for a urinary tract infection to prevent recurrence of the infection.

Discharge Teaching

Discharge teaching should include the following points:

1. explanation of side effects that could occur; physician should be notified if gastrointestinal disturbances, rash, itching, or diarrhea is noted. In order to detect the development of a blood dyscrasia the patient should be told that fever, chills, or sore throat should also be reported to the physician
2. drinking fluids, unless contraindicated because of medical problems such as heart disease, should be stressed
3. office or clinic appointments should be kept, since it is important that the physician see the patient and evaluate the progress of drug therapy. This is important because subclinical urinary tract infections may not produce symptoms noticeable by the patient, yet the bacteria will be found in urinalysis specimens. This finding might indicate the necessity of other drugs.

It is of importance that the patient fully understand the number of times per day the drug is to be taken. Sometimes the slowly excreted drugs are required only once or twice per day whereas the rapidly excreted types are taken more frequently. The patient should be warned against increasing the dose if he feels worse or stopping the medication if he feels better.

Table 17-1.
SULFONAMIDE DRUGS

Generic Name	Trade Name	Uses	Side Effects	Dose Ranges
sulfacetamide, sulfathiazole, sulfabenzamide	Sultrin Triple Sulfa	treatment of bacterial vaginitis		intravaginal application B.I.D. 4-6 days
sulfachloro-pyridazine	Sonilyn	treatment of urinary tract infections caused by bacteria susceptible to this preparation	nausea, vomiting, diarrhea, headache, tinnitus, blood dyscrasias, weakness, fatigue, Stevens-Johnson syndrome, itching, rash, joint pain	2-4 Grams daily in 3-6 divided doses orally; CHILD: 150 mg./Kg./day in 4-6 divided doses orally
sulfameter	Sulla	same as sulfachloropyridazine	same as sulfachloropyridazine	500 mg. daily orally
sulfamethizole	Thiosulfil	same as sulfachloropyridazine	same as sulfachloropyridazine	2-4 Grams daily in 3-6 divided doses orally; CHILD: 30-45 mg./Kg./day in divided doses orally
sulfamethoxazole	Gantanol	same as sulfachloropyridazine	same as sulfachloropyridazine	1 Gram B.I.D., T.I.D. orally; CHILD: 60 mg./Kg./day in 2 divided doses orally
sulfamethoxazole, trimethoprim	Septra	chronic urinary tract infections	same as sulfachloropyridazine	2 tablets q12h orally
sulfisoxazole	Gantrisin	same as sulfachloropyridazine	same as sulfachloropyridazine	2-8 Grams daily in 4-6 divided doses orally
sulfisoxazole diolamine	Gantrisin diolamine	same as sulfachloropyridazine	same as sulfachloropyridazine	adult, child: 100 mg./Kg./day S.C., I.V. in divided doses

Penicillin

The antibacterial properties of penicillin were discovered in 1928 by Sir Alexander Fleming; penicillin was first used clinically in 1941. Originally labeled a "miracle" drug, penicillin was used indiscriminately, leading to the development of bacterial mutations and drug resistance.

Types and Uses of Penicillin

There are two types of penicillin—natural penicillin and semisynthetic penicillin. One reason for the development of the semisynthetic penicillins was the increased incidence of bacterial resistance to natural penicillins.

Penicillin G (a natural penicillin) is available for parenteral use as *crystalline* penicillin G and *procaine* penicillin G. Penicillin G is also manufactured as an oral preparation, for example Pentids (potassium penicillin G). The dose of natural penicillin is expressed in *units*.

Crystalline penicillin G is given by the intramuscular or intravenous routes; procaine penicillin G is given *only* by the intramuscular route and *never* by the intravenous route. Benzathine penicillin G (Bicillin Long-Acting) is a long-acting penicillin which may be given

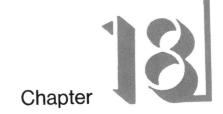

Chapter **18**   135

Penicillin, Broad-Spectrum Antibiotics, and Antifungal Agents

every 2-4 weeks. The semisynthetic penicillins are administered parenterally and orally.

SOME SYNTHETIC AND SEMISYNTHETIC
PENICILLINS
AMPICILLIN trihydrate (Amcill, Polycillin)
CARBENICILLIN indanyl sodium (Geocillin)
sodium CLOXACILLIN (Tegopen)
sodium DICLOXACILLIN (Dynapen)
sodium METHICILLIN (Staphcillin)
sodium NAFCILLIN (Unipen)
sodium OXACILLIN (Prostaphlin)

The selection of a penicillin or other antibiotic usually depends on the results of *culture* and *sensitivity* studies. Organisms which may be sensitive to the penicillins are staphylococci, streptococci, pneumococci, *Treponema pallidum* (the causative organism of syphilis), and gonococci. Penicillin is of *no* value in the treatment of viral infections, but penicillin and broad-spectrum antibiotics may be given prophylactically to patients with viral infections, to prevent secondary *bacterial* infections.

General Drug Action of Penicillin

Penicillin may be bactericidal or bacteriostatic, depending on the sensitivity of the organism and the ability of the penicillin to reach and concentrate in the area of infection. Culture and sensitivity studies indicate the resistance or sensitivity of the organism to a given antibiotic.

It appears that penicillin prevents bacteria from using a substance (muramic acid-peptide) that is essential for the maintenance of the outer cell wall. Unable to use this substance, the bacteria swell, rupture, and assume unusual shapes.

Like the sulfonamides, penicillin must attain a therapeutic blood level in order to be effective. This level varies, depending on the severity of the infection and the sensitivity of the organism to penicillin.

Side Effects of Penicillin

All antibiotics have the ability to produce side effects. The most common side effects are rash and urticaria (hives), indicating an *allergy* to the drug. If either of these side effects occurs, the next dose must be *withheld* and the physician notified immediately.

A rash does not always mean that the patient is allergic to penicillin. (The patient may be allergic to something else, such as bath soap, bed linen, or other drugs.) Even so, the drug must be withheld until the cause of the rash or urticaria is determined and the physician sees the patient.

An anaphylactoid reaction (anaphylactic shock) is an extremely serious manifestation of drug allergy. This severe reaction could follow the appearance of a rash or urticaria, especially if the dose is repeated. Anaphylactoid reactions may also occur without warning.

Symptoms of anaphylactic shock occur rapidly. The patient becomes pale, diaphoretic, hypotensive, and severely dyspneic; the patient may lose consciousness rapidly. In some cases circulatory collapse may occur immediately and cardiopulmonary resuscitation (CPR measures) may be necessary. Swelling of the larynx, pharynx, and bronchi may also be seen, with death resulting from asphyxia unless an emergency tracheostomy is performed. Anaphylactoid reactions require *immediate* emergency treatment.

Another side effect of penicillin is the occurrence of *superimposed infections.* Antibiotics not only affect pathogenic (disease-producing) organisms, but may also affect nonpathogenic organisms that normally inhabit the body. An alteration of normal bacterial flora allows an overgrowth of other organisms such as fungi and pathogenic bacteria.

Occasionally, hematological changes may be associated with the administration of penicillin, particularly when high doses are used.

Penicillinase (Neutrapen) may be administered as part of the treatment of severe penicillin allergy. This drug is given with extreme caution, since allergic reactions to penicillinase are also possible.

Clinical Considerations

The rash associated with a penicillin allergy may or may not be accompanied by itching. A rash might be detected during morning care, or the patient may mention it during morning rounds or at the time medication is administered. The patient may not even think it is important. The appearance of a rash should be reported to the physician immediately and the patient observed for other side effects.

Taking allergy histories of patients is recommended at the time of admission. The patient and/or family should be questioned regarding any problem that has been encountered with drugs. For some patients, this may require a lengthy questioning period but is well worth the effort when viewed in light of the serious reactions that can occur.

Listen carefully to any comments patients make regarding drugs. Comments such as, "It makes me sick to my stomach" or "I got bumps all over when I took the drug" require in-depth questioning plus relating all this information to the physician. Patients should also be asked if they have seasonal allergies such as hay fever or are allergic to things in the house (dust, cotton, kapok, etc.) and this should also be noted in the allergy history. Patients who are either under treatment for their allergies or who seem to have an allergy to many different pollens, objects, or animals should have this noted on their chart. The physician should also be informed of these facts. Patients who have multi-allergies are more prone to develop an allergy to penicillin, hence the necessity of caution in administering these drugs to individuals who appear to be hypersensitive. On the other hand, a patient with *no* allergy history can also develop a penicillin allergy.

If the patient has a known allergy to penicillin, warnings should be posted on the patient's chart, Kardex, and if possible at the patient's bedside. Although there may be objections to the labeling of a patient problem at the bedside, posting this information for "all to see" must be weighed against the possibility of a patient's accidentally receiving a drug that could cause death from an anaphylactoid reaction.

Some parenteral forms of penicillin are packaged as a crystal-like powder that must be reconstituted before use. Since manufacturers vary, the label should be checked as to the amount of diluent required. After addition of the diluent to *multi-dose* vials, the bottle must be labeled with the *date* and *number of units per milliliter* of solution. After the diluent has been added, the bottle should be shaken vigorously.

Patients sensitive to one penicillin should *not* receive any other type of penicillin. Since there are hundreds of drugs used in a hospital each day, reliable references should be consulted before any drug which is unfamiliar is administered, since trade names may not reveal the *type* of drug. If references are not available a phone call to the hospital pharmacist is indicated. Other antibiotics, for example the *cephalosporins*, are not to be given or are given with *caution* to patients with penicillin allergies. These antibiotics are chemically similar to penicillin; therefore patients sensitive to penicillin can also be sensitive to them.

Before receiving penicillin for the first time, the patient should be asked:

1. Have you ever received penicillin before?
2. Have you ever gotten "sick" or noticed anything unusual while you took penicillin? (Were hives, a rash, or other phenomena noted?)
3. Are you allergic to any drugs? (If so, which ones?)
4. Are you allergic to anything? (If so, what?)

"Yes" to number 2 necessitates withholding the drug. "Yes" to 3 and 4 should raise the question as to a *possible* allergy to penicillin, and the physician should be consulted prior to the administration of the drug.

Discharge Teaching

Sometimes penicillin is given prophylactically and the patient may have to take this drug after discharge from the hospital. The patient should be told that the appearance of a rash, hives, nausea, fatigue, or any other unusual occurrence necessitates stopping the drug and calling the physician.

It is also important that the patient understand that the drug is to be taken as directed. Stopping the drug or decreasing or increasing the dose because of feeling better or worse should *not* be done. When this point is stressed, the reason *why* the physician's orders are to be followed can also be stated. In this instance, stopping or decreasing the drug could cause a flare-up of the infection which may then be more difficult to treat. Increasing the dose could lead to serious side effects. Even more importantly, the patient is treating himself for something he knows nothing about; chances are great that he has "misdiagnosed" the illness.

Those experienced in clinics, outpatient departments, emergency rooms, etc. have seen many patients who have "diagnosed" their illness, taking antacids for "stomach distress" which is later found to be stomach cancer, treating a "cold" which instead is pneumonia, or applying hot compresses to a back pain which is found to be a kidney infection. One can do a great service by informing patients that *self-treatment is dangerous* and that when they are ill or have any apparent problem, professional help should be sought before treatment or drugs are instituted.

Another problem that is evident in some situations is the use of prescriptions by other members of the family for what appears to be the "same" illness. There are two problems here: (1) the medication may have been kept in the medicine chest for months (and even years!) and is no longer safe for use and (2) the family members are self-diagnosing. Patients also may use a previous prescription—or what remains of the prescription—for what is believed to be a recurrence of a previous condition.

Even though the physician orders a specific amount of liquid or number of tablets on the prescription, some patients stop taking the medication *before* all the liquid or tablets are gone, because they "feel better." Instead of discarding the medication, they save it—just in case it is needed again. This is an extremely dangerous practice, as many drugs deteriorate, some in a very short time. As for saving medication, the dangers are many and the advantages none.

Broad-Spectrum Antibiotics

The first broad-spectrum antibiotic was tetracycline, which was soon followed by the introduction of other preparations. Like penicillin, these antibiotics were used indiscriminately when first introduced.

Types and Uses of Broad-Spectrum Antibiotics

The tetracyclines are a group of closely related drugs that are similar in potency, effect on bacterial organisms, and side effects. They are generally effective against susceptible pneumococci, beta-hemolytic streptococci, nonhemolytic streptococci, rickettsiae, staphylococci, and spirochetes. Culture and sensitivity studies reveal the type of organism causing the infection and the susceptibility of the organism to the antibiotic.

TETRACYCLINES
    CHLORTETRACYCLINE (Aureomycin)
    DEMECLOCYCLINE (Declomycin)
    DOXYCYCLINE (Vibramycin)
    METHACYCLINE (Rondomycin)
    MINOCYCLINE (Minocin)
    OXYTETRACYCLINE (Terramycin)
    TETRACYCLINE (Tetracyn)

Chloramphenicol (Chloromycetin) is active against a wide variety of organisms but because of its toxicity its use is reserved for the treatment of infections that do not respond to other antibiotics. This drug is also indicated for the treatment of typhoid fever.

Erythromycin and its salts are generally effective against beta-hemolytic streptococci, pneumococci, and some strains of staphylococci. These drugs are also used to treat intestinal amebiasis.

ERYTHROMYCIN AND ITS DERIVATIVES
    ERYTHROMYCIN (Ilotycin)
    ERYTHROMYCIN ESTOLATE (Ilosone)
    ERYTHROMYCIN ETHYLSUCCINATE
        (Erythrocin ethyl succinate)
    ERYTHROMYCIN GLUCEPTATE
        (Ilotycin gluceptate)
    ERYTHROMYCIN LACTOBIONATE
        (Erythrocin lactobionate)
    ERYTHROMYCIN STEARATE
        (Erythrocin stearate)

Bacitracin is an antibiotic more commonly used as a topical medication since it is relatively toxic when given parenterally. Topically, the drug is used to treat infections of the skin and mucous membranes, such as impetigo, dermatitis, and other superficial infections caused by gram-positive organisms susceptible to bacitracin. This drug is also used parenterally in the treatment of infections that do not respond to other antibiotics.

The cephalosporins are a group of antibiotics related to penicillin. These drugs are used to treat respiratory tract infections, urinary tract infections, and skin and soft tissue infections caused by organisms susceptible to these drugs. The specific use of each cephalosporin is given at the end of this chapter.

```
CEPHALOSPORINS
  CEPHALEXIN (Keflex)
  CEPHALOGLYCIN (Kafocin)
  CEPHALORIDINE (Loridine)
  CEPHALOTHIN (Keflin)
```

Clindamycin (Cleocin) is a semisynthetic derivative of lincomycin (Lincocin). Both drugs are used to treat infections of the respiratory and urinary tracts and skin and soft tissue infections caused by organisms susceptible to these drugs.

Colistin (Coly-Mycin S) and colistimethate (Coly-Mycin M) are related to polymyxin B. Colistimethate (Coly-Mycin M) is usually used to treat urinary tract infections caused by organisms susceptible to this drug.

Colistin sulfate (Coly-Mycin S) is used to treat acute bacterial diarrheas. Colistimethate has also been useful in treating infections caused by *Pseudomonas aeruginosa*.

Gentamicin (Garamycin) is active against gram-negative organisms and is used in the treatment of septicemia and *severe* infections of the skin and soft tissues. This includes treatment of severe burns, respiratory infections, gastrointestinal infections, and urinary tract infections caused by susceptible organisms.

Kanamycin (Kantrex) is active against gram-negative infections and staphylococcal infections of the respiratory and urinary tracts and soft tissues. This drug also may be used in the treatment of osteomyelitis and septicemia caused by susceptible organisms. Orally, this drug is used to suppress intestinal flora prior to bowel surgery. Additionally, this action can be utilized in the treatment of hepatic coma by suppressing ammonia-producing bacteria.

Lincomycin (Lincocin) is effective against respiratory and urinary tract and soft tissue infections as well as osteomyelitis and septicemia caused by susceptible organisms.

Neomycin (Mycifradin) is a potentially toxic drug, and in parenteral form is used only in the treatment of severe systemic infections caused by susceptible gram-negative organisms. Used orally, the drug is poorly absorbed and does not produce serious toxic effects. Because of its poor absorbing quality, it has no systemic effects and therefore acts locally, on the flora of the large intestine. This drug may be used to (1) prepare the large bowel for surgery ("bowel prep") by decreasing the numbers of intestinal bacteria and (2) treat diarrheas caused by susceptible organisms. The surgeon may or may not elect to suppress the numbers of bacteria in the large intestine prior to surgery on that area; some surgeons feel that use of drugs that suppress intestinal flora lessens the possibility of infections that can occur with surgery on the large bowel and anus. This drug is also used topically as a solution or ointment in the treatment of infections of the skin and/or exposed underlying tissues caused by susceptible organisms.

Polymyxin B (Aerosporin) in parenteral form is used to treat *severe* infections caused by susceptible organisms that do not respond to therapy with other antibiotics. Polymyxin B is also used orally to treat bacterial infections caused by Shigella or Pseudomonas organisms. Like neomycin, it does not produce serious toxic effects when administered by the oral route. Topically, it is used to treat superficial infections caused by susceptible organisms.

Troleandomycin (TAO) is usually used to treat infections caused by susceptible organisms, including *Diplococcus pneumoniae* and *Streptococcus pyogenes*.

Spectinomycin (Trobicin) is used to treat gonorrhea in those patients who have penicillin-resistant gonococcal infections.

Vancomycin (Vancocin) is used in the treatment of severe staphylococcal infections resistant to other forms of therapy.

General Drug Action of Broad-Spectrum Antibiotics

The broad-spectrum antibiotics have different mechanisms by which they affect bacteria:

1. some antibiotics act on the cell wall of bacteria
2. others affect protein synthesis

Although their mechanisms of action may be different, antibiotics control infections by virtue of a bacteriostatic or bactericidal ability.

Side Effects of Broad-Spectrum Antibiotics

With a large group of drugs such as the antibiotics, there are varying side effects for *each* drug. It is nearly impossible to remember all the side effects of each drug; therefore references should be consulted prior to administration of each particular antibiotic (or any drug that is unfamiliar).

THE TETRACYCLINES: All drugs in this group may cause basically the same side effects, including diarrhea, which may be severe, discoloration of teeth in children (early childhood to 8 years of age), gastric distress, hematological changes, hypersensitivity reactions, phototoxic reactions, rash, and superimposed infections.

Superimposed infections, which may occur during the use of tetracyclines as well as most antibiotics, may be first suspected by sores in the mouth, black tongue, diarrhea, or anal or vaginal itching. Diarrhea may be severe and occasionally life-threatening. The drug *must* be discontinued and the physician notified if signs of a superimposed infection are evident.

Patients should be warned to avoid direct exposure to the rays of the sun. A phototoxic reaction may give no warning and may occur after even a brief exposure to the sun. Generalized swelling and redness resembling a severe sunburn are signs of a phototoxic reaction.

Long-term administration of these drugs can result in a reduction of red and white cells and platelets; therefore, periodic hematology examinations are recommended during long-term use. Easy bruising (sign of a decrease in platelets) or fatigue (sign of a decrease in red cells) may be noted.

The tetracyclines are contraindicated in children (unless use is necessary) under the age of 8 years, since permanent discoloration of the teeth—a brownish stain —may occur. There appears to be no discoloration in children over 8 and adults.

Gastric distress can often be relieved if these drugs are taken with food. However, milk and milk products or antacids should *not* be used, as these products delay the absorption of the drug.

The tetracyclines are given with caution to patients with impaired renal function. Doxycycline (Vibramycin) is a tetracycline that can be administered to those with renal impairment.

CHLORAMPHENICOL (Chloromycetin): Side effects include bone marrow depression with the possibility of the development of serious blood dyscrasias, hypersensitivity reactions, nausea and vomiting, rash, superimposed infections, and urticaria.

Accompanying the drug's depressant effect on the bone marrow, serious and fatal blood dyscrasias have been reported, and may occur even with short-term use. Manufacturers recommend use of the drug only for severe infections and that all patients be hospitalized during the time the drug is administered. Frequent blood studies are also recommended.

THE ERYTHROMYCINS: These drugs have a low incidence of toxicity when compared to other antibiotics. Reported side effects include abdominal cramping, diarrhea, hypersensitivity reactions, nausea and vomiting, rash, superimposed infections, and urticaria.

BACITRACIN: Anorexia, hypersensitivity reactions, nausea and vomiting, nephrotoxicity, pain at the site of injection, and superimposed infections can occur.

Side effects are rare when this drug is used topically. Necrosis of renal tubules can occur during oral and parenteral use; therefore, its use is reserved for infections which do not respond to other forms of therapy.

THE CEPHALOSPORINS: *Cephalexin* (Keflex)—superimposed infections, nausea, vomiting, diarrhea, abdominal pain. *Cephaloglycin* (Kafocin)—superimposed infections. *Cephaloridine* (Loridine)—nephrotoxicity, superimposed infections, nausea, vomiting. *Cephalothin* (Keflin)—pain on injection, superimposed infections.

These drugs are to be given with *caution* to patients who have a history of allergy to penicillin. Hypersensitivity reactions may occur during use. Patients receiving these drugs for the first time should be asked if they have an allergy to penicillin. If an allergy is even suspected, the drug should be withheld and the physician notified. A false-positive reaction for glucose in the urine may be obtained with Benedict's solution and Clinitest tablets. False-positive reactions are *not* seen with the use of Tes-Tape.

CLINDAMYCIN (Cleocin): Side effects include abdominal pain, diarrhea, which may be severe, hematological changes, hypersensitivity reactions, jaundice, nausea and vomiting, and superimposed infections.

Occasionally, patients may show signs of severe gastrointestinal side effects, in which case the drug may be discontinued. If diarrhea occurs, the next dose of the drug should be withheld and the physician contacted *before* the next dose is due.

COLISTIMETHATE (Coly-Mycin M), COLISTIN (Coly-Mycin S): Serious side effects with colistimethate include nephrotoxicity and respiratory arrest. Also reported are hypersensitivity reactions, numbness of the tongue and area around the mouth, tingling of the extremities, and vertigo and dizziness. Superimposed infections may occur with the use of colistin.

These drugs are contraindicated in patients with impaired renal function. Patients should be observed for the possible development of nephrotoxicity. Periodic renal studies are recommended by the manufacturer, and intake and output measurements may be of value in detecting a decrease in renal function. Since respiratory arrest has been reported following the intramuscular use of the drug, the manufacturer recommends resuscitation materials be available. The oral form (colistin sulfate) appears to be less toxic; however, superimposed infections may be seen.

GENTAMICIN (Garamycin): Side effects include hypersensitivity reactions, nephrotoxicity, ototoxicity, and superimposed infections. Other side effects, rarely reported, include muscle twitching, numbness, and skin tingling.

Ototoxicity may begin by the appearance of tinnitus and dizziness, which may necessitate discontinuing the drug. Since this drug is nephrotoxic, the patient should be observed for signs of a decrease in renal function. Measurement of the fluid intake and output aids the physician in evaluating the patient's status.

KANAMYCIN (Kantrex): Side effects include diarrhea, nausea, vomiting, and superimposed infections with oral use; nephrotoxicity, ototoxicity, and pain at the site of injection may occur.

Injury to the eighth cranial nerve (auditory nerve) may occur with use of this drug. Dizziness and tinnitus may be the first signs of auditory nerve damage and usually necessitate discontinuing the drug. Nephrotoxicity may be manifested by microscopic hematuria, albuminuria, and a decrease in urinary output. Renal function studies (BUN, NPN, creatinine) may be ordered.

LINCOMYCIN (Lincocin): Side effects include abdominal cramps, dermatitis, diarrhea, especially with oral use, hypersensitivity reactions, nausea and vomiting, rash, superimposed infections, and urticaria. If diarrhea occurs, the next dose of the drug should be withheld and the physician contacted.

NEOMYCIN (Mycifradin): Side effects include diarrhea with oral use, hypersensitivity reactions, ototoxicity, and nephrotoxicity. As with kanamycin, the same observations for appearance of drug effect on the auditory nerve and kidney should be employed during the administration of neomycin.

POLYMYXIN B (Aerosporin): Side effects include blurred vision, dizziness, hypersensitivity reactions, nephrotoxicity, numbness of the mouth, face, and extremities, pain at the site of injection, and superimposed infections.

The patient may complain of numbness around the mouth, and in some cases this symptom may cause anxiety. On occasion, the physician may wish to continue therapy despite side effects. The patient should be assured that the numbness is only temporary and will subside when the drug is discontinued. Local use of this drug rarely produces side effects.

TROLEANDOMYCIN (TAO): Side effects include diarrhea, hypersensitivity reactions, nausea and vomiting, rash, and superimposed infections.

SPECTINOMYCIN (Trobicin): Side effects include chills and fever, dizziness, hematological changes, soreness at the site of injection, and urticaria. A decrease in urinary output has been noted with multiple-dose use. There has been no kidney damage demonstrated despite the appearance of oliguria. Decrease in hemoglobin and hematocrit also can occur with multiple-dose use, but no apparent blood dyscrasias have been reported.

VANCOMYCIN (Vancocin): Side effects include chills, drug fever, nausea, nephrotoxicity, ototoxicity, rash, superimposed infections, and thrombophlebitis. Thrombophlebitis can be avoided by rotating intravenous injection sites. Inspection of the vein used for drug administration should be made at least once daily. Old sites should also be inspected for signs of thrombophlebitis, that is, redness, tenderness, and/or pain along the pathway of the vein.

It should be noted that anaphylactoid reactions can occur during the use of the antibiotics as well as *any* drug. Some drugs appear to have a higher incidence of severe reactions than others.

Superimposed infections can also occur during the use of any antibiotic.

Clinical Considerations

Some individuals believe that antibiotics are "safe" drugs. Creation of a false sense of security may lead to taking fewer precautions when administering these drugs.

Antibiotics are *not* safe drugs. Some can cause serious side effects, such as permanent hearing loss or renal damage. Patients receiving these drugs deserve careful observation for:

1. response to drug therapy; that is, does the infection appear to be controlled with the use of the drug? Signs of improvement may be manifested by: decrease in purulent drainage from a wound, decrease in temperature, improved appearance of the pa-

tient, who also feels better, decrease in pain or discomfort. Signs of improvement vary, according to the original signs of infection
2. appearance of side effects. Some side effects are extremely serious. Others, though not as serious, may be a warning of more serious side effects if the drug is continued

"Listen" to the patient's complaints. For example, a patient may complain of back pain or discomfort. While this could be due to confinement to bed, it may also be due to renal involvement. *All* patient complaints as well as the obvious side effects should be reported to the physician, who will then evaluate the relationship of the complaint or side effect to the drug prescribed.

Antibiotics *must* be administered as ordered, especially at the time interval ordered. Omitting or delaying a dose can, in some instances, affect the therapeutic value of the drug by decreasing blood levels. If the blood level of the drug is allowed to drop, as it can with the omission of a dose, the bacteriostatic or bactericidal effect may be lost.

Discharge Teaching

Occasionally, patients may be required to take antibiotics after discharge from the hospital. The importance of taking the drugs *exactly* as directed should be stressed. Warnings regarding the reuse of a drug at a later date, giving the drug to others, and stopping the medication before the time stipulated should be emphasized.

Table 18-1.
USES OF TOPICAL ANTIFUNGAL AGENTS

Generic Name	Trade Name	Use
acrisorcin	Akrinol	tinea versicolor
amphotericin B	Fungizone	monilial infections
candiciden	Candeptin	vaginal monilial infections
chlordantoin	Sporostacin	vaginal monilial infections
haloprogin	Halotex	tinea pedis, cruris, corporis, manuum
methylrosaniline (gentian violet)		vaginal yeast infections, monilial infections, Vincent's angina, impetigo
nystatin	Mycostatin	topical monilial infections of the mouth, vagina, labia
propionate compound	Propion Gel	vulvovaginal monilial infections
tolnaftate	Tinactin	same as haloprogin
undecylenic acid and zinc undecylenate	Desenex	tinea pedis, otomycosis, monilial infections

Antifungal Agents

A fungus is a colorless plant lacking chlorophyll. Fungi that cause disease in humans may be yeast-like or mold-like. Infections caused by fungi are called **mycotic** infections or fungal infections.

Mycotic infections may be of two types: (1) *superficial* mycotic infections and (2) *deep* mycotic infections.

Mycotic infections have become more prominent since the advent of antibiotic therapy, since antibiotics can destroy the normal flora (bacteria) of the body, resulting in superimposed infections.

Types and Uses of Antifungal Agents

Amphotericin B (Fungizone) is an antibiotic fungicide that is used in the treatment of **deep** mycotic infections caused by Blastomyces, Candida, Cryptococcus, and Histoplasma. This drug is effective only against fungi—it has no effect on bacteria and viruses. Amphotericin B is also available in combination with tetracycline (Mysteclin F), formulated to reduce the possibility of monilial overgrowth—a superimposed infection—during tetracycline administration. The value of this combination has been questioned.

Flucytosine (Ancobon) is used in the treatment of serious infections caused by Cryptococcus or Candida.

Griseofulvin (Fulvicin) is an antibiotic fungicide used in the treatment of superficial mycotic infections.

Nystatin (Mycostatin) is an antibiotic fungicide used in the treatment of Candida. Nystatin is available in combination with tetracycline (Tetrex-F). As noted above, the efficacy of combinations of tetracycline with an antifungal agent is questionable, although suppression of monilial growth may be accomplished with use of combination agents.

A group of topical drugs is used to treat superficial fungal infections. Amphotercin B and nystatin are also used topically; other agents including dyes, acids, and chemicals have antifungal activity (Table 18-1).

General Drug Action of Antifungal Agents

The exact mechanism of action of antifungal agents is unknown. Amphotericin B (Fungizone) and nystatin are thought to affect the permeability of bacterial cell walls, similar to the action of penicillin. The action of flucytosine (Ancobon) and griseofulvin (Fulvicin) is unknown.

Side Effects of Antifungal Agents

Amphotericin B (Fungizone) is a highly toxic drug and is used only in the treatment of severe systemic mycotic infections. This drug is administered intravenously, and daily therapy may extend over several months. Headache, nausea, vomiting, diarrhea and muscle and joint pain may occur. Abnormal kidney function is seen, and liver and bone marrow studies are recommended because of the effects of this drug on these areas. Local inflammation at the intravenous needle site and thrombophlebitis have also been reported.

Flucytosine (Ancobon), like amphotericin B, is a toxic drug whose use is reserved for severe systemic mycotic infections. Nausea, vomiting, diarrhea, and rash may be seen. This drug may have toxic effects on the bone marrow, liver, and kidney, and routine studies to detect drug toxicity are recommended.

The side effects of griseofulvin (Fulvicin) are nausea, vomiting, epigastric discomfort, and headache. Sensitivity reactions have also been reported.

Nystatin has few side effects, but diarrhea, nausea, and vomiting may occasionally occur.

Side effects are rare during the use of topical antifungal agents. Occasionally rashes or signs of local irritation or skin sensitivity may be apparent during use.

Clinical Considerations

Amphotericin B is administered daily by the intravenous route. The physician will compute the dose according to the patient's weight. Usually, the drug is administered over a period of 6 hours. The needle site should be checked not only at the time of drug administration but also after. Previous venipuncture sites should also be checked at the same time, as thrombophlebitis—if it does occur—may not be apparent for several days.

The intravenous solution containing amphotericin B is administered *slowly*. Since movement or change in position can alter the rate of infusion, the infusion should be checked every 15-30 minutes. *Any* side effects or unusual occurrences should be reported immediately. Intake and output measurement may also be advisable on these patients, especially if renal function studies appear abnormal.

Flucytosine (Ancobon) is administered orally. Nausea and vomiting appear to be relatively common side effects and may possibly be relieved by the administration of a few capsules at a time over a 15-minute period. Since this drug may affect the bone marrow, liver, and kidney, the patient requires close supervision as well as periodic laboratory studies. Any unusual or vague complaints may be meaningful and may relate to the toxic effects of the drug.

Discharge Teaching

When topical antifungal agents are prescribed, it may be necessary to demonstrate *how* to apply the drug. In some cases, the physician may desire a liberal application, whereas in others it should be applied in a thin layer. Whichever type of application is required, the fact should be stressed that only when the drug is applied in this manner can results be expected. Some patients, in an effort to save money, may be inclined to use the prescription sparingly. The reverse is also true, in that some patients may believe that the more drug applied, the quicker the infection will be cured.

Table 18-2.
PENICILLIN PREPARATIONS

Generic Name	Trade Name	Uses	Side Effects	Dose Ranges
NATURAL PENICILLINS				
benzathine penicillin G	Bicillin Long-Acting	treatment of infections caused by susceptible organisms	skin rash, urticaria, anaphylactoid reactions, superimposed infections, nausea, vomiting, diarrhea, hematological changes	300,000-3 million units I.M. per dose
penicillin G, crystalline as the potassium or sodium salt		same as benzathine penicillin G	same as benzathine penicillin G	1-12 million units daily in divided doses q2-4h I.M., I.V., S.C.
procaine penicillin G	Wycillin	same as benzathine penicillin G	same as benzathine penicillin G	300,000-1 million units in single or divided doses I.M. daily
SYNTHETIC AND SEMISYNTHETIC PENICILLINS				
sodium ampicillin	Amcill-S, Polycillin-N	same as benzathine penicillin G	same as benzathine penicillin G	250-500 mg. q6-8h I.M., I.V.; CHILD: 25-50 mg./ Kg./ day in divided doses; in severe infections doses may be higher
ampicillin trihydrate	Amcill, Polycillin	same as benzathine penicillin G	same as benzathine penicillin G	250-500 mg. q6h orally; CHILD: 50-100 mg./ Kg./ day in divided doses at 6-8 hour intervals
ampicillin and probenecid	Amcill-GC	treatment of gonorrhea	same as benzathine penicillin G	1 single-dose bottle orally
carbenicillin indanyl sodium	Geocillin	same as benzathine penicillin G	same as benzathine penicillin G	1-2 tablets Q.I.D. orally

Generic Name	Trade Name	Uses	Side Effects	Dose Ranges
disodium carbenicillin	Pyopen, Geopen	same as benzathine penicillin G	same as benzathine penicillin G	200-500 mg./Kg./day I.V. in divided doses or by continuous drip; also, 1-2 Grams q4-8h I.V., 1-2 Grams q6h I.M.; CHILD: 50-500 mg./Kg./day I.V. in divided doses or continuous drip; 50-400 mg./Kg./day I.M. in divided doses
sodium cloxacillin	Tegopen	same as benzathine penicillin G	same as benzathine penicillin G	250-500 mg. q6h orally; CHILD: 50-100 mg./Kg./day in divided doses orally
sodium dicloxacillin	Dynapen	same as benzathine penicillin G	same as benzathine penicillin G	125-250 mg. q6h orally; CHILD: 12.5-25 mg./Kg./day in divided doses orally
hetacillin, potassium hetacillin	Versapen, Versapen-K	same as benzathine penicillin G	same as benzathine penicillin G	225-450 mg. Q.I.D. I.M., I.V., orally; CHILD: 22.5-45 mg./Kg./day I.M., I.V., orally; in severe infections doses may be higher
sodium methicillin	Staphcillin	same as benzathine penicillin G	same as benzathine penicillin G	1 Gram q4-6h I.M. or q6h I.V.; CHILD: 25 mg./Kg. q6h I.M.

Table 18-2. (*Continued*)

Generic Name	Trade Name	Uses	Side Effects	Dose Ranges
sodium nafcillin	Unipen	same as benzathine penicillin G	same as benzathine penicillin G	500 mg. q4-6h I.M.; 500 mg.-1 Gram q4h I.V.; 250 mg.-1 Gram q4-6h orally; CHILD: 250 mg. T.I.D. orally or 25-50 mg./Kg./day in 4 divided doses orally; 25 mg./Kg. B.I.D. I.M.
sodium oxacillin	Prostaphlin	same as benzathine penicillin G	same as benzathine penicillin G	500 mg.-1 Gram q4-6h orally; 250 mg.-1 Gram q4-6h I.M., I.V.; CHILD: 50 mg./Kg./day in divided doses q6h orally, I.M., I.V.
potassium phenoxymethyl penicillin	Compocillin-VK	same as benzathine penicillin G	same as benzathine penicillin G	200,000-600,000 units q6-8h orally

Table 18-3.
BROAD-SPECTRUM ANTIBIOTICS

Generic Name	Trade Name	Uses	Side Effects	Dose Ranges
bacitracin		topical: superficial infections of eye, ear, nose, throat due to susceptible organisms; oral and parenteral: intestinal amebiasis, infections caused by susceptible organisms not responding to other drugs	nephrotoxicity, nausea, vomiting, anorexia, hypersensitivity reactions, superimposed infections, pain at site of injection; topical: rare	10,000-25,000 units q6-8h I.M.; 80,000-120,000 units in divided doses q6h orally; CHILD: 200-400 units/Kg. q6-8h I.M.

Generic Name	Trade Name	Uses	Side Effects	Dose Ranges
cephalexin	Keflex	respiratory tract infections, skin and soft tissue infections, urinary tract infections caused by susceptible organisms	superimposed infections, nausea, vomiting, diarrhea, abdominal discomfort, hypersensitivity reactions	1-4 Grams daily in divided doses orally; CHILD: 25-50 mg./Kg./day in 4 divided doses orally
cephaloglycin	Kafocin	acute and chronic infections of the urinary tract	superimposed infections, hypersensitivity reactions	250-500 mg. Q.I.D. orally; CHILD: 25-50 mg./Kg./day orally
cephaloridine	Loridine	serious infections of respiratory and urinary tracts, bones, joints, bloodstream, soft tissue, skin due to susceptible organisms; also for early syphilis and gonorrhea	nephrotoxicity, superimposed infections, nausea, vomiting, hypersensitivity reactions	250 mg.-1 Gram T.I.D. I.M.; single dose of 2 Grams I.M. for gonorrhea; 500 mg.-1 Gram I.M. daily × 10-14 days for syphilis; also given I.V. 500 mg.-4 Grams daily
cephalothin	Keflin	treatment of serious infections of respiratory and urinary tract, skin and soft tissue infections, septicemia, bone and joint infections, meningitis, gastrointestinal infections caused by susceptible organisms	pain at site of injection, superimposed infections, hypersensitivity reactions	500 mg.-1 Gram q4-6h I.M., I.V.; in more serious infections doses may be higher
chloramphenicol	Chloromycetin	typhoid fever, serious infections caused by susceptible organisms that do not respond to other antibiotics	nausea, vomiting, blood dyscrasias, headache, depression, mental confusion, rash, urticaria, superimposed infections, hypersensitivity reactions	50-100 mg./Kg./day in divided doses q6h I.V. orally; CHILD: 50 mg./Kg./day in divided doses q6h orally I.V.

Table 18-3. (*Continued*)

GENERIC NAME	TRADE NAME	USES	SIDE EFFECTS	DOSE RANGES
chlortetracycline	Aureomycin	treatment of infections caused by susceptible organisms	diarrhea, gastric distress, rash, phototoxic reactions, superimposed infections, hematological changes, discoloration of teeth in children, hypersensitivity reactions	1-2 Grams in 4 divided doses orally; 250-500 mg. q6-12h I.V.; CHILD: 10-20 mg./lb./day in 4 divided doses orally
clindamycin	Cleocin	treatment of infections caused by susceptible organisms	superimposed infections, diarrhea (may be severe), nausea, vomiting, abdominal pain, jaundice, hematological changes, hypersensitivity reactions	150-450 mg. q6h orally; CHILD: 8-20 mg./Kg./day in 3-4 divided doses orally
colistimethate	Coly-Mycin M	treatment of infections caused by susceptible organisms	circumoral paresthesia, tingling of extremities, dizziness, vertigo, nephrotoxicity, respiratory arrest, hypersensitivity reactions	adult, child: 2.5-5 mg./Kg./day in 2-4 divided doses I.V., I.M.
colistin	Coly-Mycin S	acute bacterial diarrheas	superimposed infections	5-15 mg./Kg./day in 3 divided doses orally
demeclocycline	Declomycin	treatment of infections caused by susceptible organisms	same as chlortetracycline	600 mg. daily in 2-4 divided doses orally; CHILD: 3-6 mg./lb./day in 2-4 divided doses orally
doxycycline	Vibramycin	treatment of infections caused by susceptible organisms	same as chlortetracycline	initially 100 mg. q12h on first day, then 100 mg. daily orally; 100 mg. daily or 200 mg. B.I.D. I.V.; CHILD: 2 mg./lb./day orally, I.V.

Generic Name	Trade Name	Uses	Side Effects	Dose Ranges
erythromycin	Ilotycin	treatment of infections caused by susceptible organisms	nausea, vomiting, rash, diarrhea, urticaria, superimposed infections, hypersensitivity reactions	250 mg. q6h orally; CHILD: 30-50 mg./Kg./day in divided doses orally
erythromycin ethylsuccinate	Erythrocin ethyl succinate	treatment of infections caused by susceptible organisms	same as erythromycin	400 mg.-1 Gram q6h orally; 100 mg. q4-8h deep I.M.; CHILD: 30-50 mg./Kg./day in divided doses orally; 12 mg./Kg./day I.M.
erythromycin gluceptate	Ilotycin gluceptate	treatment of infections caused by susceptible organisms	same as erythromycin	15-20 mg./Kg./day I.V.
erythromycin lactobionate	Erythrocin lactobionate	treatment of infections caused by susceptible organisms	same as erythromycin	adult, child: 10-20 mg./Kg./day I.V.
erythromycin stearate	Erythrocin stearate	treatment of infections caused by susceptible organisms	same as erythromycin	250 mg. q6h orally; CHILD: 30-50 mg./Kg./day in divided doses orally
gentamicin	Garamycin	treatment of infections caused by susceptible organisms	ototoxicity, nephrotoxicity, superimposed infections, hypersensitivity reactions, muscle twitching, skin tingling, numbness	3-5 mg./Kg./day q8h I.M., I.V.; CHILD: 3-6 mg./Kg./day in divided doses I.M., I.V.; patients with impaired renal function require dose adjustment according to renal function tests

Table 18-3. *(Continued)*

Generic Name	Trade Name	Uses	Side Effects	Dose Ranges
kanamycin	Kantrex	oral: suppression of intestinal flora; parenteral: treatment of infections caused by susceptible organisms, hepatic coma	oral: nausea, vomiting, diarrhea; parenteral: ototoxicity, nephrotoxicity, pain at site of injection, superimposed infections, hypersensitivity reactions	suppression of intestinal flora: 1 Gram q1h × 4, then 1 Gram q6h for 36-72 hours orally; adult, child: 7.5-15 mg./Kg./day in divided doses I.M., I.V.; hepatic coma: 8-12 Grams daily in divided doses orally
lincomycin	Lincocin	treatment of infections caused by susceptible organisms	superimposed infections, hypersensitivity reactions, nausea, vomiting, diarrhea, abdominal pain	500 mg. q6-8h orally; 600 mg. q12-24h I.M.; 600 mg.-1 Gram q8-12h I.V.; CHILD: 30-60 mg./Kg./day in 3-4 divided doses orally; 10 mg./Kg./day q12-24h I.M.; 10-20 mg./Kg./day in divided doses I.V.
methacycline	Rondomycin	treatment of infections caused by susceptible organisms	same as chlortetracycline	600 mg. daily in 2-4 divided doses orally; CHILD: 3-6 mg./lb./day in 2-4 divided doses orally
minocycline	Minocin	treatment of infections caused by susceptible organisms	same as chlortetracycline	200 mg. initially, then 100 mg. q12h I.V., orally; CHILD: 4 mg./Kg. initially then 2 mg./Kg. q12h I.V. orally

Generic Name	Trade Name	Uses	Side Effects	Dose Ranges
neomycin	Mycifradin	oral: suppression of intestinal flora, hepatic coma, infectious diarrhea; parenteral: treatment of infections caused by susceptible organisms	ototoxicity, nephrotoxicity, hypersensitivity reactions; oral: diarrhea	infectious diarrhea: 50 mg./Kg./day in divided doses orally; 15 mg./Kg./day in 4 divided doses I.M.; hepatic coma: 4-12 Grams per day in divided doses; bowel preparation: 40 mg./lb./day in 6 divided doses orally
oxytetracycline	Terramycin	treatment of infections caused by susceptible organisms	same as chlortetracycline	250 mg. q6h orally; 250-500 mg. q6-12h I.V.; 100-250 mg. q8-12h I.M.; CHILD: 25-50 mg./Kg./day in divided doses orally; 12 mg./Kg./day q12h I.V.; 15-25 mg./Kg./day in divided doses I.M.
polymyxin B	Aerosporin	treatment of infections caused by susceptible organisms	nephrotoxicity, superimposed infections, hypersensitivity reactions, dizziness, blurred vision, numbness of mouth, face, extremities	adult, child: 15,000-25,000 units/Kg./day I.V.; 25,000-30,000 units/Kg./day I.M.

Table 18-3. (Continued)

Generic Name	Trade Name	Uses	Side Effects	Dose Ranges
tetracycline	Tetracyn	treatment of infections caused by susceptible organisms	same as chlortetracycline	1-2 Grams daily in 2-4 divided doses orally; 250 mg. daily I.M.; 250-500 mg. q12h I.V.; CHILD: 10-20 mg./lb./day in 4 divided doses orally; 15-25 mg./Kg./day in single or divided doses I.M.; 12 mg./Kg./day in 2 divided doses I.V.
vancomycin	Vancocin	severe staphylococcal infections	chills, rash, drug fever, ototoxicity, nephrotoxicity, superimposed infections, hypersensitivity reactions, thrombophlebitis	500 mg. q6h or 1 Gram q12h I.V.; CHILD: 20 mg./lb./day I.V.

Table 18-4.
ANTIFUNGAL AGENTS

Generic Name	Trade Name	Uses	Side Effects	Dose Ranges
acrisorcin	Akrinol	treatment of tinea versicolor	local irritation	cream applied topically B.I.D. A.M. and P.M.
amphotericin B	Fungizone	treatment of deep mycotic infections	headache, nausea, vomiting, diarrhea, joint and muscle pain, abnormal renal function, pain and/or thrombophlebitis at site of infusion	0.25 mg./Kg./day I.V. for 6 hours; dose is gradually increased as tolerance permits; maximum limit is 1.5 mg./Kg./day
amphotericin B (cream)	Fungizone	superficial monilial infections	local irritation	cream, ointment, or lotion applied topically B.I.D. to Q.I.D.

Generic Name	Trade Name	Uses	Side Effects	Dose Ranges
candicidin	Candeptin	vaginal moniliasis	local irritation	1 applicator full or 1 vaginal tablet or capsule B.I.D. in A.M. and P.M.
chlordantoin	Sporostacin	vaginal moniliasis	local irritation	1 applicator full B.I.D. A.M. and P.M.
flucytosine	Ancobon	treatment of serious infections caused by susceptible strains of Candida or Cryptococcus	toxic to bone marrow, liver, kidney; rash, nausea, vomiting, diarrhea	50-150 mg./Kg./day in divided doses orally
griseofulvin	Fulvicin	treatment of superficial mycotic infections	headache, rash, nausea, diarrhea	500 mg.-1 Gram daily in single or divided doses orally; CHILD: 5 mg./lb./day orally
haloprogin	Halotex	treatment of tinea pedis, cruris, corporis, manuum	local irritation	apply liberally to affected area B.I.D.
methylrosaniline (gentian violet)		treatment of infections due to yeasts and molds	local irritation	apply topically B.I.D.
nystatin	Mycostatin	treatment of Candida albicans	nausea, vomiting, diarrhea	500,000-1 million units T.I.D. orally; also as an ointment applied B.I.D.
propionate compound	Propion Gel	vulvovaginal moniliasis	local irritation	applied topically B.I.D. A.M. and P.M.
tolnaftate	Tinactin	treatment of tinea pedis, cruris, manuum	local irritation	apply topically B.I.D.
undecylenic acid and zinc undecylenate	Desenex	superficial dermatomycosis		apply powder B.I.D.

Tuberculosis is caused by the *Mycobacterium tuberculosis* bacillus and infects both animals and humans. Identified by Robert Koch in 1882, treatment of this disease was generally ineffective until the advent of streptomycin in 1947.

Types and Uses of Antitubercular Drugs

Aminosalicylic acid (PAS, Parasal) is an oral antitubercular agent that is bacteriostatic and is usually administered in conjunction with other antitubercular agents. Most commonly, this drug is given with isoniazid (INH) and/or streptomycin. It is of little value when used alone.

Capreomycin (Capastat) is given by the intramuscular route, usually with other antitubercular agents. This drug is recommended for use in those who have developed resistance to other antitubercular agents.

Cycloserine (Seromycin), an oral antitubercular agent, may be given alone or in combination with other antitubercular agents. Choice of this drug is made upon results of sensitivity studies. This drug may also be used when bacterial resistance to aminosalicylic acid (PAS), isoniazid (INH) or streptomycin develops, or when the patient cannot

Chapter **12**

Drugs Used in the Treatment of Tuberculosis

tolerate these agents due to the development of side effects. This drug may also be employed in the treatment of nontubercular urinary tract infections caused by susceptible organisms.

Ethambutol (Myambutol) is administered orally, either alone or in combination with other antitubercular agents. Resistance appears to develop rapidly when this drug is used alone; consequently it is usually combined with isoniazid (INH) or other agents.

Ethionamide (Trecator) is an oral antitubercular agent utilized when bacterial resistance develops or the patient cannot tolerate other agents.

Isoniazid (INH) is administered orally. This drug is used along with other agents in the treatment of active tuberculosis. It may also be used alone as preventative therapy in the following instances:

1. household contacts—those living in the household of an active tubercular patient
2. persons who have had tuberculosis which now is inactive, but who have not had adequate antitubercular therapy
3. those whose skin tests have become positive (increased by 6 mm. or more) within two years
4. those with positive skin tests and abnormal pulmonary findings seen on chest X-ray
5. positive skin tests in those (a) younger than twenty years (b) in close association with tubercular patients, and (c) receiving other drugs such as corticosteroids or having conditions which might lower body resistance to tuberculosis

Rifampin (Rimactane) is an oral antitubercular agent used in conjunction with other antitubercular agents.

Streptomycin and dihydrostreptomycin are used in conjunction with aminosalicylic acid (PAS) and/or isoniazid (INH). These antibiotics are also used to treat infections other than tuberculosis, caused by bacteria sensitive to the streptomycins.

General Drug Action

The exact mode of action of aminosalicylic acid (PAS), capreomycin (Capastat), and ethionamide (Trecator) is unknown. The action of other antitubercular agents is still not clear, but they may (1) inhibit the multiplication of microorganisms (2) interfere with bacterial metabolism, or (3) inhibit protein synthesis.

Side Effects of Antitubercular Drugs

One main problem encountered during the administration of antitubercular agents is the development of bacterial resistance. Although not a side effect in the strict sense, this problem occurs frequently, and in some cases rapidly. Once bacterial resistance develops, another antitubercular agent must be employed.

The side effects most commonly seen with each agent are as follows:

Aminosalicylic acid (PAS): gastrointestinal disturbances are the most common side effects of this drug; they may disappear during the first week or two of therapy. Giving the drug with meals and/or antacids may alleviate the nausea, vomiting, and diarrhea in some patients. If these side effects continue despite these measures, the drug may have to be discontinued and other agents employed. Occasionally blood dyscrasias and liver damage occur.

Capreomycin (Capastat) is capable of producing eighth cranial nerve (auditory) damage with resultant loss of hearing, dizziness, and tinnitus. Renal damage has also been reported. This drug is given by *deep* intramuscular injection. Pain, excessive bleeding, induration, and sterile abscesses at injection sites may be seen.

Cycloserine (Seromycin), when given in doses of 1 Gram or more daily, may produce a variety of side effects, namely drowsiness, headache, mental confusion, psychotic reactions, convulsions, and allergic dermatitis. In smaller doses the incidence of these side effects is reduced.

Ethambutol (Myambutol) is capable of causing a variety of visual disturbances, ranging from a loss of color discrimination (usually green and occasionally red) to blurred vision and loss of vision. In most instances these symptoms disappear several weeks to several months after the drug is discontinued. Other side effects are rash, headache, nausea, and numbness and tingling of the extremities.

The most common side effects of ethionamide (Trecator) are related to the gastrointestinal tract: nausea, anorexia, vomiting, diarrhea, and a metallic taste in the mouth. Mental depression, peripheral neuritis, jaundice, headache, rash, and dermatitis may also occur.

The side effects of isoniazid (INH) appear to be dose-related. The most common side effect is numbness with tingling of the extremities. Nervous system side effects may be relieved by the administration of pyridoxine. Other side effects include jaundice, rash, blood dyscrasias, gastrointestinal distress, headache, and dryness of the mouth.

Rifampin (Rimactane) side effects are mainly gastrointestinal in nature, including anorexia, nausea, vomiting, diarrhea, and abdominal cramps. Headache, fatigue, dizziness, mental confusion, muscle weakness, and numbness of the extremities may also be noted.

Streptomycin and dihydrostreptomycin are ototoxic drugs. Damage to the auditory and vestibular branches of the eighth cranial (auditory) nerve results in hearing loss, tinnitus, dizziness, and vertigo. The hearing loss may be permanent. Pain and tenderness at the site of injection commonly occur. Hypersensitivity reactions (anaphylactic shock) have also been reported.

Clinical Considerations and Discharge Teaching

Antitubercular drugs are administered for long periods of time; therefore careful patient instruction and close medical supervision are necessary. Many patients receiving these drugs may be outpatients of a hospital clinic or public health department. Those receiving injectable drugs may also be at home, with injections given by the public health nurse.

When a patient is first placed on an antitubercular drug, the following points should be incorporated into a teaching plan: the importance of drug therapy and the importance of medical supervision.

Depending on circumstances, teaching can be done with groups or with individuals. There is a distinct advantage in teaching a small group of patients, since the questions raised by the group often cover more areas than questions from one individual. This also gives the patient, who may be reticent about asking questions, the opportunity of learning from others.

In discussing the importance of drug therapy, the following points should be mentioned:

1. antitubercular drugs are of value only if taken as prescribed by the physician. Omission of the drug is serious. The only way tuberculosis can be controlled by drug therapy is by strict adherence to the physician's orders regarding medication
2. antitubercular drugs can cause side effects, and the physician must be notified immediately if they occur

During discussion of the importance of medical supervision, the patient must understand the importance of keeping clinic or private physician appointments. Drug therapy is based on the patient's response.

X-rays, sputum tests, and physical examination are tools used by the physican to determine the therapeutic response. In some cases, drugs will have to be discontinued and different drugs prescribed due to the development of bacterial resistance. This can be determined only by routine visits to a physician.

Some antitubercular agents are toxic to the eye, kidney, liver, and central nervous system. Periodic hearing and eye tests, blood studies, and liver and renal studies may be ordered. Any problem the patient experiences should be reported, since some toxic manifestations are preceded by tinnitus, dizziness, and fatigue. Some of these manifestations may be in the form of vague and nonspecific complaints.

Parenteral antitubercular drugs such as capreomycin (Capastat) and the streptomycins are painful on injection. Pain may persist for hours or days. The buttocks should be inspected for induration of tissue and the possible development of sterile abscesses. Injection sites should also be rotated, but even this measure may fail to prevent discomfort.

Table 19-1.

ANTITUBERCULAR AGENTS

Generic Name	Trade Name	Uses	Side Effects	Dose Ranges
aminosalicylic acid (PAS)	Parasal	treatment of tuberculosis, along with other antitubercular agents	nausea, vomiting, diarrhea, abdominal pain, epigastric distress, hepatic damage, blood dyscrasias	10-15 Grams daily in divided doses orally
capreomycin	Capastat	treatment of tuberculosis, usually given with other antitubercular agents	pain at site of injection, ototoxicity, nephrotoxicity; induration, excessive bleeding, sterile abscesses may be noted at injection sites	1 Gram daily to 2-3 ×/week I.M.
cycloserine	Seromycin	treatment of tuberculosis; may be used alone or with other antitubercular agents	drowsiness dizziness, headache, psychotic reactions, confusion, convulsions, allergic dermatitis	250 mg. q8-12h and up to 1 Gram daily in 4 divided doses orally
ethambutol	Myambutol	treatment of tuberculosis; may be used alone or with other antitubercular agents	blurred vision, inability to perceive green and red colors, rash, headache, nausea, numbness and tingling of extremities	15-25 mg./Kg./day orally
ethionamide	Trecator	treatment of tuberculosis; used when resistance develops to other agents or patient cannot tolerate other drugs	anorexia, nausea, vomiting, metallic taste, diarrhea, headache, rash, dermatitis	500 mg.-1 Gram daily in divided doses orally

Table 19-1. (*Continued*)

GENERIC NAME	TRADE NAME	USES	SIDE EFFECTS	DOSE RANGES
isoniazid	INH	treatment of tuberculosis; may be used alone or with other agents	rash, dryness of mouth, headache, nausea, vomiting, numbness and tingling of extremities, jaundice, blood dyscrasias, fever	PREVENTIVE THERAPY: 300 mg. daily in single or divided doses orally; CHILD: 10 mg./Kg./day in single or divided doses orally TREATMENT: 5 mg./Kg./day in single or divided doses, orally; CHILD: 10-30 mg./Kg./day in single or divided doses orally
rifampin	Rimactane	treatment of tuberculosis; used with other antitubercular agents	anorexia, nausea, vomiting, gastric distress, abdominal cramps, headache, fatigue, dizziness, mental confusion, muscle weakness, numbness of extremities	600 mg. daily orally; CHILD: 10-20 mg./Kg./day orally
streptomycin, dihydrostreptomycin		treatment of tuberculosis; used in conjunction with other antitubercular agents; also used in infections due to susceptible organisms	ototoxicity, hypersensitivity reactions, pain at site of injection	AS ANTITUBERCULAR: 1 Gram 2-3 ×/week I.M.; CHILD: 20-40 mg./Kg./day I.M.

Malaria has been and still is a worldwide health problem. This disease was recorded in early Greek and Roman writings; some historians feel that the decline of some ancient cultures might have been due to epidemics of smallpox, typhus, and malaria.

Invasion by helminths (**helminthiasis**) is worldwide, affecting both humans and animals. Although social stigma is attached to parasitic infestations, they may be seen in all levels of society.

Amebiasis is the invasion of the body by the amoeba—*Entamoeba histolytica.* This disease also has worldwide distribution.

Malaria

Cases of malaria are relatively rare in residents of the United States; this disease may be seen by health-care professionals practicing in countries where malaria is prevalent. Malaria may also be seen in the United States in those who have traveled to, or lived in, countries where this disease is a health problem.

Malaria is transmitted by certain species of the *anopheles* mosquito. The four different protozoans causing malaria are:

Chapter **20**

Drugs Used in the Treatment of Parasitic Diseases

LIFE CYCLE OF THE PLASMODIUM

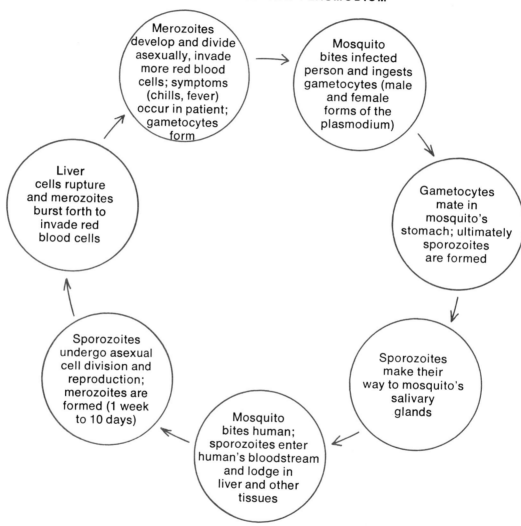

Merozoites develop and divide asexually, invade more red blood cells; symptoms (chills, fever) occur in patient; gametocytes form

Mosquito bites infected person and ingests gametocytes (male and female forms of the plasmodium)

Gametocytes mate in mosquito's stomach; ultimately sporozoites are formed

Sporozoites make their way to mosquito's salivary glands

Mosquito bites human; sporozoites enter human's bloodstream and lodge in liver and other tissues

Sporozoites undergo asexual cell division and reproduction; merozoites are formed (1 week to 10 days)

Liver cells rupture and merozoites burst forth to invade red blood cells

1. *Plasmodium falciparum:* falciparum malaria, also called malignant tertian malaria
2. *Plasmodium malariae:* malariae malaria, also called quartan malaria
3. *Plasmodium ovale:* ovale malaria
4. *Plasmodium vivax:* vivax malaria, also called benign tertian malaria

Types and Actions of Antimalarial Drugs

Different kinds of antimalarial drugs affect different phases of the malarial cycle.

CAUSAL PROPHYLAXIS. An antimalarial drug with causal prophylactic activity destroys the malarial parasites prior to their entrance into red blood cells (pre-erythrocyte stage). Although there are antimalarial drugs capable of causal prophylaxis, relatively high doses are required, resulting in the appearance of side effects.

SUPPRESSIVE PROPHYLAXIS. This mode of action prevents the completion of asexual reproduction in the red blood cells, thus keeping the individual free of malarial symptoms.

CLINICAL CURE. Drugs effecting a clinical cure relieve the symptoms of a malarial attack.

RADICAL CURE. Antimalarial agents that eradicate the parasites in both the blood cells and the bloodstream are capable of a radical cure. This type of cure also relieves the symptoms of malaria.

SUPPRESSIVE CURE. This type of drug effect eliminates malarial parasites by eradicating the asexual forms present in red blood cells or inhibiting the further development of the parasites present in the bloodstream.

Table 20-1.
EFFECTS OF ANTIMALARIAL DRUGS

Generic Name	Trade Name	Type of Effect
amodiaquin	Camoquin	suppressive prophylaxis, clinical cure, true causal prophylaxis and cure of *P. falciparum*
chloroquine	Aralen	same as amodiaquin
hydroxychloroquine	Plaquenil	same as amodiaquin
primaquine		radical cure of relapsing *P. vivax*, radical cure of a suppressed infection
pyrimethamine	Daraprim	radical cure of *P. falciparum*, suppressive prophylaxis
quinine		clinical cure, suppression of *P. vivax*

The development of resistant strains of plasmodia has made some cases of malaria difficult to treat; consequently the drugs in Table 20-1 may be used in manners other than those stated.

The prevention of malaria is not only drug-oriented, but is also aimed at eliminating areas where the mosquito breeds.

Side Effects of Antimalarial Drugs

In doses used to treat malaria, the side effects of antimalarial agents are mild. This applies of course to those patients who are taking the drug *as prescribed by the physician.*

Occasionally, epigastric distress, nausea, vomiting, and diarrhea may be seen. Taking the drug with meals may minimize these side effects. Excessive doses can cause severe epigastric distress resulting in extreme weakness and serious fluid and electrolyte imbalance.

Clinical Considerations and Discharge Teaching

People needing instruction may include military service personnel going to, or residing in, malaria-infected areas as well as patients discharged from the hospital who are required to take antimalarial agents at home. The following points should be stressed:

1. take the drug *only* as directed by the physician
2. *do not omit* scheduled doses
3. *do not exceed* the dose ordered. Taking more of the drug will not lessen the chance of contacting malaria. In some cases an increase in dose can result in the appearance of side effects which can be serious

Usually, antimalarials are taken weekly *on the same day each week.* The patient should decide which day of the week is best, if possible, since it might be easier to remember to take the drug every week if it fits into a routine schedule.

Helminthiasis

Helminthiasis is an invasion of the body by helminths (worms). An anthelmintic is a drug used to treat helminthiasis. Roundworms, pinworms, whipworms, hookworms, and tapeworms are examples of helminths.

Types and Uses of Anthelmintic Agents

The finding and identification of the ova (eggs), larvae, and adult worms is essential in the treatment of helminthiasis. Once the helminth has been eliminated, measures must be taken to prevent reinfection. It should also be noted that an individual can harbor more than one type of helminth, for example, infestation with hookworm *and* roundworm.

HELMINTHS

Nematodes
  hookworm (*Necator americanus*)
  pinworm (*Enterobius vermicularis*)
  roundworm (*Ascaris lumbricoides*)
  whipworm (*Trichuris trichura*)

Cestodes
  beef tapeworm (*Taenia saginata*)
  dwarf tapeworm (*Hymenolepis nana*)
  fish tapeworm (*Diphyllobothrium latum*)
  pork tapeworm (*Taenia solium*)

The drugs used to treat helminthiasis are shown in Table 20-2.

Table 20-2.
DRUGS USED TO TREAT HELMINTHIASIS

Generic Name	Trade Name	Type of Helminth
aspidium oleoresin (male fern)		tapeworm (beef, pork, fish, dwarf)
bephenium hydroxynaphthoate	Alcopara	hookworm, roundworm
hexylresorcinol	Crystoids	roundworm, hookworm; may also be used in the treatment of pinworm, tapeworm, and whipworm, although other drugs are considered more effective
methylrosaniline chloride (gentian violet)		pinworm
piperazine	Antepar	pinworm, roundworm
pyrantel pamoate	Antiminth	pinworm, roundworm
pyrvinium pamoate	Povan	pinworm
thiabendazole	Mintezol	pinworm, roundworm, hookworm, whipworm

Side Effects of Anthelmintic Agents

The side effects of most anthelmintic agents are minimal when drugs are used in recommended doses. Aspidium oleoresin (male fern) is rarely used today since it causes more side effects and possible serious toxic effects than other equally effective anthelmintics.

Hexylresorcinol (Crystoids) is a local irritant; the drug must be *swallowed whole* and *not chewed.* Methylrosaniline (gentian violet), when taken orally, may cause mild gastrointestinal upset with nausea, vomiting, diarrhea, and abdominal pain. These side effects may also be seen with pyrantel pamoate (Antiminth).

Clinical Considerations and Discharge Teaching

Many cases of helminthiasis may be treated in outpatient clinics or physicians' offices. Teaching is an important part of clinical efforts to prevent reinfection, in that the patient possibly requires careful instruction regarding the medications prescribed.

Pyrvinium (Povan) is administered as a single dose which usually eliminates the pinworm. Piperazine (Antepar), also used to treat pinworms, is given daily for seven days.

PYRVINIUM
(Povan)

Directions:
1. take one dose only
2. liquid form will stain if spilled on furniture, clothes, etc.
3. stools will be bright red
4. the tablet form *must* be swallowed whole

Patient teaching should include the following points:

1. pinworm infestation can recur
2. showers are recommended instead of tub baths during the time family members are being treated, as well as after treatment, until no repeat infestation is apparent
3. particular attention should be paid to cleaning the bathroom, which should be thoroughly cleaned and scrubbed daily; toilet seat, bathtub, and bathroom floor must be cleaned
4. children should be taught to thoroughly wash their hands; adult supervision may be necessary
5. the nails should be kept *short* and *clean* since the worms and eggs can get under the nails when children touch or scratch the anal area; a good nail brush is necessary for proper cleaning
6. the hands should not be placed in the mouth, as this is the most common original route of infection and reinfection
7. anal itching may be a sign of reinfection

In clinics or offices where pinworm-infested patients are seen, it may be of value to write out directions for drug administration and suggestions for elimination of sources of infection. Copies given to the patient in this format may serve as a reminder.

In the treatment of whipworm, hexylresorcinol (Crystoids) may be prescribed. As noted above, the tablets must be *swallowed whole* and *not chewed* since the drug can burn the oral mucosa. When tablets are given to a small child, an adult should check to see if the medication has been swallowed. The buccal areas should be inspected for irritation with a flashlight and tongue blade. At home, the parent can use the handle of a spoon instead of a tongue blade.

Health teaching for whipworm, roundworm, and hookworm may present a difficult problem. These helminths are more prevalent in areas of poor sanitary facilities. It is easy to say "improve sanitary facilities" but for many reasons this may be impossible. Adequate sewer facilities may not be available or the cost of obtaining same may not be within the financial reach of these patients. Consultation with the public health department may be of value.

Amebiasis

Amebiasis, an invasion of the body by the amoeba *Entamoeba histolytica*, has worldwide distribution. When the amoeba occupies the intestine the disease is termed **intestinal amebiasis.** When the amoeba is found in body organs or tissues it is termed **extraintestinal amebiasis.** The amoeba, in this case, may be found in the liver, lungs, heart, and skin.

VARIOUS FORMS OF AMEBIASIS
1. asymptomatic
2. mild amebic colitis
3. amebic dysentery
4. amebic hepatitis, hepatic abscess, invasion of other organs by the amoeba

---

Drug therapy is aimed at the type of amoebic infection as well as the severity of the infection.

Types and Uses of Amebacide Agents

Amodiaquin (Camoquin) is used in the treatment of extraintestinal amebiasis and is usually administered along with an intestinal amebacide.

Carbarsone is useful in treating mild to moderately severe forms of intestinal amebiasis. This drug is an arsenic compound and therefore interrupted therapy is necessary to avoid cumulative arsenic poisoning, due to the slow excretion of the drug. Carbarsone is given twice daily for ten days. If a repeat course of therapy is necessary, a two-week rest period is recommended before reinstitution of therapy.

Chloroquine (Aralen), which is also used in the treatment of malaria, is effective in the treatment of extraintestinal amebiasis. This drug is usually used in conjunction with an intestinal amebacide.

Diiodohydroxyquin (Diodoquin) is useful in the treatment of intestinal amebiasis.

Emetine is used in the treatment of intestinal and extraintestinal amebiasis. Emetine is a toxic drug, and the patient must be under close medical supervision during and after therapy.

Glycobiarsol (Milibis), like carbarsone, is an arsenic compound. This drug is used to treat intestinal amebiasis.

Iodochlorhydroxyquin (Vioform) is used to treat the intestinal form of amebiasis. In severe forms of the disease emetine is usually given first.

Antibiotics are also used to treat amebiasis. Erythromycin (Ilotycin), oxytetracycline (Terramycin), and paromomycin (Humatin) are used to prevent relapses of the disease. Paromomycin is amebacidal and is used to treat intestinal amebiasis. Erythromycin and oxytetracycline are not amebacidal but decrease the numbers of normal intestinal flora, which are apparently essential for the existence of the amoeba.

Side Effects of the Amebacides

Emetine produces toxic symptoms and must be administered with caution. Diarrhea, nausea, vomiting, marked prostration, vertigo, and tachycardia may occur during therapy. Cardiac failure and cellular degeneration of the liver, heart, kidney, skeletal muscles, and intestinal tract may occur. Therapy with this drug consists of deep subcutaneous injection daily for 4-9 days.

Chloroquine (Aralen) is relatively nontoxic when used in doses for amebiasis. Carbarsone may produce signs of arsenic toxicity; BAL (dimercaprol) may be used as an antidote.

Diiodohydroxyquin (Diodoquin) and iodochlorhydroxquin (Vioform) contain iodine and must not be given to those allergic to iodine. Both drugs are usually well tolerated; however, symptoms of iodism may occasionally occur in some patients. Diarrhea, constipation, abdominal pain, and pruritus may also occur.

SYMPTOMS OF IODISM
chills, fever
dermatitis
furunculosis
headache
rhinitis

The side effects of erythromycin (Ilotycin) and oxytetracycline (Terramycin) when used in the treatment of amebiasis are the same as when these drugs are used for bacterial infections. Paromomycin (Humatin) side effects are nausea, vomiting, and diarrhea.

Clinical Considerations

Patients with amebiasis may appear chronically or acutely ill or may be asymptomatic. Asymptomatic patients may be the most difficult to treat since they have no symptoms and may not fully understand the importance of eliminating the amoeba. Also to be considered in these patients is the fact that a drug may cause discomforting gastrointestinal distress, whereas *no* symptoms were present prior to therapy. It is rather difficult to ask an apparently "well" patient to take a drug that will make him sick, and athough not all patients develop side effects to amebacidal drugs, some do.

Patients receiving emetine require close supervision. Blood pressure, pulse, and respirations should be taken before administration of the drug as well as every 3-4 hours during the day. If tachycardia and/or hypotension occur, the physician should be notified immediately.

These patients should also be on bedrest. The physician may desire limitation of activities for several weeks after a course of therapy. This should be explained thoroughly to the patient, with specific instructions as to how much activity the physician deems advisable.

Discharge Teaching

Health teaching is important in patients with amebiasis. Patients should be instructed to thoroughly wash their hands before leaving a restroom. Poor sanitary conditions lead to the transmission of amebiasis but may be almost impossible to correct.

Above all, patients must be encouraged to continue with therapy and periodic check-ups, which will involve the collection of stool specimens or rectal smears. In some instances it may be necessary to reinforce teaching by explaining that others may become infected and could become seriously ill if those with amebiasis do not seek proper treatment and medical supervision. This approach may also be of value in teaching the asymptomatic patient.

Table 20-3.
ANTIPARASITIC DRUGS

GENERIC NAME	TRADE NAME	USES	SIDE EFFECTS	DOSE RANGES
ANTIMALARIAL DRUGS				
amodiaquin	Camoquin	prevention and treatment of malaria	usually mild in low doses; anorexia, nausea, vomiting, diarrhea, abdominal cramps may occur	PREVENTION: 400-600 mg. weekly orally; CHILD: 100-400 mg. weekly orally TREATMENT: 600 mg.-1 Gram orally; CHILD: 10 mg./Kg. in a single or divided dose orally
chloroquine	Aralen	prevention, treatment, and cure (*P. falciparum* only) of malaria	same as amodiaquin	PREVENTION: 500 mg. weekly orally TREATMENT: 1 Gram initially followed by 500 mg. q6-8h later, then 500 mg. daily × 2 days orally; CHILD: dose based on age
hydroxychloroquine	Plaquenil	prevention, treatment, and cure (*P. falciparum* only) of malaria	same as amodiaquin	PREVENTION: 400 mg. weekly orally TREATMENT: 800 mg. initially, followed by 400 mg. q6-8h later, then 400 mg. daily × 2 days orally; CHILD: dose based on age
primaquine		cure of malaria	usually mild; abdominal cramps, epigastric distress, hematological changes may be seen	26.3-52.6 mg. daily × 14 days orally
pyrimethamine	Daraprim	prevention and cure (*P. falciparum* only) of malaria	usually mild in low doses	PREVENTION: 25 mg. weekly orally CURE: 25 mg. daily × 2 days

173

Table 20-3. *(Continued)*

Generic Name	Trade Name	Uses	Side Effects	Dose Ranges
quinine		prevention and treatment of malaria	usually mild but tinnitus, hearing difficulty, dizziness may occur	TREATMENT: 1 Gram q8h × 3 days then 600 mg. q8h × 5-6 days orally
ANTHELMINTIC DRUGS				
aspidium oleoresin (male fern)		tapeworms (beef, pork, fish, dwarf)	colic, diarrhea, headache, dizziness	4-5 Grams in 2 divided doses given 1 hour apart orally; fat-free diet given 24-48h prior to therapy
bephenium hydroxy- naphthoate	Alcopara	hookworms, roundworms	occasionally gastrointestinal disturbances	ROUNDWORM: 1 packet (2.5 Grams) B.I.D. × 1 day HOOKWORM: same dose × 3 or more days
hexylresorcinol	Crystoids	roundworms, hookworms; also pinworms, tapeworms, whipworms	occasionally gastrointestinal disturbances, oral mucosa irritation if tablets are chewed	1 Gram orally; CHILD: 400-800 mg. orally. Saline cathartic h.s. before and patient kept N.P.O. 4 hours after. 24 hours after taking drug another saline cathartic is given
methylrosaniline chloride (gentian violet)		pinworms	mild nausea, vomiting, diarrhea	60 mg. T.I.D. × 8-10 days orally; CHILD: 3 mg. for each year of age T.I.D. × 8-10 days orally
piperazine	Antepar	pinworms, roundworms	occasionally nausea, vomiting, diarrhea, headache	PINWORMS: 50 mg./ Kg./day, up to 2 Grams orally × 7 days ROUNDWORM: drug given 2, 5, or 7 days; ADULT: 3.5 Grams daily orally; CHILD: 2-3 Grams daily orally. If given for 5 or 7 days the dose is the same as for pinworms

Generic Name	Trade Name	Uses	Side Effects	Dose Ranges
pyrantel pamoate	Antiminth	pinworms, roundworms	gastrointestinal disturbances	5 mg./lb., up to 1 Gram × 1 dose orally
pyrvinium pamoate	Povan	pinworms	drug stains clothing or objects if spilled; occasionally nausea, vomiting; stools will be bright red	5 mg./Kg. × 1 dose orally
quinacrine hydrochloride	Atabrine	tapeworms (beef, pork, fish)	occasionally gastrointestinal symptoms	500 mg. orally × 1 dose with sodium bicarbonate. Fat-free diet 24-48 hours prior to therapy. A cathartic should be given h.s. and 1 hour after drug is given. Soapsuds enema is then given 1 hour+ after the cathartic
thiabendazole	Mintezol	pinworms, roundworms, hookworms, whipworms	gastrointestinal disturbances, dizziness, itching, headache, drowsiness	PINWORMS: 22 mg./Kg. B.I.D. × 1 day orally ROUNDWORM, HOOKWORM, WHIPWORM: 22 mg./Kg. B.I.D. × 1-2 days orally
Amebacides amodiaquin	Camoquin	extraintestinal amebiasis	usually mild	600 mg. daily × 10 days orally followed by a rest period of 8-10 days and a repeat of therapy for 8 days
carbarsone		intestinal amebiasis	signs of arsenic poisoning may occur	250 mg. B.I.D. × 10 days orally; may be repeated after 14 days rest

Table 20-3. (*Continued*)

Generic Name	Trade Name	Uses	Side Effects	Dose Ranges
chloroquine	Aralen	extraintestinal amebiasis	usually mild	1 Gram daily orally × 2 days, then 500 mg. daily × 2-3 weeks. When used with another amebacide dose is lower
diiodohydroxyquin	Diodoquin	intestinal amebiasis	symptoms of iodism may occur	650 mg. T.I.D. × 20 days orally; may be repeated after 2-3 week rest period
emetine		intestinal and extraintestinal amebiasis	diarrhea, nausea, vomiting, marked prostration, vertigo, tachycardia, cardiac failure, cellular degeneration of liver, heart, kidney, skeletal muscles, and intestinal tract may occur	up to 60 mg. daily S.C. × 4-6 days; CHILD: 5-20 mg. daily S.C. × 4-6 days. In amebic hepatitis drug is given for 9 days with a rest period of 1 week followed by 6 more days of therapy
glycobiarsol	Milibis	intestinal amebiasis	occasionally gastrointestinal symptoms	500 mg. T.I.D. × 7-10 days orally
iodochlorhydroxyquin	Vioform	intestinal amebiasis	usually mild	250 mg. T.I.D. × 10 days orally, followed by a rest period of 8-10 days with a repeat 10-day course
ANTIBIOTICS				
erythromycin	Ilotycin	intestinal amebiasis	see Chapter 18	1 Gram daily orally
oxytetracycline	Terramycin	intestinal amebiasis	see Chapter 18	250 mg. Q.I.D. orally
paromomycin	Humatin	intestinal amebiasis	nausea, vomiting, diarrhea	25 mg./Kg./day in divided doses × 5 days orally

Pituitary Hormones

The pituitary gland lies deep within the cranial vault, connected to the brain by a stalk. The pituitary is protected by an indentation of the sphenoid bone—the sella turcica. There are two parts to the pituitary gland: the **anterior** pituitary or **adenohypophysis** and the **posterior** pituitary or **neurohypophysis.** The hormones of the pituitary and the organs or structures influenced by these hormones are shown in the chart on the following page.

Pituitary hormones regulate growth, metabolism, the reproductive cycle, electrolyte balance, water retention and loss. They initiate labor in the gravid female and control secretions of various glands.

Types, Actions, and Uses of Pituitary Hormones

ANTERIOR PITUITARY HORMONES

The **gonadotropins** are FSH (*follicle stim-*ulating *hormone*), LH (*luteinizing hormone*), and LTH (*luteotropic hormone*). Only two of these hormones are used medically—LH and FSH, available as menotropins (Pergonal). This drug has been useful in the treatment of infertility due to a failure to ovulate.

Pituitary Hormones and Adrenal Cortical Hormones

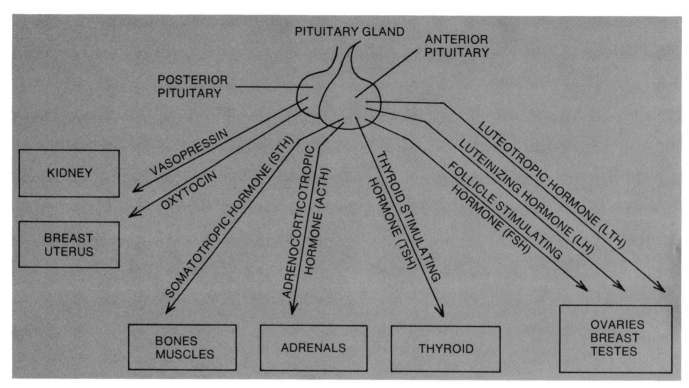

Growth hormone or STH (*somatotropic hormone*) is difficult to obtain, since it must be extracted from human cadaver pituitaries. STH is used to induce growth in hypopituitary dwarfism. Since treatment must extend over many years, clinics for the purpose of treating this form of dwarfism have been established in several large medical centers.

There is little need for *thyroid stimulating hormone* (TSH) since thyroid hormones—thyroxine and triiodothyronine—are easier and cheaper to produce either as synthetic products or as extracts from animal thyroids.

Adrenocorticotropic hormone (ACTH) stimulates the cortex of the adrenal gland. The adrenal cortex secretes three types of hormones: glucocorticoids, mineralocorticoids, and small amounts of sex hormones. Adrenal cortex hormones are called adrenocorticosteroids, corticosteroids, or steroids.

ACTH that is administered to the patient is of *no value* if the adrenal glands are incapable of secreting a sufficient amount of hormone, or if the adrenal glands have been surgically removed. In many instances, the use of corticosteroid hormones (i.e., hormones of the adrenal gland) is preferred to the use of the pituitary hormone ACTH. ACTH can be administered only parenterally and is unpredictable since it is dependent on the ability of the adrenals to secrete hormones to produce a desired effect.

ACTH may occasionally be used as a diagnostic agent to determine pituitary function, as well as in the treatment of collagen diseases, dermatological diseases, allergic states, neoplastic diseases, respiratory diseases, and hematological disorders. Since corticosteroids are usually preferred, this drug has limited therapeutic use in conditions responding to corticosteroid therapy.

ACTH may be used during withdrawal from corticosteroid therapy. As the dose of corticosteroids is reduced (or tapered), ACTH is given to reactivate the adrenal glands. This method of withdrawal is not usually necessary in short-term therapy, but occasionally is employed during withdrawal from long-term therapy.

POSTERIOR PITUITARY HORMONES

Vasopressin, also called *antidiuretic hormone* or ADH, affects the distal convoluted tubules of the kidney nephron, resulting in a conservation of body fluids. Vasopressin (ADH) is secreted by the posterior pituitary when water must be conserved. An example of the need for water conservation may be seen in severe diarrhea and/or vomiting with little or no fluid intake. When this and similar conditions are present, vasopressin is released. Water is then reabsorbed into the bloodstream (i.e., conserved) and the urine secreted becomes more concentrated.

Vasopressin is given in the treatment of *diabetes insipidus*, a disease due to failure of the pituitary gland to secrete vasopressin or to surgical removal of the pituitary (hypophysectomy). Occasionally, this drug may be used to treat postoperative abdominal distention. Lypressin (Diapid) is a synthetic preparation related to vasopressin and can be applied topically in the form of a nasal spray when urinary frequency and excessive thirst develop in these patients.

Oxytocin's only known role is in the female, although this hormone is produced by the posterior pituitary of both sexes. Oxytocin initiates labor in the gravid female at term. The action and uses of this hormone are covered in more detail in Chapter 24.

Side Effects of Pituitary Hormones Used in Medicine

Menotropins (Pergonal), a combination of FSH and LH, is a potent gonadotropin capable of mild to severe reactions. Ovarian enlargement, collection of fluid or blood in the abdomen, abdominal distention, and arterial thromboembolism have been reported during use. Menotropins is usually administered in the physician's office or clinics, although the appearance of adverse reactions may require hospitalization.

Use of ACTH (adrenocorticotropic hormone) can result in many undesirable side effects, most of which are the same as the side effects of steroid therapy. (See Tables 21-1 and 21-2.) Some patients may be sensitive to pork, from which ACTH is obtained, and therefore exhibit an allergic reaction: dizziness, nausea, vomiting, skin reactions, and possibly shock.

The use of vasopressin (ADH) may cause water intoxication unless the dose is carefully regulated. Symptoms are listlessness, headache, and drowsiness. Late symptoms are coma and convulsions. Other side effects that may be noted are vertigo, sweating, tremors, "pounding" sensation in the head, abdominal cramps, nausea, vomiting, urticaria, and anaphylactic shock.

Clinical Considerations

Menotropins (Pergonal) is usually administered on an outpatient basis. The patient will supply a preliminary gynecological history and will have a physical and tests prior to the institution of therapy. The patient should be advised to contact the physician's office should any unusual symptoms occur.

Patients receiving ACTH require close supervision during therapy. Since the side effects are numerous and affect many body organs and systems any complaint or symptom must be considered a side effect until ruled otherwise.

Two factors must be considered in planning the care of patients receiving ACTH: (1) the disease and (2) the effect of this drug on various body organs and structures. The plan of care will contain specific measures pertinent to the patient's disease plus observation for a therapeutic affect of the drug (i.e., does the patient appear to be improved?) and observation for drug side effects. Since some side effects of ACTH therapy may have to be tolerated and the drug continued, the physician should be alerted to any side effects that appear. A decision will then be made as to future therapy with this hormone.

Patients receiving vasopressin should be placed on accurate intake and output measurement during the early phases of therapy as this is one determinant used to measure drug effectiveness. A continued excessive output may indicate that the dose is too *low*, whereas a decrease in output—when compared to the intake—may indicate that the dose is too *high*.

The patient should also be observed for signs of water intoxication, especially when the urinary output is *decreased*. If water intoxication becomes apparent, it may be necessary to measure the urinary output every 2-4 hours rather than at the end of each shift.

Hormones of the Adrenal Cortex— the Corticosteroids

As noted above, the adrenal cortex manufactures three types of hormones: (1) **glucocorticoids** (2) **mineralocorticoids,** and (3) small amounts of **sex hormones.** Collectively, these hormones are called **corticosteroids.**

Glucocorticoids and mineralocorticoids are essential to life and influence many organs and structures of the body, such as blood-forming cells (hematopoietic system), the kidney, and the immune response system.

Types, Actions, and Uses of Corticosteroids

Two glucocorticoids found in the body are cortisone and hydrocortisone (cortisol). Both hormones plus synthetic corticosteroids are used medically. Synthetic glucocorticoids were developed in an effort to produce more potent and more selective corticosteroid compounds, as well as eliminate the sodium-retaining properties of cortisone and hydrocortisone. Prednisone and prednisolone are examples of synthetic corticosteroids which have increased anti-inflammatory activity and fewer sodium-retaining qualities.

Because of the wide variety of effects exhibited by the corticosteroids, major clinical uses may be grouped as follows:

ANTI-INFLAMMATORY RESPONSE—corticosteroids have the ability to reduce inflammation and the symptoms of inflammation (redness, swelling, heat, and pain). This drug action is useful in the treatment of arthritis, asthma, dermatitis, inflammatory diseases of the eye, and ulcerative colitis.

HEMATOLOGICAL RESPONSE—corticosteroids affect lymphoid tissue. They also affect eosinophils by a mechanism not fully understood. Corticosteroids are capable of reducing the number of lymphocytes and eosinophils. This drug action is useful in the treatment of certain forms of leukemia.

CONNECTIVE TISSUE RESPONSE—corticosteroids affect connective tissue and connective tissue protein (collagen). Cartilage, tendons, ligaments, bone, fat, blood cells, and reticuloendothelial cells contain connective tissue. This action is useful in the treatment of gout, collagen diseases, bursitis, and connective tissue injuries.

GENERAL OVERALL RESPONSE—since corticosteroids affect many organs and structures, they are helpful adjuncts when the body incurs an acute emergency state. This action is useful in the treatment of the nephrotic syndrome, rheumatic carditis, profound shock, fulminating infections, cerebral edema, and increased intracranial pressure.

Corticosteroids may be used topically, intramuscularly, orally, and intravenously. They may also be injected into joints and bursae.

In some cases corticosteroid *replacement therapy* is necessary. Patients with *adrenal insufficiency* are incapable of producing an adequate amount of adrenal hormones. Adrenal insufficiency may be due to Addison's disease or result from *prolonged* corticosteroid drug therapy. Total absence of adrenal hormones also requires replacement therapy. Adrenalectomized patients will require lifetime corticosteroid replacement. Surgical removal of the pituitary (hypophysectomy) also requires lifetime replacement therapy, since removal of the pituitary results in the absence of ACTH, which is necessary for adrenal hormone production.

Prolonged therapy with the corticosteroids is capable of causing adrenal insufficiency. The pituitary secretes ACTH which in turn stimulates the adrenal cortex to produce corticosteroids. When there is a sufficient amount of corticosteroids, the pituitary *ceases* ACTH secretion. When corticosteroids are needed, the pituitary again secretes ACTH. This can be compared to a furnace thermostat. When the room is warm, the furnace, under the control of the thermostat, turns off. When the room becomes cool, the furnace turns on. Administration of corticosteroid *drugs* results in a decrease in ACTH secretion. The adrenals, no longer stimulated to produce their own hormones, may begin to atrophy due to prolonged inactivity. Once corticosteroid therapy is discontinued, the patient's own adrenal glands may be unable to secrete sufficient amounts of hormones.

The mineralocorticoids, aldosterone and desoxycorticosterone, have sodium-retaining and potassium-excreting abilities. The mineralocorticoids control salt and water balance. Of these two hormones, aldosterone is the more potent. Deficiency of these hormones results in a loss of sodium and water.

Patients with severe adrenal insufficiency require replacement with mineralocorticoids as well as with glucocorticoids. One synthetic glucocorticoid—fludrocortisone acetate (Florinef)—has both glucocorticoid and mineralocorticoid activity. Desoxycorticosterone (Percorten), available as an intramuscular preparation or as pellets surgically implanted under the skin, is also used in mineralocorticoid replacement therapy.

Side Effects of Corticosteroids

Corticosteroids have a profound effect on the body; side effects during therapy may be numerous. Side effects are also more likely to occur with long-term therapy or at higher doses, rather than short-term therapy.

The patient on long-term therapy may develop a cushingoid appearance (the appearance of one with Cushing's disease—an *excess* of corticosteroid hormones). Other side effects are numerous, and some patients may develop more side effects than others. These side effects may also develop at varying times during therapy, and not all patients necessarily develop a great number of symptoms. However, some signs of a cushingoid appearance may be the first side effects noted. These include "buffalo" hump, moon face, oily skin and acne, osteoporosis, purple striae on abdomen and hips, skin pigmentation, and weight gain. Such patients may also bruise easily or show poor healing of cuts, mental changes, or carbohydrate intolerance.

Other side effects include:

FLUID AND ELECTROLYTE DISTURBANCES—sodium retention, edema, potassium loss, hypertension

GASTROINTESTINAL—abdominal distention, peptic ulcer with possible hemorrhage and perforation

SKIN—thin, fragile skin, petechiae, ecchymosis, increased sweating

MUSCULOSKELETAL—weakness, loss of muscle mass, compression fractures of the vertebrae, fractures of long bones

NEUROLOGICAL—vertigo, headache, convulsions, increased intracranial pressure

ENDOCRINE—menstrual irregularities, suppression of growth in children

EYES—posterior subcapsular cataracts, glaucoma

OTHER—manifestations of latent diabetes mellitus, negative nitrogen balance, poor resistance to infections

Side effects of the mineralocorticoids are edema, cardiac failure, pulmonary congestion, and hypertension. There may also be an excessive loss of potassium resulting in signs of hypokalemia—muscle weakness and cramping.

Clinical Considerations

Corticosteroids are given in a wide variety of situations; patient care must be planned according to the individual patient and the circumstances under which the drug is given.

Patients on short-term therapy, for example, two or three weeks, require an explanation of how to taper the drug dose at the end of therapy. Although this information will be printed on the prescription container by the pharmacist, the nurse may have to stress that these directions must be followed. Since printed instructions may be brief, it may be of value if the patient writes the tapering dose schedule on a calendar by noting the number of tablets to be taken each day, as shown below:

10	11	12	13	14	15	16
2 TABS	2 TABS	2 TABS	2 TABS	1 TAB	1 TAB	1 TAB
17	18	19	20	21	22	23
1 TAB	NONE					

Patients receiving large doses of corticosteroids, or those taking steroids for a long period of time, require specific nursing measures. Obviously, a long list of side effects is difficult to remember, but a list could be included in the Kardex on a separate card or posted in the medicine room. Some units use a small notebook listing the side effects of drugs requiring special observations of the patient. The notebook can be indexed and kept in the medicine room or nurses' station.

Physical changes, for example, the development of acne, facial hair, and moon face, may have an emotional impact on the patient. Any time an adverse physical change occurs, remember that this change is capable of producing varying levels of anxiety. Some patients may be so acutely ill that they are unaware of these changes. Yet there are many other patients who are aware. Some patients, once they understand that these changes may have to be tolerated, may accept the alteration of body image. Others may require encouragement in changing their style of clothes; some may need counseling. Each patient is different, and each time a problem is encountered careful consideration must be given to approaching the problem. In such cases team conferences are of value.

Another problem that may be seen is the mental changes that can be evident during corticosteroid therapy. Some patients may be euphoric, others depressed. Depression can become a serious problem; although not common, a few patients may express suicidal tendencies. This must be reported to the physician, and the patient must be observed frequently. Any unusual behavior or expression of suicide may require suicide precautions. These drugs are given with caution to those with a history of mental depressive states.

Since glycosuria (glucose in the urine) may occur during therapy, the patient's urine should be checked daily or several times per week. The physician may feel that it is unnecessary to perform this test or may order urine testing three or four times per day. If there is any doubt as to whether urine testing should be continued, the physician should be consulted. Some diabetics who are taking insulin and/or oral hypoglycemic agents may require an increase in their medication during corticosteroid therapy. Some well-controlled diabetics may find it necessary to check their urine more frequently. Special instructions regarding the management of diabetes are often necessary.

Fluid and electrolyte disturbances may cause a loss of potassium and retention of sodium. Muscle cramps are usually indicative of potassium loss, whereas edema indicates sodium retention. During morning care, the extremities should be checked for early signs of edema. Tight rings, slippers, or shoes as well as swelling of the ankles might be apparent. The patient may also complain of swelling of the extremities or a "tight feeling" in the hands, feet, or ankles.

Peptic ulcers with bleeding can develop during prolonged corticosteroid therapy. Tarry stools and abdominal or epigastric pain or discomfort may indicate formation of an ulcer. Any occurrence of these symptoms requires immediate attention, as ulcer perforation is always a possibility.

It is important to remember that *at no time is corticosteroid therapy abruptly discontinued*. This applies to short-term as well as long-term therapy. Abrupt stoppage can precipitate adrenal insufficiency and adrenal crisis. In some cases, death could result. There are several implications here. (1) Drug histories on new admissions must be taken. If the patient has been taking corticosteroids at home, the use of this drug must continue during hospitalization. (2) Patients who are on oral corticosteroid preparations and who are unable to take this form of the drug due to nausea, vomiting, surgery, etc. must be given the parenteral form until oral therapy can be resumed. (3) Medicine cards can and do get lost or misplaced and unless all personnel are aware of the patient's drug therapy and the implications of that therapy, doses could be omitted. It may be of value if the chart, Kardex, and even the patient's bedside has a notice "corticosteroid therapy." Emergency room personnel must try to obtain a drug history or look for identification tags on all admissions—especially unconscious patients. The family, if present, should also be asked about the patient's drug history.

Infections and poor wound healing may be a problem during drug therapy. Surgical patients should be watched closely for wound infections, wound separations, and evisceration. Some patients may require reverse isolation techniques if the white blood cell count drops to low levels. Personnel with infections, including upper respiratory infections, should avoid contact with patients who may be in danger of infection. It may also be necessary to warn the patient to avoid exposure to infections after discharge from the hospital. If the patient is in a semiprivate (or larger) room, patients with infections should *not* be placed in this room. If it is necessary to do so, and the patient is known to have a low white blood cell count, the physician should be notified as soon as possible.

Patients receiving mineralocorticoids will be required

to regulate their intake of sodium, potassium, and water.

When these drugs are injected into joints, bursae, or connective tissues side effects are rare. Since this procedure can be uncomfortable and even painful for a short time, the patient may need emotional support during the procedure. Staying with the patient and giving reassurance will often be of great help. Fear of the unknown—especially if this is the first time the procedure has been performed—often creates a great deal of anxiety, which in turn can increase the amount of pain.

The patient with carcinoma receiving corticosteroids may often show marked improvement for a period of time. An increase in appetite, weight gain, and a feeling of well-being may be noted. Occasionally a terminally ill patient may believe that the cancer has been "cured." Here again, team conferences (including the physician if possible) may help to decide on an approach if such patients should inquire about their condition. Since patients are different, there is no one answer; consequently each situation is handled individually.

Discharge Teaching

Discharge teaching may require several sessions, especially if the patient must take these drugs for a long period of time or a lifetime. The following points should be included in the discharge teaching plan:

1. doses are *not to be omitted.* If for some reason the medication cannot be taken—for example, if nausea and vomiting should occur—the physician must be contacted *immediately.* If the patient is on lifetime replacement therapy and cannot contact the physician, the patient should go to the emergency room of a hospital (preferably the hospital where he was treated), as it might be necessary to give the drug in parenteral form until the oral form can be taken. Adrenalectomized and hypophysectomized patients must never go without medication!

2. any occurrence of illness or infection should be reported to the physician immediately since an increase in dose may be necessary

3. these drugs are potent, and close medical supervision is important. Physican appointments must be kept

4. patients should be encouraged to discuss *any* questions or problems with the physician no matter how minor or unimportant they seem. Since patients have a tendency to "forget" some points of instruction or questions they may wish to ask the physician, they can be advised to write down their questions and take these notes with them when they are scheduled for office or clinic visits

5. those on long-term or lifetime therapy should carry identification, such as Medic-Alert tags. The wearing of tags at all times should be stressed. Some hospitals and/or physicians provide adrenalectomized or hypo-

physectomized patients with instruction booklets regarding points of care, warnings, and dose schedules. Since these patients must take corticosteroids for the rest of their lives, there are usually many instructions, which can be overwhelming when given orally. If booklets are not available, the patient should be encouraged to obtain a small notebook for taking notes during teaching sessions

6. patients on long-term therapy should be encouraged to develop a confidence in their physician. They should be told that the physician wants to and must know about any changes that may occur. If their disease or condition appears to improve, the physician should be made aware of this improvement. On the other hand, if the condition worsens or if side effects develop, the physician also must be made aware of these changes

During a teaching program, the patient should be allowed sufficient time to ask questions. Giving only a small amount of information each day will not only give the patient time to think about the material presented and possibly ask questions, but also make the teaching program appear to be somewhat less overwhelming. It sometimes helps to try to imagine what it would be like to be a patient!

Be alert to other problems the patient may have but may not fully express. Some patients find it difficult, financially, to purchase their medications and may need referral to the social service worker. Others may seem to be unable to care for themselves after discharge or appear to be confused about the directions given to them. Referral to the Public Health Nurse or other agencies may be necessary.

When corticosteroid agents are used topically, the patient may need instruction as to the application of the drug. Like any other topical agent, the physician may want the ointment, cream, or liquid applied in a certain way—liberally, sparingly, or in moderate amounts.

Table 21-1.

ANTERIOR AND POSTERIOR PITUITARY HORMONES

Generic Name	Trade Name	Uses	Side Effects	Dose Ranges
ANTERIOR PITUITARY HORMONES				
corticotropin (adrenocorticotropic hormone, ACTH)	Acthar	diagnosis of pituitary function, allergic states, neoplastic diseases, inflammatory skin conditions, nephrotic syndrome, blood dyscrasias, respiratory diseases; corticosteroids usually preferred to ACTH in many conditions	fluid and electrolyte disturbances, musculoskeletal changes; gastrointestinal, dermatological, cardiovascular, metabolic, ophthalmic effects and allergic reactions	varies with reason for use; may be given I.M., S.C., slow I.V. drip (label must indicate preparation can be used by this route)
menotropins	Pergonal	treatment of infertility in women	ovarian enlargement, collection of blood in abdominal cavity, fever, nausea, vomiting, thromboembolism, diarrhea, abdominal distention	1-2 ampules daily for 9-12 days I.M.
POSTERIOR PITUITARY HORMONES				
lypressin	Diapid	treatment of diabetes insipidus	occasionally nasal congestion, irritation, and ulceration, headache	spray once or twice in one or both nostrils when urinary frequency or excessive thirst develops
vasopressin tannate	Pitressin	same as lypressin	vertigo, sweating, tremors, water intoxication, pounding in the head, cramps, nausea, vomiting, urticaria, anaphylactic shock	0.3-1 ml. as required I.M.

Table 21-2.
THE ADRENOCORTICOSTEROIDS*

GLUCOCORTICOID PREPARATIONS

betamethasone—Celestone
betamethasone sodium phosphate and betamethasone acetate—Celestone Soluspan
cortisone acetate
dexamethasone—Gammacorten
fludrocortisone acetate—Florinef
hydrocortisone—Cortef, Hydrocortone
methylprednisolone—Medrol
methylprednisolone sodium succinate—Solu-Medrol
meprednisone—Betapar
paramethasone acetate—Haldrone
prednisolone—Delta-Cortef, Hydeltra
prednisone—Deltasone, Meticorten
triamcinolone—Aristocort, Kenacort
triamcinolone diacetate—Aristocort, Kenacort diacetate
triamcinolone hexacetonide—Aristospan

MINERALOCORTICOID PREPARATIONS

desoxycorticosterone—Doca acetate, Percorten acetate

USES OF CORTICOSTEROID PREPARATIONS

GLUCOCORTICOIDS: acute allergic rhinitis, acute gouty arthritis, acute leukemia (children), acute rheumatic carditis, acute and subacute thyroiditis, Addison's disease, adrenogenital syndrome, angioneurotic edema, ankylosing spondylitis, asthma, atopic dermatitis, breast cancer (metastatic), bursitis, chronic lymphatic leukemia, contact dermatitis, eczema, erythema multiforme, exfoliative dermatitis, Hodgkin's disease, hypercalcemia associated with cancer, idiopathic thrombocytopenic purpura, inflammatory diseases of the eye, lymphosarcoma, nephrosis, panhypopituitarism, pemphigus, psoriasis, psoriatic arthritis, rheumatoid arthritis, serum sickness, status asthmaticus, Stevens-Johnson syndrome, systemic lupus erythematosus, systemic sarcoidosis, ulcerative colitis

MINERALOCORTICOIDS: adrenal insufficiency which produces Addison's disease

SIDE EFFECTS OF GLUCOCORTICOIDS

ENDOCRINE: menstrual irregularities, suppression of growth in children

EYES: posterior subcapsular cataracts, glaucoma

FLUID AND ELECTROLYTE DISTURBANCES: sodium retention, edema, hypokalemia, hypertension, weight gain

GASTROINTESTINAL: abdominal distention, peptic ulcer (with possible perforation, hemorrhage)

MUSCULOSKELETAL: weakness, loss of muscle mass, osteoporosis, compression fractures of vertebrae, fractures of long bones, "buffalo" hump, moon face

NEUROLOGICAL: vertigo, headache, convulsions, increased intracranial pressure, mental changes

SKIN: thin, fragile skin, petechiae, ecchymosis, increased sweating, easy bruising, pigmentation, acne, oily skin, purple striae on abdomen and hips, cuts heal poorly

OTHER: carbohydrate intolerance, manifestations of latent diabetes mellitus, negative nitrogen balance, poor resistance to infections

SIDE EFFECTS OF MINERALOCORTICOIDS

edema, cardiac dilatation and failure, pulmonary congestion, hypertension, hypokalemia

---

* NOTE: The uses and dose ranges of adrenocorticosteroids vary widely with the reason(s) for use, planned length of therapy, and the patient's response to therapy. Commonly available preparations, along with the uses and side effects of this class of drugs, are shown above. References should be consulted for recommended doses. In some cases the physician may elect to use doses higher or lower than those recommended.

Male hormones—testosterone and its derivatives—are called **androgens.** Androgen secretion is under the influence of the anterior portion of the pituitary gland.

Estrogens and **progesterone** are female hormones, and like the androgens, their production is under the influence of the anterior pituitary.

Androgens

Androgens actuate the reproductive potential in the adolescent male. From puberty onward, androgens continue to aid in the development of secondary sex characteristics: facial hair, deep voice, body hair, body fat distribution, and muscle development.

Uses of Androgens

Testosterone and its derivatives are used in medicine in androgen therapy in males, androgen therapy in females, and as anabolic agents (agents that aid in the building and repairing of body tissues).

In the male, androgen therapy may be employed as substitution therapy for testosterone deficiency. Deficiency states such as the male climacteric, impotence (due to androgen deficiency), delayed puberty, hypogonadism,

Male and Female Hormones

and any other condition in which testosterone is deficient or absent may respond to androgen therapy.

In the female, androgen therapy may be used as part of the chemotherapeutic management of inoperable carcinoma of the breast in those who are more than one year but less than five years past menopause. Postpartum breast engorgement and pain in the non-nursing mother may also be relieved with androgens. Androgens may also be used to treat menorrhagia (heavy or excessive menstrual flow), metrorrhagia (bleeding between menstrual periods), premenstrual tension, and endometriosis. Some physicians prefer drugs other than androgens to treat these disorders.

Some androgens are probably effective as anabolic agents; that is, they may be useful in creating a positive nitrogen balance. Patients in a debilitated state may benefit from androgen therapy; however, diet and general health measures should also be considered and should accompany androgen therapy.

Side Effects of Androgen Therapy

In the adult male, androgen side effects are minimal when the optimum dose is administered. Redness and pain may be noted at injection sites. A decreased ejaculatory volume and sodium and water retention may also occur.

In the prepuberty male, precocious sexual development may occur and require discontinuing therapy. Early epiphyseal closure may also be seen, resulting in a retardation of growth.

In the female, masculinizing effects frequently occur when androgens are administered for long periods of time. This will usually not occur when these drugs are used briefly to treat postpartum breast engorgement.

Edema, jaundice, and elevation of blood calcium levels may also be seen in both sexes during androgen therapy. Androgens are contraindicated in males with prostatic cancer, serious cardiorenal disease, and severe liver damage. These drugs are also contraindicated in pregnant women.

Female Hormones

Estrogens are hormones secreted primarily by the ovarian follicle but are also secreted by the adrenal cortex, the corpus luteum (the yellow body remaining on or near the surface of the ovary after the ovum has been released), and the placenta. Estradiol, estrone, estriol, equilin, and equilenin are naturally occurring (endogenous) estrogens. Of these, estradiol, estrone, and estriol are the most significant.

Progesterone is a hormone secreted by the corpus luteum, adrenal cortex, and placenta. Progestogens (synthetic progesterones) were developed and are often preferred for medical use because of the decreased effectiveness of progesterone when administered orally.

Estrogens are responsible for the development of secondary sex characteristics in the female, cyclic changes in the vaginal lining, and endometrial development.

Progesterone is responsible for endometrial changes in the second half of the menstrual cycle and is also necessary for the development of the placenta.

Estrogen increases the thickness of the endometrium, and progesterone prepares the endometrium for implantation of the fertilized ovum.

Types and Uses of Female Hormones

ESTROGENS

There are three types of estrogens available: (1) the natural steroids, for example, estradiol and estriol (2) nonsteroid synthetics that are capable of producing essentially the same effects as the natural steroids, for example, dienestrol and diethylstilbestrol, and (3) conjugated estrogenic substances which are a mixture of natural estrogens.

Estrogen therapy is employed in the treatment of menopausal symptoms, e.g., hot flashes, headaches, dizziness, and sweating. Treatment of postmenopausal disorders such as osteoporosis and atrophic changes of the genitalia and pruritus vulvae and vaginitis due to decreased estrogen levels may be treated with estrogens.

Estrogens may also be employed in the treatment of underdeveloped ovaries, hypopituitarism, dysmenorrhea (painful menses), postpartum breast engorgement, and, in combination with progesterone, delayed menses. *Surgical* menopause—that is, the ovaries are removed from premenopausal women for reasons other than carcinoma—may also be treated with estrogens.

Prostatic carcinoma may respond to estrogen therapy, resulting in a relief of pain, tumor regression, and delay of metastasis. Some of these patients respond well to therapy whereas others do not. Estrogens are also used in the palliative treatment of carcinoma of the breast in patients five or more years past menopause.

Combinations of estrogens and progestogens are used as oral contraceptives. These same drugs can also be used to treat endometriosis and hypermenorrhea (increase in the frequency, amount, and duration of the menstrual flow). The oral contraceptives are of two types: combination and sequential. A list of oral contraceptive preparations is given in Table 22-2.

These drugs are usually available in inserts, which are placed in a reusable case. Once a month the empty inserts are removed and replaced with a new supply. The 20- and 21-tablet preparations contain this same number of tablets in the inserts. Tablets are taken for 20 or 21 days per month, and there is a 6- or 7-day rest period each month during which no tablets are taken. The 28-day tablet preparations contain 28 tablets, 21 of which are estrogen/progestogen combinations. The remaining 7 tablets are either inert or contain ferrous fumarate (Norlestrin $\boxed{Fe}$), an iron preparation. For identification of the inert or iron-containing preparations a coloring is added.

Most sequential preparations contain 14 tablets of estrogen and 7 tablets of estrogen and progestogen—a total of 21 tablets. These drugs are taken for 20 or 21 days per month, that is, three weeks of medication and one week without medication. There is a variety of preparations, as well as different strengths; the physician selects the type of preparation that best suits the patient. Table 22-2 shows the amount of hormones in each preparation.

PROGESTOGENS AND PROGESTERONE

As noted above, progesterone is the hormone secreted by the corpus luteum, adrenal cortex, and placenta. It is available as an oral preparation, but this is considered less effective than the parenteral form. The synthetic progestogens are more effective than progesterone when given orally, and therefore are often preferred.

These female hormones are useful in the treatment of amenorrhea, abnormal uterine bleeding due to hormone imbalance, dysmenorrhea, endometriosis, and in oral contraception.

Special Note

Since female hormones are contraindicated in women with malignancies, with the exception of women five or more years past menopause, a thorough physical examination including a gynecological examination is performed prior to the institution of therapy. Examinations are also scheduled periodically during therapy.

Actions of Female Hormones

As contraceptives, female hormones suppress the secretion of pituitary gonadotropins. Without the stimulation of these hormones, there is no follicular development and ovulation does not occur. In a manner not clearly understood, these drugs may also have other actions that contribute to their ability to prevent conception.

Estrogen/progestogen therapy can also be employed to *promote* conception in some women who are having difficulty in becoming pregnant. Although conception does not occur during therapy with these drugs, the chances of conceiving appear to increase once therapy is discontinued. Multiple pregnancies also appear to be statistically greater in those who have taken oral contraceptives and then discontinued the medication.

Side Effects of Female Hormone Therapy

ESTROGENS

The most frequent side effects of estrogen therapy mimic pregnancy—nausea, vomiting, abdominal cramps, headache, and breast engorgement and tenderness. These side effects usually disappear with the continuance of therapy. Other side effects that may be encountered are fluid retention, increase in size of existing fibroid tumors, breakthrough bleeding, spotting, mental depression, increase in blood pressure, jaundice, and migraine.

Much research has been done regarding the association between oral contraceptives and thromboembolic disease. Because of the possible causal relationship, these drugs are contraindicated in those with thrombophlebitis, a history of thrombophlebitis or a history or presence of any vascular or clotting disorder.

Diabetics taking oral contraceptives should be carefully followed by the physician. In some cases it may be necessary to change insulin doses and dietary allowances.

When estrogens are given to males, breast enlargement and reduced libido may be seen. When drugs are given in low doses these changes—if they appear—do so slowly.

Clinical Considerations

Prolonged androgen therapy in the female patient with carcinoma requires special consideration. Masculinizing changes often occur and it is important to be alert to the patient's response to these physical changes in body image. Team conferences are of value in order to explore the patient's response to therapy and the intervention of health-care personnel. Each patient is different and there is no one (or two or three) approach that is best. In some instances, the patient may not seem to care about the masculinization or she may be too ill to notice. Yet another patient may show a great deal of anxiety.

What is important is that the patient's reaction is accepted, be it one of depression, open hostility, or any other response. Try to give, in return, understanding plus an extra dose of T.L.C., T.I.D. *and* h.s. *and* P.R.N.!

Prescriptions for the administration of androgens for the male are most commonly seen in physicians' offices and outpatient clinics. Some males may be embarrassed if female *or* male personnel administer the parenteral form of the drug, since they may (wrongly) believe that taking male hormones is an open admission of sexual inadequacy. Although it may not be practical in some instances, some of these patients feel more at ease if the physician prescribing the drug also administers the drug. If the patient appears unduly upset, the physician should be told.

The male patient receiving female hormones should have a thorough explanation of physical changes that may possibly occur, especially if the dose is high enough to make such changes likely; this explanation is best given by the physician. Be prepared to answer any questions the patient may have during office or clinic visits. In some instances, the physician may prefer to withhold an explanation at the beginning of therapy and introduce information to the patient over a period of time. It is important to know how much has and will be told to the patient so that questions, if need be, can be answered.

When androgens are used as anabolic agents, drug effects should be noted. Since anabolic effects usually occur over a period of time rather than a few days, drug effects might be difficult to assess. The patient may appear to feel better, the appetite may improve, and weight gain noted. Daily or weekly weights, daily observation of eating patterns, and assessment of the patient's mood will add to the value of drug therapy.

It is important to discourage the *illegal* purchase and use of oral contraceptives; encourage those who obtain them by these means to consult a physician or free clinic. There have been incidents of unnecessary illnesses and deaths from the use of oral contraceptives by those not under the supervision of a physician.

Discharge Teaching

When patient teaching is planned, there must be sufficient time allowed for questions. The taking of hormones by the male or female patient may raise many questions, some of which may have to be referred to the physician. Patients taking oral contraceptives should be told to take the drug at approximately the same time each day. It must also be stressed that doses of the drug are not to be omitted. Some clinics may do group teaching for those using these preparations for the first time. This allows for group learning and group sharing of experiences. Patients may also ask questions that may not occur to other patients, thus enhancing group learning.

Patients must also be encouraged to report the occurrence of side effects. Side effects such as vomiting and nausea will prompt a patient to call a physician, but other side effects, such as mild leg cramps or fatigue, may not be considered important by the patient and therefore not be reported. The patient should be told that the physician is interested in *all* problems that might occur, no matter how minor they seem to be.

Patients taking estrogen/progestogen combinations may do so to prevent or promote conception. Thus there are two different kinds of patients. One wants to *prevent* pregnancy, the other *desires* pregnancy; both situations may well have an emotional overlay. Both kinds of patients may need to express their desires, fears, and anxieties. The nurse may have to act as an intermediary, as the patient may be reticent about asking questions of the physician. While talking to the patient the nurse can mentally summarize questions she herself cannot answer and present these questions to the physician, thus saving time. The nurse's own views regarding these drugs must never alter teaching plans or be used to influence a patient's decision regarding the taking of these preparations.

Table 22-1.

MALE AND FEMALE HORMONES

Generic Name	Trade Name	Uses	Side Effects	Dose Ranges
Androgens				
dromostanolone	Drolban	palliative treatment of advanced breast carcinoma in women 1-5 years past menopause	facial hair, deepening of voice, enlargement of clitoris (all signs of virilization), acne, edema, hypercalcemia	100 mg. 3 × week I.M.
fluoxymesterone	Halotestin	MALE: replacement therapy in conditions associated with absence or deficiency of testosterone; FEMALE: postmenopausal osteoporosis, prevention of postpartum breast engorgement and pain, palliative treatment of advanced breast carcinoma in women 1-5 years past menopause	MALE: hypercalcemia, jaundice, priapism, gynecomastia, oligospermia; FEMALE: signs of virilization, jaundice, hypercalcemia	2-30 mg. daily in single or divided doses orally
methandrostenolone	Dianabol	osteoporosis, as anabolic agent for acute and chronic diseases	MALES: same as fluoxymesterone; FEMALES: same as fluoxymesterone + menstrual irregularities, postmenopausal bleeding, swelling of breasts; BOTH SEXES: nausea, vomiting, diarrhea, increased or decreased libido, edema, insomnia	2.5-5 mg. daily orally

Table 22-1. (*Continued*)

GENERIC NAME	TRADE NAME	USES	SIDE EFFECTS	DOSE RANGES
methyltestosterone	Oreton methyl	same as fluoxymesterone	same as fluoxymesterone	males: 5-20 mg. (as buccal tablets) daily; 10-40 mg. (tablets) daily orally; females: POSTPARTUM—40 mg. buccal tablets daily orally; for BREAST CARCINOMA—200 mg. daily (as buccal or oral tablets)
nandrolone	Durabolin	palliative treatment of advanced breast carcinoma, anabolic agent	same as fluoxymesterone	AS ANABOLIC AGENT: 25-50 mg. weekly I.M.; BREAST CANCER: 50-100 mg. weekly I.M.
testosterone	Oreton	same as methyltestosterone	same as methyltestosterone	males: 10-25 mg. 2-3 × week I.M.; females: POSTPARTUM—25-50 mg. × 3-4 days I.M.; BREAST CARCINOMA—100 mg. 3 × week I.M.
FEMALE HORMONES ESTROGENS				
chlorotrianisene	Tace	prevention of pospartum breast engorgement	usually none	1 capsule (72 mg.) B.I.D. × 2 days orally
diethylstilbestrol* U.S.P.		estrogen deficiency states associated with menopausal syndrome, postpartum breast engorgement, carcinoma of prostate, breast cancer 5+ years past menopause	nausea, vomiting, uterine bleeding, abdominal distress, breast tenderness, anorexia, diarrhea, vertigo, paresthesias, headache, anxiety, insomnia, thirst, rash, purpura	MENOPAUSAL SYMPTOMS: 0.2-0.5 mg. daily orally; POSTPARTUM: 5 mg. daily to T.I.D. for a total of 30 mg. orally; BREAST CANCER: 15 mg. daily orally; PROSTATIC CANCER: 1-3 mg. daily orally

* NOTE: Current investigation indicates that the use of diethylstilbestrol (DES) be limited to treatment of senile vaginitis (0.5 to 2 mg., oral, daily) and prostatic carcinoma in light of its possible carcinogenic properties.

Generic Name	Trade Name	Uses	Side Effects	Dose Ranges
estradiol	Progynon	same as diethylstilbestrol	nausea, vomiting, edema, breast soreness, vertigo, jaundice, rash, mental depression, amenorrhea, hypercalcemia, endometrial bleeding, uterine fibroids may increase in size, thromboembolitic episodes, diabetic patients may need regulation; MALES: decrease in libido, gynecomastia	MENOPAUSAL SYMPTOMS: 0.5-1.5 mg. 2-3 × week I.M.; BREAST and PROSTATIC CANCERS: 1.5 mg. 2-3 × week I.M.; other conditions: doses vary
estrogenic substances, conjugated	Premarin	treatment of abnormal uterine bleeding (parenteral form)+ same as diethylstilbestrol	same as diethylstilbestrol	MENOPAUSAL SYMPTOMS: 1.25 mg. daily orally; BREAST CARCINOMA: 10 mg. T.I.D. orally; PROSTATIC CARCINOMA: 1.25-2.5 mg. T.I.D., orally; other conditions: doses vary
piperazine estrone sulfate	Ogen	prevention of postpartum breast engorgement, estrogen deficiency states, prostatic carcinoma, management of abnormal uterine bleeding, female hypogonadism	same as diethylstilbestrol	MENOPAUSAL SYMPTOMS: 1.25-2.5 mg. daily orally; POSTPARTUM: 3 1.25 mg. tablets q4h during first 20 hours after delivery; other conditions: doses vary
PROGESTOGENS dydrogesterone	Duphaston	amenorrhea, abnormal uterine bleeding, endometriosis, dysmenorrhea	thromboembolitic disorders, rise in blood pressure, change in libido, headache, nervousness, dizziness, fatigue, fluid retention	10-20 mg. daily orally; in some instances doses may be higher

Table 22-1. (*Continued*)

GENERIC NAME	TRADE NAME	USES	SIDE EFFECTS	DOSE RANGES
medroxyproges-terone	Depo-Provera (parenteral), Provera (oral)	same as dydrogesterone	same as dydrogesterone	UTERINE BLEEDING: 5-10 mg. daily orally, 50 mg. weekly, or 100 mg. q2 weeks I.M.
norethindrone	Norlutate	same as dydrogesterone	same as dydrogesterone	dose varies as to reason for use and patient response
progesterone	Proluton	threatened and habitual abortion, functional uterine bleeding, premenstrual tension, amenorrhea, female hypogonadism, premature labor	edema, urticaria, pruritus vulvae, gastrointestinal disturbances, weight gain, thromboembolitic disease	HABITUAL ABORTION: 5-20 mg. 3 × week I.M.; THREATENED ABORTION: 25-50 mg. daily I.M.; FUNCTIONAL UTERINE BLEEDING: 5-10 mg. daily I.M.; DYSMENORRHEA, PREMENSTRUAL TENSION: 10-25 mg. I.M. daily

Table 22-2.
ORAL CONTRACEPTIVE AGENTS*

GENERIC NAME AND DOSE	TRADE NAME	TYPE
ethynodiol diacetate 1 mg. ethinyl estradiol 50 mcg.	Demulen Demulen-28	COMBINATION (21 tablets) COMBINATION (28 tablets; 7 are inert)
ethynodiol diacetate 1 mg. mestranol 0.1 mg.	Ovulen Ovulen-28	COMBINATION (21 tablets) COMBINATION (28 tablets; 7 are inert)
mestranol 0.08 mg. (14 tablets) mestranol 0.08 mg. + norethindrone 2 mg. (6 tablets)	Norquen Ortho-Novum SQ	SEQUENTIAL (20 tablets) SEQUENTIAL (20 tablets)

Generic Name and Dose	Trade Name	Type
norethindrone 1 mg. ethinyl estradiol 0.05 mg.	Norlestrin 21 1 mg. Norlestrin 28 1 mg. Norlestrin Fe 1 mg.	COMBINATION (21 tablets) COMBINATION (28 tablets; 7 are inert) COMBINATION (28 tablets; 7 contain ferrous fumarate 75 mg.)
norethindrone 2.5 mg. ethinyl estradiol 0.05 mg.	Norlestrin 21 2.5 mg. Norlestrin Fe 2.5 mg.	COMBINATION (21 tablets) COMBINATION (28 tablets; 7 contain ferrous fumarate 75 mg.)
norethindrone 1 mg. mestranol 0.05 mg.	Norinyl 1 + 50 21-day Norinyl 1 + 50 28-day Ortho-Novum 1/50 □ 20 Ortho-Novum 1/50 □ 21 Ortho-Novum 1/50 □ 28	COMBINATION (21 tablets) COMBINATION (28 tablets; 7 are inert) COMBINATION (20 tablets) COMBINATION (21 tablets) COMBINATION (28 tablets; 7 are inert)
norethindrone 1 mg. mestranol 0.08 mg.	Norinyl 1 + 80 21-day Norinyl 1 + 80 28-day Ortho-Novum 1/80 □ 21 Ortho-Novum 1/80 □ 28	COMBINATION (21 tablets) COMBINATION (28 tablets; 7 are inert) COMBINATION (21 tablets) COMBINATION (28 tablets; 7 are inert)
norethindrone 2 mg. mestranol 0.1 mg.	Norinyl 2 mg.	COMBINATION (20 tablets)
norethynodrel 2.5 mg. mestranol 0.1 mg.	Enovid-E Enovid-E 21	COMBINATION (20 tablets) COMBINATION (21 tablets)
norethynodrel 5 mg. mestranol 0.075 mg.	Enovid 5 mg.	COMBINATION (20 tablets)
norgestrel 0.5 mg. ethinyl estradiol 0.05 mg.	Ovral	COMBINATION (21 tablets)

* NOTE: These drugs are started on the fifth day (also called day 5) of the menstrual cycle. The first day of menstruation is counted as day 1. A new course begins 7 or 8 days after the last tablet has been taken. Some preparations are also available as 28 tablets (7 of which are inert tablets, or contain iron) and are taken every day, with therapy beginning on the fifth day (day 5) of the menstrual cycle.

An enlarged thyroid gland, or goiter, is mentioned in the writings of ancient Rome and Egypt. It wasn't until the middle of the nineteenth century that the thyroid gland was associated with cretinism, myxedema, and hyperthyroidism.

The thyroid gland is located in the neck, in front of the trachea. This highly vascular gland manufactures and secretes two hormones: thyroxine or tetraiodothyronine (T-4) and triiodothyronine or liothyronine (T-3). Iodine is essential for the manufacture of both these hormones. The activity of the thyroid gland is regulated by the anterior pituitary hormone TSH (thyroid stimulating hormone). When the level of circulating thyroid hormones drops, the anterior pituitary secretes TSH which activates cells of the thyroid to release stored thyroid hormones.

Diseases of the thyroid involve two categories: (1) **hypothyroidism,** a decrease in the amount of thyroid hormones manufactured and secreted, and (2) **hyperthyroidism,** an increase in the amount of thyroid hormones manufactured and secreted.

Cretinism is a state of hypothyroidism from infancy up to and through the growth years. This hypothyroid state is due to a lack of iodine in the diet or a failure in the fetal development of the thyroid gland. With the

Chapter **23**

Thyroid and Antithyroid Agents

Table 23-1.
SIGNS OF THYROID DYSFUNCTION

BODY SYSTEM OR FUNCTION	HYPOTHYROIDISM	HYPERTHYROIDISM
METABOLISM	*decreased*, with symptoms of anorexia, intolerance to cold, low body temperature, weight gain despite anorexia	*increased*, with symptoms of increased appetite, intolerance to heat, elevated body temperature, weight loss despite increased appetite
CARDIOVASCULAR SYSTEM	bradycardia, moderate hypotension	tachycardia, moderate hypertension
CENTRAL NERVOUS SYSTEM	lethargy, sleepiness	nervousness, anxiety, insomnia, tremors
SKIN AND SKIN STRUCTURES	pale, cool, dry, face appears puffy, hair coarse, nails thick and hard	flushed, warm, moist
OVARIAN FUNCTION	heavy menses, may be unable to conceive, loss of fetus also possible	irregular or scant menses
TESTICULAR FUNCTION	low sperm count	

use of *iodized* table salt there are fewer instances of cretinism due to a lack of iodine in the diet in areas where this form of salt is available.

Myxedema results from an inability of the thyroid to manufacture thyroid hormones or a failure of the pituitary to secrete TSH. Borderline hypothyroidism may also be seen in some individuals, and although they do not exhibit all the symptoms of myxedema, vague symptoms of fatigue, headaches, muscle weakness, and emotional upsets may be noted.

The cause of hyperthyroidism is unknown, but the signs and symptoms are obvious to the patient, are often distressing, and may be dangerous.

Types and Uses of Thyroid Preparations

Drug therapy for hypothyroidism is aimed at supplying additional amounts of thyroid hormone, thereby creating a *euthyroid* (normal thyroid) state. Thyroid hormones in common use are shown in Table 23-2.

Table 23-2.
DRUGS USED IN HYPOTHYROIDISM

GENERIC NAME	TRADE NAME	THYROID HORMONES
levothyroxine	Letter	thyroxine (T-4)
liothyronine	Cytomel	triiodothyronine (T-3)
liotrix	Euthroid	levothyroxine (T-4) liothyronine (T-3)
thyroglobulin	Proloid	levothyroxine (T-4) liothyronine (T-3) (animal sources)
thyroid U.S.P.		levothyroxine (T-4) triiodothyronine (T-3) (animal sources)

The dose of thyroid preparations is adjusted to the patient's response to the drug.

Side Effects of Thyroid Preparations

The side effects of thyroid preparations are the signs of *hyper*thyroidism, since in effect a state of hyperthyroidism occurs if the dose is too high. (See Table 23-1.) In most instances, side effects will disappear once the dose is reduced.

Patients receiving thyroid preparations must have the dose adjusted until a proper balance is reached. The physician usually prescribes the smallest dose and then increases the dose gradually until the desired effect—a euthyroid (normal thyroid) state—is reached. During the adjustment period the patient may experience side effects, that is, symptoms of hyperthyroidism.

Types and Uses of Antithyroid Preparations

Hyperthyroidism may be treated by surgical removal of some or most of the thyroid gland, radiation therapy using radioactive ^{131}I, or administration of antithyroid agents.

Antithyroid agents are indicated prior to surgery on the hyperactive thyroid gland and in the medical management of those who cannot tolerate thyroid surgery.

The types of antithyroid preparations are shown in Table 23-3.

Prior to surgery on the thyroid gland, iodine plus one of the thiouracils may be administered for two or three weeks.

Radioactive iodine (sodium iodine^{131}) may also be used to treat hyperthyroidism. ^{131}I is a heavy element that undergoes disintegration, losing a charged particle from the nucleus of the atom. Electromagnetic radiation in the form of alpha, beta, and gamma rays occurs. The beta rays given off destroy some of the thyroid tissue without harming surrounding tissues. The thyroid cells that remain will usually be sufficient to carry on normal activity.

The patient may require more than one treatment with radioactive iodine if an insufficient amount of cells was destroyed the first time. Although careful calculations and measurements are made, there may be an occasional patient who receives a dose that destroys more than the expected number of thyroid cells. These patients will then experience signs of *hypo*thyroidism, and will require treatment with thyroid agents.

Table 23-3.
DRUGS USED IN HYPERTHYROIDISM

GENERIC NAME	TRADE NAME
IODINE	
iodine U.S.P. as iodine solution, strong (Lugol's solution)	
THIOURACILS	
methylthiouracil	Methacil
propylthiouracil	
OTHER	
methimazole	Tapazole

General Drug Action

Iodine, when used with other antithyroid agents prior to surgery, reduces the vascularity of the gland and makes it less friable. This reduces the risk of bleeding during the surgical procedure. Antithyroid agents also inhibit the synthesis of thyroid hormones, thereby reducing hormonal activity of the thyroid gland and partially or totally eliminating the symptoms of hyperthyroidism.

Side Effects of Antithyroid Preparations

Some patients may be allergic to iodine and therefore cannot be given iodine. Symptoms of iodine allergy may also develop during therapy and require stopping the drug. Symptoms of rash, sinus pain, pain and/or swelling of the parotid gland, and increased salivation are signs of iodine allergy. Severe iodism can result in circulatory collapse and death.

Agranulocytosis (a decrease in the number of agranulocytes, a type of white blood cell) is the most serious side effect of therapy with the thiouracils and methimazole (Tapazole). This is manifested by susceptibility to infections, ulcerations of the mouth, fever, and sore throat. This side effect is most likely to occur during long-term therapy rather than the brief period of therapy instituted prior to surgery.

Other side effects of the thiouracils and methimazole (Tapazole) therapy are rash, urticaria, nausea, vomiting, arthralgia (joint pain), headache, and vertigo.

Clinical Considerations and Discharge Teaching

Patients receiving thyroid preparations should have special instruction regarding these drugs, especially when taking them for the first time. A dose increment schedule, used when the drug dose is increased every 1-2 or more weeks, must be followed exactly in order to obtain maximum benefits. Even though the patient is closely supervised by routine visits to the physician it must be understood that signs of *hyper*thyroidism may become apparent. This means then that the patient should know what side effects to look for and what to do if they occur. The severe hypothyroid patient may show signs of mental dullness (due to the disease and *not* to a lack of intelligence), and may forget what has been explained. Printed sheets explaining dose schedules and side effects are of definite value and serve as a reminder for dose increases.

Antithyroid drugs may be prescribed for the patient who is scheduled for surgery. These drugs will be taken at home as well as when the patient is admitted for surgery. Iodine is given as a liquid preparation, in water. Other antithyroid preparations are oral tablets. The patient taking two antithyroid drugs will have to have the dose schedule explained, and in some instances it may have to be written so the patient fully understands. The hyperthyroid patient may show a great deal of anxiety and therefore may not listen carefully to directions.

Patients should also be told to contact their physician should any unusual symptoms occur. Some physicians may explain the symptoms of iodism (if iodine is included in the preoperative regimen), since this phenomenon may begin with symptoms (headache, salivation) that the patient may not know are drug-related.

The nurse should not cause undue alarm when explaining the importance of telling the physician of side effects should they occur. This applies to antithyroids as well as *any* drug. There are many ways to explain side effects to a patient; one way is to tell the patient that "drugs act differently in different people. Some take a drug and have no problem, while others may become allergic to the drug. When a person is allergic to a drug, the drug must be stopped. Very often other drugs can then be given that may not cause an allergy." The patient can also be told that "side effects also occur when some people take drugs. Sometimes the doctor has to prescribe another drug or change the dose of the medication. This is why the physician should be told when anything unusual occurs. In some instances, it may be necessary to call the physician to see if the drug should be stopped."

Patients receiving radioactive iodine for the destruction of thyroid cells usually require specific care, since the dose of radioactive iodine is much higher than for diagnostic studies. Hospital policies vary; therefore the department of radiation therapy should be consulted regarding precautions that are to be taken.

Table 23-4.
THYROID AND ANTITHYROID AGENTS

GENERIC NAME	TRADE NAME	USES	SIDE EFFECTS	DOSE RANGES°
THYROID PREPARATIONS				
levothyroxine	Letter	treatment of hypothyroid states	overdose produces symptoms of *hyper*thyroidism: palpitation, weight loss, diarrhea, abdominal cramps, tachycardia, cardiac arrhythmias, angina, headache, insomnia, intolerance to heat, fever, nervousness, menstrual irregularities	0.025-1 mg. daily orally
liothyronine	Cytomel	same as levothyroxine	same as levothyroxine	5-100 mcg. daily orally
liotrix	Euthroid	same as levothyroxine	same as levothyroxine	tablets numbered according to amount of thyroid hormone in each; one tablet of Euthroid 1, 2, or 3 daily
thyroglobulin	Proloid	same as levothyroxine	same as levothyroxine	0.5-3 grains daily orally
thyroid U.S.P.		same as levothyroxine	same as levothyroxine	gr. ¼ to gr. 3 daily orally

Table 23-4. (*Continued*)

GENERIC NAME	TRADE NAME	USES	SIDE EFFECTS	DOSE RANGES
ANTITHYROID PREPARATIONS				
iodine U.S.P. (Lugol's solution)		preoperative preparation for thyroidectomy	symptoms of iodism: rash, sinus pain, salivation, pain or swelling of the parotids, circulatory collapse	0.1-0.3 ml. in water T.I.D. 2-3 weeks prior to surgery
methimazole	Tapazole	same as iothiouracil	agranulocytosis, rash, urticaria, gastrointestinal disturbances, headache, arthralgia, vertigo	5-60 mg. daily in divided doses orally
methylthiouracil	Methiacil	same as iothiouracil	same as methimazole	200-300 mg. daily in divided doses orally
prophylthiouracil		same as iothiouracil	same as methimazole	50-600 mg. daily in divided doses orally

°NOTE: The dose of thyroid preparations is adjusted according to the need and response of the patient.

A drug that *stimulates* the uterus is called an **oxytoxic** drug. The oldest known oxytoxic is ergot—a chemical present in a fungus that grows on rye and other cereal grains. The effect of ergot on the pregnant uterus has been known for 2000 years, but this drug was not used as an oxytoxic agent until approximately 400 years ago. It is still used today in the form of the ergot alkaloid—ergonovine, and the semisynthetic—methylergonovine.

Other drugs used for their effect on the uterus are uterine *relaxants*. These agents have the opposite effect of oxytoxics.

Types and Uses of Drugs Acting on the Uterus

There are three oxytoxic agents: (1) ergot derivatives, (2) oxytocin (natural or synthetic), and (3) sparteine. The ergot preparations include ergonovine maleate (Ergotrate) and methylergonovine maleate (Methergine). Ergonovine is used for the prevention and treatment of postpartum hemorrhage. The drug may be given parenterally after delivery, followed by oral administration until danger of uterine relaxation has passed—usually about 48 hours. This drug also hastens uterine involution.

Methylergonovine (Methergine) has the

Drugs That Act on the Uterus

same use as ergonovine. In addition, the drug can be administered during the second stage of labor, following delivery of the anterior shoulder. The drug acts in 30-60 seconds after intravenous administration and 2-5 minutes after intramuscular administration. Methylergonovine may also be administered after the third stage of labor.

Oxytocin (Pitocin, Syntocinon) is a posterior pituitary hormone whose only known role is in the female. This drug has a powerful effect on uterine muscle and is used in the following instances:

1. to artificially begin labor. This is called induction of labor. One reason for artificial induction of labor is a larger than normal fetus
2. to stimulate the uterus after normal labor has begun. Occasionally a patient may have uterine inertia—that is, labor contractions that are slowed, ceased, or of decreased intensity
3. to stimulate immediate contraction of the uterus *after* delivery of the infant, thereby aiding in the delivery of the placenta, as well as in preventing uterine hemorrhage
4. to control bleeding after the delivery of the placenta

Oxytocin is also used in the form of a nasal spray (Syntocinon) for the relief of breast engorgement and to aid in breast-feeding. The nasal spray is used 2-3 minutes prior to breast-feeding as the drug has a short duration of action.

Sparteine (Spartocin) has the same uses as oxytocin, although it appears to be less potent than oxytocin.

Lututrin (Lutrexin) is a uterine-relaxing agent, and is used to treat dysmenorrhea (painful menses), premature labor, and threatened abortion occurring in the second or third trimester. In the treatment of dysmenorrhea, the drug is taken before the onset of symptoms, when possible.

Antispasmodics (cholinergic blocking agents) are also used to relax the uterus, principally in the treatment of dysmenorrhea. Their value appears to be limited, although they have helped some patients.

General Drug Action

The ergot derivatives act on the smooth muscle of the uterus resulting in an increase in (1) muscle *tone* (the tension or contracting ability of a muscle) (2) the *rate* of uterine contractions, and (3) the *amplitude* (strength or force) of uterine contraction.

Oxytocin and sparteine also act on uterine muscle, producing *rhythmic* contraction, that is, alternate contraction and relaxation.

Lututrin is a corpus luteum hormone that relaxes uterine muscle by either direct action on uterine muscle fibers or by blocking pituitary stimulation.

The cholinergic blocking agents block the action of parasympathetic nerve fibers. The uterus is innervated by parasympathetic nerve fibers, and these drugs should therefore be capable of blocking the action of these fibers, thereby aiding in the relief of painful menses. However, the action of cholinergic blocking agents on the nerves innervating the uterus is somewhat unpredictable, and relief may only be temporary.

Side Effects of Drugs Acting on the Uterus

Side effects of ergonovine (Ergotrate) appear to be minimal when it is used in short-term therapy. Nausea and vomiting occasionally occur and hypertension has been reported in patients who have had caudal or spinal anesthesia. Methylergonovine (Methergine) side effects are the same as seen during the use of ergonovine, but headache, dizziness, tinnitus, diaphoresis, dyspnea, and chest pain may also occur. *Prolonged* use of ergot derivatives can result in gangrene; however in the short-term obstetrical use of these drugs, this is not a problem.

Oxytocin (Pitocin, Syntocinon) is a potent drug and must be administered with caution and constant observation of the patient's response. Side effects include:

Oral form (as buccal tablets)—cardiac arrhythmias (mother: premature ventricular contractions [P.V.C.'s], fetus: bradycardia, tachycardia), local vasoconstriction of oral mucosa, nausea and vomiting, tetanic contractions, and uterine rupture and fetal death

Parenteral form—anxiety, chest pain, cyanosis, dyspnea, fetal bradycardia, flushing of skin, hypotension, severe water intoxication (with prolonged use), tachycardia, and uterine rupture and fetal death

The side effects of sparteine (Spartocin) are the same as those of oxytocin, although this drug also has quinidine-like effects and bradycardia may be seen when large doses are used.

There appear to be no side effects associated with the use of lututrin (Lutrexin).

Clinical Considerations

The ergot derivatives may be administered in the delivery room as well as on the postpartum unit. Physicians usually have a preference as to agents used during and after delivery, and the materials necessary (drug, needles, syringe, tourniquet) should be placed in a special area for easy access and immediate use. The blood pressure should be taken after these drugs are given—2-3 minutes after intravenous administration and 5-10 minutes after intramuscular administration. Any appreciable rise requires further monitoring of the blood pressure, as well as watching for excess bleeding.

When drugs are administered orally during the postpartum period, the patient may complain of abdominal cramping. The physician should be notified, as it may be necessary to discontinue the medication, especially if the cramping becomes severe.

When oxytocin is administered *intravenously* for induction of labor or uterine inertia, the drug is added to an intravenous solution and given *slowly*. The rate of infusion (as drops/minute) is regulated according to the patient's response to the drug. The physician's order will indicate this, as shown on page 212.

The rate of infusion may be *slowed* should the patient experience *severe* uterine contractions. In some instances a "Y"-tubing infusion set may be used—one tubing for the intravenous solution containing the medication (oxytocin) and the other for an intravenous

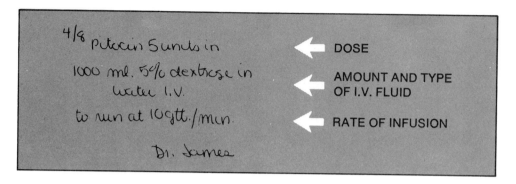

4/8 pitocin 5 units in
1000 ml. 5% dextrose in
water I.V.
to run at 10gtt./min.

Dr. James

DOSE

AMOUNT AND TYPE
OF I.V. FLUID

RATE OF INFUSION

solution (usually the same as ordered for the dilution of the oxytoxic agent) without medication. If it becomes necessary to discontinue drug administration, the *slow* administration of the solution without the oxytoxic agent keeps the needle available for further use.

When oxytocin is administered intravenously, the following measures should be employed:

1. monitoring of vital signs. Blood pressure and pulse should be taken every half hour, or more frequently if unstable
2. the rate of infusion should be checked and adjusted (when necessary) to the rate of flow prescribed by the physician. Depending on the patient and the response to the medication, this can be done every half hour. Restless patients should be observed more frequently, as arm movements can alter the rate of infusion
3. the infusion site should be checked for possible leakage of fluid into surrounding tissues

4. the frequency, length, and intensity of uterine contractions should be checked and recorded according to the physician's preference or hospital policy
5. fetal heart sounds must also be taken, again according to physician's preference or hospital policy

Hospital policy or professional judgment may alter the above implementations.

The physician should be notified immediately if *any* toxic effects are noted. Should prolonged uterine contractions occur, the rate of infusion should be slowed *or* discontinued until the physician examines the patient.

Oral administration of oxytocin, as a buccal tablet, may require patient instruction and supervision regarding the use of the tablet. The patient should be shown where the tablet is to be placed. Accidental swallowing does not harm the patient, as the drug is rendered ineffective by gastric juices. The patient will require the same supervision as is required in the intravenous administration of the drug.

Use of oxytocin as a nasal spray may also have to be explained and demonstrated to the nursing mother. Occasionally it may be necessary to stay with the patient while the drug is being self-administered.

Patients receiving sparteine (Spartocin) require the same supervision as those receiving oxytocin. Special attention should be paid to the pulse rate and quality, as the quinidine-like effect of this drug is capable of creating cardiac arrhythmias. If the drug must be discontinued, several hours must elapse before another oxytoxic agent can be given, as sparteine is slowly excreted. Giving another drug immediately may result in severe uterine contractions.

If uterine-relaxing agents are used to treat a threatened abortion, the patient will most likely be on bedrest. There appear to be no side effects associated with the use of lututrin (Lutrexin), but the nurse should be alert to changes in the patient's condition, namely excessive bleeding, signs of shock, passage of the fetus, and abdominal pain.

Table 24-1.
DRUGS ACTING ON THE UTERUS

GENERIC NAME	TRADE NAME	USES	SIDE EFFECTS	DOSE RANGES
OXYTOXIC AGENTS				
ergonovine maleate	Ergotrate	prevention and treatment of postpartum hemorrhage, hastening of uterine involution	nausea, vomiting, hypertension, cramping	0.2-0.4 mg. per dose I.M., I.V., orally
methylergonovine maleate	Methergine	same as ergonovine + stimulation of uterine contractions during delivery	nausea, vomiting, headache, hypertension, cramping, dizziness, tinnitus, diaphoresis, dyspnea, chest pain	0.2 mg. I.M., I.V. after delivery of shoulder or placenta; 0.2 mg. T.I.D., Q.I.D. orally
oxytocin	Pitocin Syntocinon	induction of labor, uterine inertia, control of hemorrhage or bleeding	hypotension, fetal bradycardia, tachycardia, anxiety, dyspnea, chest pain, cyanosis, flushing, water intoxication, uterine rupture, fetal death	0.3-1 ml. I.M. for postpartum bleeding; 1 ampul added to intravenous solution as I.V. infusion

Table 24-1. (*Continued*)

Generic Name	Trade Name	Uses	Side Effects	Dose Ranges
oxytocin	Pitocin buccal tablets	same as oxytocin	nausea, vomiting, cardiac arrhythmias in mother and fetus, tetanic contractions, local vasoconstriction of oral mucosa, uterine rupture, fetal death	1 tablet given according to patient response; usually given q1/2h until response is obtained
oxytocin	Syntocinon nasal spray	aid in ejection of milk in breast-feeding		1 spray into 1 or both nostrils 2-3 minutes before nursing
sparteine	Spartocin	same as oxytocin	same as oxytocin + cardiac arrhythmias	150 mg. per dose I.M., may be repeated
Uterine-Relaxing Agent				
lututrin	Lutrexin	functional dysmenorrhea, premature labor, threatened or habitual abortion		DYSMENORRHEA: 6000 to 9000 units q3-4h orally; PREMATURE LABOR, THREATENED or HABITUAL ABORTION: initially 12,000-24,000 units followed by 3,000-12,000 units orally

Antineoplastic agents are those used to treat malignant diseases. Although these drugs rarely effect a complete cure, they are one of the tools that can be used in the treatment of carcinomas.

Types and Uses of Antineoplastic Agents

Several kinds of chemicals are used in the treatment of cancer. One of the problems in the use of chemotherapeutic agents (drugs) in cancer therapy is that while these drugs may halt the growth of malignant cells, they also may affect *normal* cells.

Alkylating agents interfere with cell division. These drugs will slow the cell division of malignant cells as well as normal cells; however, malignant cells appear to be more susceptible. Names and uses of the alkylating agents are shown in Table 25-1. On occasion, these drugs may be used in the treatment of neoplasms other than those listed.

The **antimetabolites** interfere with cell growth by preventing the use of materials necessary for cell growth. Antimetabolites and their uses are shown in Table 25-2.

Natural products include plant alkaloids and antibiotics with antineoplastic activity. A list of natural products and their uses is given in Table 25-3.

Chapter **25**

Antineoplastic Agents

Table 25-1.
ALKYLATING AGENTS

Generic Name	Trade Name	Uses	Generic Name	Trade Name	Uses
busulfan	Myleran	chronic myelocytic leukemia	melphalan	Alkeran	multiple myeloma
chlorambucil	Leukeran	chronic lymphocytic leukemia, Hodgkin's disease, other malignant lymphomas	thiotepa U.S.P.		advanced carcinoma of breast, ovary, and lung, cerebral metastatic lesions, chronic granulocytic and lymphocytic leukemias, control of serous effusions of pleura, pericardial, and peritoneal cavities, Hodgkin's disease; other solid tumors have occasionally responded
cyclophosphamide	Cytoxan	malignant lymphomas including Hodgkin's disease and reticulum cell sarcoma, multiple myeloma, neuroblastoma, ovarian cancer, acute and chronic leukemias, retinoblastoma	triethylenemelamine	TEM	Hodgkin's disease, chronic lymphocytic and myelogenous leukemia, lymphosarcoma
mechlorethamine	Mustargen	Hodgkin's disease, lymphosarcomas, Wilms's tumor, tumors of breast, ovary, nasopharynx, stomach, uterus, and kidney, neuroblastomas, chronic myelocytic and lymphocytic leukemia, seminomas	uracil mustard		chronic lymphocytic and granulocytic leukemia, Hodgkin's disease, lymphosarcoma, giant follicular lymphoma, reticulum cell sarcoma

Vincristine and vinblastine are extracted from the periwinkle plant, vincristine being an analog (a compound structurally similar to another compound) of vinblastine.

Miscellaneous agents are (1) mitotane (Lysodren), which is used in the palliative treatment of inoperable adrenocortical carcinoma and (2) quinacrine (Atabrine), a drug used in the treatment of malaria and also employed in the management of recurring effusions of the peritoneal and pleural cavities. This drug is administered directly into these cavities.

Hormones and **hormone-like** agents are also employed in the treatment of neoplastic diseases. Steroids are used in the management of some leukemias,

Table 25-2.
ANTIMETABOLITES

Generic Name	Trade Name	Uses
cytarabine	Cytosar	acute leukemias in adults and children, solid tumors, lymphomas, Hodgkin's disease
floxuridine	FUDR	intra-arterial infusions in the palliative management of tumors
fluorouracil	5-FU	palliative treatment of solid tumors not amenable to surgery or radiation
hydroxyurea	Hydrea	melanoma, chronic myelocytic leukemia, ovarian carcinoma
mercaptopurine	6-MP, Purinethol	acute leukemia
methotrexate		choriocarcinoma, palliative treatment of acute leukemia, intra-arterial infusion of solid tumors
procarbazine	Matulane	Hodgkin's disease, treatment of solid tumors
thioguanine		acute leukemia, chronic myelocytic leukemia

Table 25-3.
NATURAL PRODUCTS

Generic Name	Trade Name	Uses
bleomycin sulfate	Blenoxane	malignant lymphomas, squamous cell carcinomas of the skin, penis, vulva, cervix, larynx, head, and neck, embryonal cell carcinoma, choriocarcinoma, teratocarcinoma, renal carcinoma, soft tissue sarcomas. Intra-arterially in the treatment of otorhinolaryngeal tumors, intrapleurally in the prevention of pleural fluid accumulation
dactinomycin	Cosmegen	Wilms's tumor, metastatic tumors of the testes, choriocarcinoma, neuroblastoma, malignant melanoma, some lymphomas
mithramycin	Mithracin	malignant testicular tumors
vinblastine	Velban	Hodgkin's disease and other malignant lymphomas, choriocarcinoma, carcinoma of the breast
vincristine	Oncovin	acute leukemia

Hodgkin's disease, and lymphosarcoma. Androgens (male hormones) may be used in the palliative management of metastatic carcinoma of the breast in women one to five years past menopause. Estrogens are used in the treatment of prostatic carcinoma and carcinoma of the breast in women five or more years past menopause. Testolactone (Teslac) is an antineoplastic drug chemically similar to androgens and is employed in the management of advanced carcinoma of the breast.

General Drug Action

Generally, antineoplastic agents affect cells that rapidly divide (proliferate) to form new cells. Neoplasms are generally rapidly proliferating cells, but so too are the cells lining the oral cavity and gastrointestinal tract and cells of the gonads, bone marrow, hair follicles, and lymph tissue. Thus, antineoplastic drugs affect not only the division of neoplastic cells but also normal cells.

While their action is not clearly understood, they appear to inhibit or slow cell division by various methods.

Side Effects of Antineoplastic Drugs

Antineoplastic agents are potentially toxic drugs and most patients experience varying degrees of side effects during therapy. There are times when side effects must be tolerated, in order to obtain optimum therapeutic results.

Those administering these drugs must be aware of the side effects of *each*, because in some instances the physician may wish to increase or decrease the dose according to the response of the patient.

Some side effects are desirable, such as bone marrow depression in the treatment of leukemia, as this is the purpose of using a specific antineoplastic agent. One patient may experience more side effects with a particular drug than another patient. And some patients may experience a greater intensity of one or more side effects than other patients.

There are also side effects that can be distressing regarding the appearance rather than the physical well-being. Loss of hair (alopecia) or skin pigmentation, while not a threat to life, is, in most instances, distressing to the patient.

The side effects for each antineoplastic agent are listed in Table 25-4.

Clinical Considerations

Patients diagnosed as having a malignancy may be treated with surgery, radiation therapy, or drugs. For some patients, a combination of two or all three measures may be employed in an attempt to cure or halt the progression of the disease. Antineoplastic drugs can also be used as palliative agents.

Patients receiving these agents may or may *not* know their diagnosis, what results can be expected from the use of these agents, or some or any of the drug side effects.

In order for health care personnel to effectively participate in the chemotherapeutic regimen for a patient, the amount of information *given to the patient* by the physician(s) and/or nurses must be made known. These patients may be in the hospital or may be attending clinics for long periods; therefore, questions regarding these drugs are bound to arise.

It is important to know the side effects and toxic effects that may occur during therapy. Since these may be numerous, reference sources should be consulted. It may be of value to make cards listing the side effects for each particular agent and to insert these cards into the patient's Kardex or post them in the medicine room. The physician must always be made aware of *any* side effects that occur during therapy.

Many of these drugs have a profound effect on the hematopoietic system. Occurrence of thrombocytopenia (decrease in platelets) can result in easy bruising and bleeding tendencies. Venipuncture sites may require prolonged pressure when the needle is removed from the vein. Direct pressure with the thumb (or fingers) is required to eliminate the possibility of hematoma. It is important that all bleeding has stopped before pressure is finally released. The patient may also experience bleeding of the gums (gingiva) during or after oral care. Soft toothbrushes, extra rinses with a mouth wash, cleaning the teeth with hydrogen peroxide, or use of a water pick may be necessary. The physician should be consulted for approval of the last two measures. Shaving with safety razors may provoke bleeding; consequently use of an electric razor should be considered.

The urine, stool, and oral cavity should be watched for signs of bleeding—this must be reported immediately. Patients who are restless or incoherent may need special padding around the side rails to prevent bruising that can occur even with minor injury. At all times, precautions must be taken to prevent injury to the skin, such as in the removing of adhesive tape, changing the patient's position in bed, oral care, and other measures which under normal circumstances rarely cause injury.

When the number of white blood cells is severely decreased, there is always the possibility of severe infections. Some hospitals institute reverse isolation techniques or utilize germ-free units. Extra precautions *must* be taken to prevent introduction of bacteria since the patient's own defense mechanisms are incapable of controlling bacterial invasions. Even bacteria normally found in the air may prove fatal to some of these patients. Personnel with *any* signs of bacterial, fungal, or viral infections should not be assigned to these patients. Despite all precautions, some patients succumb to fatal infections which cannot be controlled even with intensive antibiotic therapy.

The first signs of an impending infection—chills, fever, pharyngitis, cough, weakness—must be reported immediately. If fever occurs, the temperature must be closely monitored, as the patient may rapidly develop a life-threatening infection.

Many antineoplastic agents cause varying degrees of gastrointestinal side effects. In some instances the nausea is mild and can be relieved by antiemetics, antacids, or both. Administration of mechlorethamine (Mustargen) almost always causes nausea which may last 24 hours despite the use of antiemetics. Vomiting, which may be severe, usually occurs in ½-8 hours after administration of the drug and may be difficult to control.

This drug also has a vesicant (blistering) action on the skin. When the powder is reconstituted according to the manufacturer's directions, care must be taken not to spill the liquid on the skin. This also applies to the preparations involved with inserting the drug into the intravenous tubing, as none of the drug must spill on the *patient's* skin. Placing a piece of plastic or plastic-backed paper padding over the patient's arm will provide protection.

Mechlorethamine (Mustargen) is to be administered *immediately* after reconstitution of the powder. The drug is added to the intravenous tubing of a rapidly flowing solution of isotonic sodium chloride or 5% dextrose. In most instances the physician will administer the drug, but other personnel may be responsible for preparation of the solution. After use, syringes should be *carefully and thoroughly rinsed* under running water.

Whenever antineoplastics are given by intravenous infusion, care must be taken that the drug does not extravasate into surrounding tissues. Mechlorethamine (Mustargen) and dactinomycin (Cosmegen) are capable of severe local reactions should this occur. Patients who are restless need special attention, and various approaches can be used to avoid displacement of the intravenous needle:

1. use of veins in the hand or lower arm rather than the antecubital fossa (area in front of the elbow) usually requires fewer restraining measures
2. use of intracaths instead of needles, when possible, since these are more flexible and less likely to penetrate the vein wall

Rigid restraint of the arm of a restless patient may only *increase* restlessness!

Intravenous or intra-arterial administration of these drugs may lead to thrombophlebitis. Rotation of intravenous sites may decrease the incidence. The veins used for administration should be inspected daily, including veins currently in use *as well as those used previously.* Thrombophlebitis may not occur immediately and may take several days, hence the necessity of checking *all* areas of recent use. Any redness, swelling, pain, or induration of a vein *above* or *below* the site of use must be reported immediately.

As noted above, some side effects, though not life-threatening, are nonetheless important to the patient's self-image. Alopecia (loss of hair) and skin pigmentation are distressing and may add to the patient's discomfort and anxiety. The patient can be encouraged to wear a wig, an item which need not be expensive. Skin pigmentation can be mild to severe and sometimes little can be done cosmetically.

Before antineoplastic therapy is begun, the physician should explain to the patient and/or family the possible dangers and side effects of these agents. Some questions must be answered only by the physician; therefore, judgment must be exercised before an attempt is made to answer questions.

Ulcerations of the mouth may occur during therapy with some of the antineoplastic agents. The lips, mouth, and gums should be inspected daily during oral care. A tongue blade and flashlight will provide a good view of the oral cavity; care should be exercised in the use of a tongue blade, as the mucous membranes may have a tendency to bleed.

Discharge Teaching

Patients referred to outpatient clinics for further therapy should be encouraged to keep appointments since the antineoplastics must be administered at regular intervals for maintenance therapy and tumor control.

Team conferences regarding patient status—both mental and physical—will help meet the needs of the patient *and* the family. Since the future of many of these patients—some of whom may be very young—is uncertain, they require special care, consideration, patience, and understanding.

Table 25-4.
ANTINEOPLASTIC AGENTS*

GENERIC NAME	TRADE NAME	SIDE EFFECTS
ALKYLATING AGENTS		
busulfan	Myleran	G.I.: nausea, vomiting, diarrhea, glossitis G.U./REPRODUCTIVE: impotence, sterility, amenorrhea HEMATOPOIETIC: thrombocytopenia, pancytopenia SKIN: pigmentation, alopecia OTHER: pulmonary fibrosis
chlorambucil	Leukeran	HEMATOPOIETIC: neutropenia, lymphocytopenia
cyclophosphamide	Cytoxan	G.I.: nausea, vomiting, anorexia G.U./REPRODUCTIVE: cystitis, hematuria, amenorrhea HEMATOPOIETIC: thrombocytopenia, anemia, leukopenia SKIN: pigmentation of skin and nails, alopecia OTHER: interstitial pulmonary fibrosis
mechlorethamine	Mustargen	G.I.: nausea (may last 24 hours), vomiting (may occur in ½-8 hours), anorexia, diarrhea G.U./REPRODUCTIVE: amenorrhea HEMATOPOIETIC: lymphocytopenia, thrombocytopenia, anemia SKIN: alopecia OTHER: fever, tinnitus, deafness, metallic taste, headache. This drug has a vesicant action on the skin. Thrombophlebitis and/or thrombosis may occur in veins used for I.V. administration
melphalan	Alkeran	G.I.: nausea, vomiting HEMATOPOIETIC: anemia, neutropenia, thrombocytopenia
thiotepa U.S.P.		G.I.: nausea, vomiting, anorexia G.U./REPRODUCTIVE: amenorrhea HEMATOPOIETIC: leukopenia, anemia, thrombocytopenia SKIN: rash, urticaria OTHER: dizziness, headache, local pain

Table 25-4. (*Continued*)

GENERIC NAME	TRADE NAME	SIDE EFFECTS
triethylenemelamine	TEM	G.I.: nausea, vomiting, diarrhea, anorexia G.U./REPRODUCTIVE: albuminuria, crystalluria, hematuria HEMATOPOIETIC: leukopenia OTHER: hiccups, weakness, euphoria, headache, retrosternal burning sensation, atrophy and necrosis of lymphoid, myeloid, hepatic, adrenal, and testicular tissue, abdominal pain
uracil mustard		G.I.: nausea, vomiting, anorexia, epigastric distress, diarrhea HEMATOPOIETIC: leukopenia, thrombocytopenia, anemia SKIN: dermatitis, alopecia, pruritus OTHER: irritability, mental clouding or depression
ANTIMETABOLITES		
cytarabine	Cytosar	G.I.: nausea, vomiting, anorexia, diarrhea, oral inflammation or ulceration, hepatic dysfunction HEMATOPOIETIC: leukopenia, thrombocytopenia, anemia, bone marrow suppression SKIN: rash OTHER: fever, thrombophlebitis
floxuridine	FUDR	G.I.: gastrointestinal hemorrhage, nausea, vomiting, cramps, pain, diarrhea, enteritis, stomatitis, glossitis, gastritis, duodenal ulcer, gastroenteritis HEMATOPOIETIC: anemia, leukopenia SKIN: erythema, alopecia, dermatitis, edema, excoriation, rash, pruritus, ulcerations, abscesses OTHER: ataxia, blurred vision, convulsions, lethargy, vertigo, weakness, depression, fever, dysuria, hiccups, hemiplegia, thrombophlebitis. Laboratory abnormalities: B.S.P., prothrombin, total proteins, sedimentation rate, alkaline phosphatase, transaminase, bilirubin, lactic dehydrogenase (L.D.H.)
fluorouracil	5-FU	G.I.: stomatitis, diarrhea, anorexia, nausea, vomiting HEMATOPOIETIC: leukopenia SKIN: alopecia, dermatitis, rash, erythema, pigmentation, loss of nails OTHER: photophobia, epistaxis, euphoria

Generic Name	Trade Name	Side Effects
hydroxyurea	Hydrea	G.I.: stomatitis, anorexia, nausea, vomiting, diarrhea, constipation G.U./REPRODUCTIVE: temporary impairment of renal tubular function HEMATOPOIETIC: leukopenia, anemia, thrombocytopenia SKIN: rash, facial erythema, alopecia OTHER: drowsiness
mercaptopurine	6-MP, Purinethol	G.I.: nausea, vomiting, anorexia (may be signs of toxicity), diarrhea, jaundice, liver damage, biliary stasis HEMATOPOIETIC: leukopenia, thrombocytopenia
methotrexate		G.I.: ulcerative stomatitis, nausea, abdominal distress, gingivitis, pharyngitis, anorexia, vomiting, diarrhea, gastrointestinal ulcerations and bleeding, atrophy of the liver, cirrhosis G.U./REPRODUCTIVE: renal failure, cystitis, hematuria, menstrual dysfunction, infertility, abortion HEMATOPOIETIC: leukopenia, thrombocytopenia, anemia SKIN: rash, pruritus, urticaria, depigmentation, alopecia, ecchymosis, acne, furunculosis, telangiectasia OTHER: malaise, fatigue, chills, fever, dizziness, headache, drowsiness, blurred vision, convulsions, aphasia, hemiparesis, sudden death, pneumonitis, precipitating diabetes, osteoporosis
procarbazine	Matulane	G.I.: nausea, vomiting, anorexia, stomatitis, dry mouth, diarrhea, dysphagia, constipation, jaundice HEMATOPOIETIC: leukopenia, anemia, thrombocytopenia SKIN: petechiae, purpura, dermatitis, pruritus, pigmentation, herpes, flushing, alopecia OTHER: drugs capable of C.N.S. depression should be avoided; pain, including joint and muscle pain, chills, fever, sweating, weakness, fatigue, lethargy, drowsiness, epistaxis, bleeding tendencies, ascites, cough, edema, respiratory symptoms, headache, dizziness, paresthesias, mental depression and confusion, apprehension, nervousness, ataxia, tremors, coma, photophobia
thioguanine		G.I.: nausea, vomiting, anorexia, stomatitis, jaundice HEMATOPOIETIC: leukopenia, thrombocytopenia

Table 25-4. (*Continued*)

Generic Name	Trade Name	Side Effects
Natural Products		
bleomycin sulfate	Blenoxane	G.I.: stomatitis, oral ulcerations, nausea, vomiting, anorexia HEMATOPOIETIC: thrombocytopenia, leukopenia SKIN: hypoesthesia, hyperesthesia, paresthesia, urticaria, hyperpigmentation, alopecia, rash OTHER: interstitial pneumonitis, fever, chills, hypotension, weight loss, mental confusion
dactinomycin	Cosmegen	G.I.: nausea, vomiting, anorexia, stomatitis, pharyngitis, proctitis, diarrhea, abdominal pain HEMATOPOIETIC: leukopenia, agranulocytosis, anemia, thrombocytopenia, pancytopenia SKIN: dermatitis, acne, erythema, alopecia, increased erythema if radiation given at the same time, pigmentation of areas previously radiated OTHER: severe local reaction if extravasation occurs, thrombophlebitis
mithramycin	Mithracin	G.I.: anorexia, nausea, vomiting, diarrhea, stomatitis, abnormal liver function tests G.U./REPRODUCTIVE: abnormal renal function tests HEMATOPOIETIC: thrombocytopenia, bleeding syndrome which begins with epistaxis, elevation of bleeding and clotting time, abnormal clot retraction, anemia, leukopenia SKIN: rash, facial flushing OTHER: electrolyte imbalance, fever, drowsiness, weakness, malaise, headache, lethargy, depression, phlebitis
vinblastine	Velban	G.I.: nausea, vomiting, anorexia, constipation, diarrhea, abdominal pain, rectal bleeding, pharyngitis HEMATOPOIETIC: leukopenia OTHER: numbness, paresthesias, peripheral neuritis, mental depression, headache, convulsions, malaise, dizziness. Extravasation during I.V. administration may cause cellulitis, phlebitis, sloughing

224

Generic Name	Trade Name	Side Effects
vincristine	Oncovin	G.I.: constipation, abdominal cramps, oral ulcerations, vomiting, diarrhea HEMATOPOIETIC: leukopenia G.U./REPRODUCTIVE: dysuria OTHER: neuritic pain, difficulty in walking, paresthesias, convulsions, hypertension, ataxia, weight loss, fever, headache
MISCELLANEOUS AGENTS		
mitotane	Lysodren	G.I.: anorexia, nausea, vomiting, diarrhea SKIN: flushing G.U./REPRODUCTIVE: hematuria, albuminuria, hemorrhagic cystitis OTHER: lethargy, depression, dizziness, vertigo, blurred vision, double vision, orthostatic hypotension
male and female hormones		See Chapter 22

*NOTE: Dose ranges for neoplastic agents vary widely and because of this are not listed. References, including manufacturers' suggested dose schedules, can be used as guidelines. If there is doubt regarding the dose schedule, the physician should be consulted. Uses of antineoplastic agents can be found in Tables 25-1, 25-2, and 25-3.

The first modern drug for the treatment of epilepsy—a bromide—was used in the 1850's. The barbiturates were employed as anticonvulsants around 1912, and since the middle 1940's improved anticonvulsant agents have been developed.

Epilepsy is a word used to describe periodic attacks of disturbed cerebral function that may or may not be accompanied by convulsive movements, loss of consciousness, and abnormal behavior.

Types and Uses of Anticonvulsant Drugs

Once the diagnosis and type of epilepsy have been confirmed, the physician will select an anticonvulsant that will best suit the patient. Occasionally, a certain drug will not be effective and another must be tried. The patient may also develop side effects to one agent so that other agents of value for that particular form of epilepsy must be given.

Anticonvulsant agents and their uses are shown in Table 26-1.

Diphenylhydantoin (Dilantin) may be used prophylactically to control seizures during and after neurosurgical procedures. It may also be used to terminate attacks of status epilepticus. If it is ineffective, other anticon-

Drugs Used in the Treatment of Convulsive Disorders

vulsants, barbiturates, or other measures may be necessary.

Anticonvulsant agents should never be abruptly discontinued as seizures—including status epilepticus—may result. Patients should be made aware of the danger of stopping medications without first consulting their physician.

General Drug Action

Diphenylhydantoin (Dilantin) appears to prevent the leakage of sodium ions out of neurons into nerve cells, which reduces the hyperexcitability of neurons. In effect, this drug appears to "stabilize" neurons, thus controlling seizures. Other anticonvulsants are central nervous system depressants, for example, the anticonvulsants of the barbiturate class. Others elevate the threshold of cells in the central nervous system, thereby decreasing hyperexcitability. Regardless of the mode of action, the results are basically the same.

Side Effects of Anticonvulsants

Although these drugs do a great service in the control of epilepsy and convulsive disorders, they are not without side effects, some of which are serious.

Diphenylhydantoin (Dilantin): the most common side effects are related to the central nervous system—mental confusion, slurred speech, dizziness, insomnia, nystagmus (involuntary movement of the eyeball), nervousness, and headache. A rash, resembling measles, is the most common skin manifestation, but other types of rash may also be seen. This drug is also capable of affecting the hematopoietic system, and serious blood dyscrasias such as thrombocytopenia, leukopenia, and pancytopenia have been reported. Another problem arising from the long-term use of this drug is gingival hyperplasia (overgrowth of the gums). Dental supervision and good oral hygiene can do much to reduce the incidence of this problem. Other side effects include liver damage, toxic hepatitis, and periarteritis nodosa, which can be fatal. Diligent medical supervision and proper patient teaching can do much to reduce the incidence of side effects.

Ethosuximide (Zarontin), methsuximide (Celontin), and phensuximide (Milontin): these drugs may cause blood dyscrasias, some of which can be fatal if not detected early. Because of this, periodic blood counts are recommended. The manufacturers also recommend periodic urinalysis and liver function studies. All three drugs may cause drowsiness and/or impairment of mental and physical abilities. The patient should be cautioned against driving, operating heavy machinery, or other tasks which could be hazardous to self or others should drowsiness occur. Some patients may notice that after a period of time this impairment has diminished and they may be able to safely carry on normal activities.

Ethotoin (Peganone): chemically related to diphenylhydantoin (Dilantin) it also has hematopoietic toxicity. If nausea and vomiting occur, they may be alleviated when the drug is taken after meals. Gingival hyperplasia appears less frequently than with the use of diphenylhydantoin. Dizziness, headache, double vision, nystagmus, numbness, fever, diarrhea, and skin rash have also occurred during use.

Mephenytoin (Mesantoin): this drug is also chemically related to diphenylhydantoin (Dilantin) and shares the side effects of this compound.

Mephobarbital (Mebaral), metharbital (Gemonil), and phenobarbital (Luminal): these drugs are barbiturates and are capable of causing varying degrees of drowsiness and other side effects of barbiturate preparations (see Chapter 8).

Paramethadione (Paradione) and trimethadione (Tridione): these drugs are related anticonvulsants. Skin rash, which necessitates stopping the drugs, may progress to exfoliative dermatitis or erythema multiforme. Monthly blood and urine tests are recommended because of the possibility of adverse effects on the hematopoietic system and kidney. Jaundice may indicate liver involvement and also requires stopping the drug. Gastrointestinal side effects include nausea, vomiting, anorexia, weight loss, hiccups, and abdominal pain. The central nervous system side effects that may occur are photophobia, double vision, vertigo, insomnia, drowsiness, headache, fatigue, and personality changes.

Phenacemide (Phenurone): because of its toxicity this drug is used when other anticonvulsants have been found to be ineffective. Blood dyscrasias, hepatitis, nephritis, and personality changes have occurred.

Primidone (Mysoline): the most frequent side effects are ataxia and vertigo which may disappear with therapy. Occasionally gastrointestinal distress, double vision, emotional disturbances, drowsiness, and a measles-like rash may be seen.

The Stevens-Johnson syndrome (see Chapter 17) may occur during the use of some anticonvulsant agents. The appearance of *any* type of rash needs to be investigated and closely observed.

Clinical Considerations

Anticonvulsant agents may be given alone or in combination with other anticonvulsant agents, and the results of therapy must be known in order to raise, lower, or maintain the dose. If seizures are not controlled by one drug, another may be tried. It is important to observe the patient's response, namely the *effectiveness* and the *side effects* (if any), of the drug(s) administered.

If a patient has a seizure, all information regarding the seizure must be observed and charted. The duration of the seizure, a description, the aura (if any), and the patient's condition after the seizure must be accurately documented, as this will confirm the patient's response to therapy. Knowing this information aids the physician in selecting the drug(s) and dose(s) that will provide optimum benefit.

Sedation will occur with some of these drugs, and depending on the degree, the patient may have to be helped in and out of bed. Extreme sedation necessitates keeping the patient in bed until the dose is adjusted.

The patient should receive thorough instruction as to the importance of medication in the control of seizures. Occasionally, a patient who is seizure-free for a period of time may feel that the drug is no longer necessary and stop taking medication. Seizures can recur if the medication is stopped. It must be impressed on the patient that anticonvulsants must be taken exactly as ordered and that the medication is *never* discontinued unless by order of the physician. The patient should also be told that some anticonvulsants take several days to a week or more before they take effect, and therefore seizures may occur *early* during therapy.

There are some patients who will continue to have

seizures—although they may be decreased in number or intensity—despite medication.

Neurosurgical patients may receive diphenylhydantoin (Dilantin) during and after neurosurgical procedures. When a patient is scheduled for neurosurgery there should be a sufficient amount of the drug stocked on the unit for use during the postoperative period. Since status epilepticus could occur, the drug may be administered intravenously as an emergency measure.

Discharge Teaching

Patient teaching should include facts about epilepsy as well as the role of drug therapy in the control of epilepsy. Thorough understanding of the disease and its treatment is essential. Some patients or the parents of children with epilepsy may have erroneous preconceived notions, and it may be of value to ask what is known about epilepsy before teaching is begun. This gives an opportunity to correct any false impressions, which may cloud the receptiveness of the patient and/or parents during teaching sessions. A positive approach plus stressing the importance of the physician in treatment may help the patient and/or family overcome the fears and anxieties that often occur when the patient is first informed of the diagnosis.

The following points should be included in the teaching plan. Additional facts that apply to a particular patient or situation may be necessary.

1. the physician must be kept informed of progress after discharge. When information is *accurately* related, drugs and/or doses can be changed as necessary. All facts, whether they appear important or not, should be told to the physician. Mutual cooperation and the sharing of information between the physician and patient will contribute to the control of epilepsy

2. any side effects must be reported, even if they are transient. The physician should be consulted to determine what side effects should be told to the patient. In some instances, presentation of the more serious side effects may only add to patient anxiety and are best presented at a later time

3. the importance of clinic, office, or laboratory appointments should be stressed. The patient can be told that laboratory tests are often ordered on patients receiving these drugs and this is one way the physician can determine the effectiveness of drug therapy

4. it is very important that the patient and/or family realize that doses must *not* be omitted, even though there have been no seizures. Also, doses are *not* to be increased if the patient is having more seizures; instead, the physician should be notified

5. identification tags, such as Medic-Alert, should be carried or preferably worn. Should such patients be admitted to an emergency room in an unconscious state, medical personnel will be able to institute effective treatment if the diagnosis is known

Understanding the epileptic and the problems that must be faced is important. Education of the public as to the truth and fallacies of epilepsy may help to dispel the stigma that has unfortunately been attached to this disease.

Table 26-1.
ANTICONVULSANT AGENTS

Generic Name	Trade Name	Uses	Side Effects	Dose Ranges
diphenylhy-dantoin	Dilantin	grand mal, psychomotor seizures	ataxia, nystagmus, mental confusion, slurred speech, dizziness, insomnia, nervousness, headache, nausea, vomiting, fever, constipation, rash, blood dyscrasias, gingival hyperplasia, toxic hepatitis, liver damage, periarteritis nodosa, lymphadenopathy, Stevens-Johnson syndrome (see Chapter 17)	100 mg. T.I.D., Q.I.D. orally, 100-200 mg. q4h I.M.; CHILD: 4-8 mg./Kg./day in divided doses orally STATUS EPILEPTICUS: 150-250 mg. I.V. then 100-150 mg. 30 minutes later if necessary; CHILD: I.V. dose according to weight
ethosuximide	Zarontin	petit mal	blood dyscrasias, liver and renal toxicity, anorexia, nausea, vomiting, cramps, diarrhea, weight loss, abdominal pain, drowsiness, rash, Stevens-Johnson syndrome, myopia, vaginal bleeding, swelling of tongue, hirsutism, gum hypertrophy	initially 2 capsules (0.5 Gram) daily orally and increased as necessary up to 1.5 Grams daily; CHILD: 1 capsule daily and increased if necessary
ethotoin	Peganone	grand mal, psychomotor seizures	blood dyscrasias, liver damage, nausea, vomiting, fatigue, insomnia, headache, dizziness, double vision, nystagmus, rash, numbness, diarrhea, fever, chest pain, gingival hyperplasia	initially up to 1 Gram daily in divided doses p.c. orally; increased to 2-3 Grams daily if needed; CHILD: initially up to 750 mg. daily in divided doses p.c. orally; increased to 2-3 Grams daily if needed

Table 26-1. (*Continued*)

Generic Name	Trade Name	Uses	Side Effects	Dose Ranges
mephenytoin	Mesantoin	grand mal, focal, Jacksonian, psychomotor seizures in those not controlled by other agents	blood dyscrasias, rash, other skin manifestations, ataxia, double vision, nystagmus, fatigue, irritability, nausea, vomiting, nervousness, insomnia, dizziness, mental confusion, psychotic disturbances, hepatitis, jaundice, alopecia, weight gain, edema, photophobia, conjunctivitis, gum hyperplasia, lupus syndrome, pulmonary fibrosis, lymphadenopathy	initially 50-100 mg. daily orally; increased to 0.2-0.6 Grams daily if needed; CHILD: 0.1-0.4 Grams daily orally
mephobarbital	Mebaral	grand mal, petit mal	side effects of barbiturates (see Chapter 8)	400-600 mg. daily orally; CHILD: 16-64 mg. T.I.D., Q.I.D. orally
metharbital	Gemonil	grand mal, petit mal, myoclonic and mixed types of seizures	same as mephobarbital	initially 100 mg. daily to T.I.D. orally; increased to 800 mg. daily if needed; CHILD: 5-15 mg./Kg./day orally
methsuximide	Celontin	petit mal not controlled by other agents	blood dyscrasias, nausea, vomiting, anorexia, weight loss, diarrhea, constipation, epigastric and abdominal pain, drowsiness, ataxia, nervousness, headache, blurred vision, photophobia, insomnia, hiccups, confusion, psychological changes, rash, Stevens-Johnson syndrome	initially 0.3 Gram daily orally; increased up to 1.2 Grams daily if needed

Generic Name	Trade Name	Uses	Side Effects	Dose Ranges
paramethadione	Paradione	petit mal not controlled by other agents	rash, hiccups, nausea, vomiting, abdominal pain, gastric distress, anorexia, weight loss, photophobia, vertigo, double vision, insomnia, drowsiness, headache, paresthesias, malaise, personality changes, bleeding gums, blood dyscrasias, jaundice, hepatitis, nephrosis, alopecia	0.9-2.4 Grams daily in 3-4 divided doses orally; CHILD: 0.3-0.9 Grams in 3-4 divided doses orally
phenacemide	Phenurone	mixed forms of psychomotor seizures not controlled by other agents, grand mal, petit mal	blood dyscrasias, hepatitis, nephritis, personality changes	initially 1.5 Grams daily in 3 divided doses orally; increased to 2-5 Grams daily if needed; CHILD: ½ adult dose
phenobarbital	Luminal	grand mal, petit mal	same as barbiturates	50-120 mg. daily orally; larger doses may be necessary
phensuximide	Milontin	petit mal	nausea, vomiting, anorexia, blood dyscrasias, ataxia, dizziness, headache, lethargy, rash, urinary frequency, renal damage, hematuria, alopecia, muscle weakness	0.5-1 Gram B.I.D., T.I.D.
primidone	Mysoline	grand mal, focal, psychomotor seizures	ataxia, vertigo, nausea, vomiting, fatigue, irritability, double vision, nystagmus, rash, drowsiness	0.75-1.5 Grams daily orally; CHILD: usually ½ adult dose
trimethadione	Tridione	same as paramethadione	same as paramethadione	same as paramethadione

NOTE: Doses of anticonvulsants are individualized and may be higher or lower than average doses.

In 1817 Dr. James Parkinson accurately described the symptoms of a disease then called the "shaking palsy." Atropine was probably the first drug used to treat Parkinson's disease, and when synthetic cholinergic blocking agents were introduced, several of these agents proved effective. Levodopa, a more recent drug, has also been shown to be of value.

Parkinson's disease—also called paralysis agitans—is characterized by fine tremors and rigidity of some muscle groups and weakness of others. As the disease progresses, the speech becomes slurred, there is a mask-like and emotionless expression to the face, the patient may drool, and the gait is shuffling with the upper part of the body bent forward.

Types and Action of Drugs Used in the Treatment of Parkinson's Disease

Parkinson's disease may be treated with several different types of drugs. "Parkinson-like" syndromes can occur, for example, during the use of drugs such as the phenothiazines and after encephalitis. When the cause is due to a drug, the drug may be discontinued, but if drug therapy is deemed essential, an antiparkinsonism agent may be administered simultaneously.

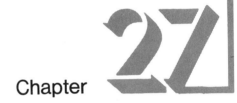

Chapter

Agents Used in the Treatment of Parkinson's Disease

> ANTIPARKINSONISM AGENTS WITH
> ANTICHOLINERGIC-LIKE ACTIVITY
>
> benztropine (Cogentin)
> biperiden (Akineton)
> cycrimine (Pagitane)
> ethopropazine (Parsidol)
> orphenadrine (Disipal)
> procyclidine (Kemadrin)
> trihexyphenidyl (Artane)

Synthetic preparations with anticholinergic-like activity are used in the treatment of Parkinson's disease. As with many other drugs, not all patients respond well to a particular agent, and the physician may need to prescribe different preparations until optimal results are obtained.

Another drug—amantadine (Symmetrel)—whose exact mechanism of action is unknown, may be used alone or in conjunction with anticholinergic-like antiparkinsonism agents or with levodopa (Larodopa, Dopar).

Antiparkinsonism agents with anticholinergic-like activity have a direct inhibitory effect on the parasympathetic nervous system, including smooth muscles. These drugs appear to have more central activity rather than peripheral activity, resulting in minimal atropine-like peripheral effects.

It is believed that Parkinson's disease may be due to a depletion of *dopamine* in the brain. Dopamine, if given as a drug, will not cross the blood/brain barrier and therefore would be ineffective. Levodopa, a *precursor of dopamine*, does cross the blood/brain barrier and therefore is useful in the treatment of Parkinson's disease.

Treatment of parkinsonism involves not only drugs but also a combined effort on the part of the medical team. Assessment of the patient's present condition, rehabilitation, physiotherapy, drugs, and good care can do much to delay the progress of the disease.

Side Effects of Antiparkinsonism Agents

Drugs with anticholinergic activity cause some of the side effects of anticholinergic agents. Some patients may note more pronounced side effects with one drug than another, and one patient may tolerate one drug better than another. These drugs are to be used with caution in those with glaucoma and benign prostatic hypertrophy, as an increase in symptoms of glaucoma or urinary retention may occur. In some cases, gastric distress can be minimized if the drug is given immediately after meals. Constipation may be relieved by increasing the fluid intake and/or laxatives, the fecal-softening type usually being preferred.

Some side effects become minimal after therapy has continued. On the other hand, the dose may have to be reduced in an effort to lessen side effects. Not all patients respond to the same dose; consequently the dose is titrated according to the patient's response. Confusion, disorientation, and other mental changes may abate in time or may require a reduction in dose or a change in medication.

Amantadine (Symmetrel) also produces some anticholinergic side effects as well as incidences of congestive heart failure, mental changes, and psychosis. As

Agents Used in the Treatment of Parkinson's Disease

with agents that have anticholinergic-like activity, some patients may note more pronounced side effects than others. This drug may also be used along with other antiparkinsonism agents, including those with anticholinergic-like activity or levodopa. Use of this drug should not be abruptly discontinued as the patient may experience a parkinsonian crisis—a sudden deterioration of the condition with a marked increase in symptoms of Parkinson's disease.

Levodopa (Larodopa, Dopar) can cause many side effects; some patients are unable to tolerate the drug. Others do very well, once the optimum dose is attained. Close medical supervision is necessary and periodic evaluation of liver, renal, and cardiovascular functions plus blood studies are recommended by the manufacturers.

Pyridoxine (vitamin B$_6$) must not be taken during therapy with levodopa as it will rapidly reverse the effects of the drug. Many vitamin preparations contain pyridoxine (a B-complex vitamin) and therefore vitamin therapy, if needed, must be selective and preparations *without* pyridoxine used.

Mental depression and suicidal tendencies have been noted during therapy with levodopa, and all patients should be carefully observed for *any* mental changes—especially depression. Other side effects may be mild, for example, dry mouth, and can be tolerated, whereas the appearance of other side effects may necessitate a change in dose or termination of therapy. This is why the physician must be made aware of all side effects that are noticed by others or experienced by the patient.

Clinical Considerations

The dose of an antiparkinsonism agent is usually tailored according to the patient's response. Several factors are considered in drug therapy: (1) are the patient's condition and/or symptoms improved? (2) what side effects are occurring? and (3) how serious are the side effects?

The hospitalized patient receiving these drugs for the first time will require observations concerning drug response, although improvement may be slow and undramatic. Discharge planning should begin immediately, and plans for discharge should be incorporated into the daily plan of care.

The patient's status before and during therapy is evaluated along with the goals the physician believes may be achieved. From this, a plan of care and of teaching for discharge can be formulated. The totally incapacitated patient who appears to show only a mild response to therapy may require long-term care either in a hospital, nursing home, or supervised home atmosphere. The family must be involved with future plans as it may be necessary to demonstrate basic care procedures (bed bath, etc.) carried out after discharge into the home setting. Every facet of daily care must be covered in detail. If possible, the family may be utilized to help give basic care to the patient, with the nurse acting as an instructor and supervisor.

Patients should be encouraged to do as much for themselves as possible and should be allowed to proceed at their own pace. The patient who will be able to perform minimal daily tasks may need supervision and/or instruction along with rehabilitation. The main goal is to prolong independence and prevent dependence.

Occasionally mental changes occur during therapy with these drugs. The confused patient may require almost constant supervision and may become difficult to manage. Reduction in dosage or a change in drug may be necessary. Sometimes the mere fact that the patient is in unfamiliar surroundings may be the cause of confusion!

Depression should prompt frequent observation of the patient as well as reporting this occurrence to the physician. Again, the disease rather than the drug may be the cause of depression. The depressed patient may or may not benefit from being with other patients, and changes in mood may be noticed. It is *most important* that those expressing suicidal ideas be carefully watched. If the patient appears confused, has difficulty in walking, or has an unsteady gait, precautions must be taken so that injury does not occur. Falls are common in those with the typical parkinsonism gait.

Discharge Teaching

Patients receiving levodopa must be warned against using any vitamin preparation that has not been first approved by the physician. In order to be sure the patient understands the full implications of this warning, it should be explained that the use of a vitamin not approved by the physician may cancel the effects of the drug. In effect, the symptoms present *before* therapy will quickly return.

The patient with severe parkinsonism will most likely be seen frequently by the physician during the early phase of therapy. All side effects—no matter how mild or unimportant they may seem—should be reported to the physician during each office visit. All these points should also be explained to the family, as they may find it necessary to reinforce this teaching after discharge or see that the patient follows and adheres to these suggestions.

Table 27-1.
DRUGS USED IN THE TREATMENT OF PARKINSON'S DISEASE

Generic Name	Trade Name	Uses	Side Effects	Dose Ranges
amantadine	Symmetrel	parkinsonism (idiopathic, postencephalitic, symptomatic)	depression, congestive heart failure, orthostatic hypotension, psychosis, urinary retention, confusion, anxiety, dry mouth, anorexia, ataxia, nausea, constipation, dizziness, vomiting, headache, fatigue, insomnia, rash, slurred speech, visual disturbances	100-400 mg. daily in 2 divided doses orally; when used with other antiparkinson agents dose is less

Generic Name	Trade Name	Uses	Side Effects	Dose Ranges
benztropine	Cogentin	all forms of parkinsonism	dry mouth, blurred vision, nausea, nervousness, vomiting, constipation, depression, numbness of fingers	0.5-6 mg. daily in single or divided doses I.M., orally
biperiden	Akineton	same as benztropine	dry mouth, blurred vision, gastric distress, transient postural hypotension, euphoria	2 mg. daily to Q.I.D. orally; 2 mg. I.M., I.V.
cycrimine	Pagitane	same as benztropine	dry mouth, blurred vision, epigastric distress, vertigo, weakness, disorientation	1.25-5 mg. T.I.D., Q.I.D.
ethopropazine	Parsidol	Parkinson's disease	drowsiness, dizziness, lassitude, blurred vision, dry mouth, epigastric distress, ataxia, paresthesias, hypotension, headache, confusion	40-600 mg. daily in divided doses orally
levodopa	Larodopa, Dopar	idiopathic, arteriosclerotic, postencephalitic, and symptomatic parkinsonism	postural hypotension, choreiform movements, cardiac irregularities, mental changes, depression, suicide tendencies, anorexia, nausea, vomiting, dry mouth, headache, dizziness, weakness, confusion, insomnia, delusions, anxiety, euphoria, fatigue, muscle twitching, burning sensation of tongue, bitter taste, diarrhea, constipation, blurred vision, diplopia, gastrointestinal bleeding in those with history of ulcer	0.5-8 Grams daily in 2 or more divided doses with food

Table 27-1. (Continued)

GENERIC NAME	TRADE NAME	USES	SIDE EFFECTS	DOSE RANGES
orphenadrine	Disipal	same as benztropine	dry mouth, blurred vision, tachycardia, urinary hesitancy or retention, headache, dizziness, urticaria, nausea, vomiting, weakness, constipation, drowsiness	50 mg. T.I.D. and up to 250 mg. per day orally
procyclidine	Kemadrin	same as benztropine	dry mouth, blurred vision, tachycardia, urinary retension, lightheadedness, nausea, vomiting, constipation	2-5 mg. T.I.D. orally; 4-5 mg. h.s. may also be given
trihexyphenidyl	Artane	same as benztropine	dry mouth, blurred vision, dizziness, mental confusion, nausea, vomiting	1-15 mg. daily orally

The introduction of chlorpromazine (Thorazine) and the reserpine alkaloids in the mid-1950's radically changed psychiatric care and opened a new frontier in psychiatry. Just as antibiotics were miracle drugs for infections, so were psychotherapeutic agents the miracle drugs of the mind.

Types and Uses of Psychotherapeutic Agents

A drug that affects the functioning of the mind is called a **psychotropic** agent. Narcotics, sedatives, alcohol, hallucinogens, and psychotherapeutic agents are examples of psychotropic drugs. The degree of mind change depends on the drug, the dose, and the patient.

There are two basic types of psychotherapeutic drugs: the **tranquilizers** and the **antidepressants**. Tranquilizers can be further subdivided into the **major tranquilizers** and the **minor tranquilizers**. Tranquilizers are also called **ataractic** agents, the word taken from the Greek—ataraxia—meaning peace of mind.

Tranquilizers are used to treat varying degrees of anxiety. Minor tranquilizers are usually employed in the treatment of mild anxiety states, neurosis, and management of

Chapter **28**

Psychotherapeutic Agents

psychosomatic conditions. Major tranquilizers are usually used in the treatment of psychosis. Some of the major tranquilizers in smaller doses may be used to treat some of the conditions usually reserved for the minor tranquilizers.

THE TRANQUILIZERS

THE MAJOR TRANQUILIZERS

The **rauwolfia alkaloids** are probably the oldest tranquilizers since they were used in India centuries ago. These drugs are used for agitated psychotic states,

---

RAUWOLFIA ALKALOIDS
rauwolfia serpentina (Raudixin)
reserpine (Rau-Sed, Serpasil)

---

especially in those patients who cannot tolerate the phenothiazines. These drugs are also used to treat hypertension, often in combination with diuretic agents.

THE PHENOTHIAZINES
dimethylamine subgroup
　　chlorpromazine (Thorazine)
　　triflupromazine (Vesprin)
piperazine subgroup
　　acetophenazine (Tindal)
　　butaperazine (Repoise)
　　fluphenazine (Permitil)
　　perphenazine (Trilafon)
　　piperacetazine (Quide)
　　prochlorperazine (Compazine)
　　trifluoperazine (Stelazine)
piperidyl subgroup
　　thioridazine (Mellaril)

The **phenothiazines**, the first of which was chlorpromazine (Thorazine), were introduced in the early 1950's and have been widely used in the treatment of various psychotic disorders. These drugs can be used to quiet a severely disturbed and agitated patient, in the manic phase of manic-depressive psychosis, and in toxic states where the patient is confused, disoriented and agitated. Alcoholic intoxication, withdrawal states from alcohol or drugs, and chronic brain disorders are examples of toxic states.

Some of these drugs, for example, perphenazine (Trilafon) and prochlorperazine (Compazine), are also used as antiemetics. The antiemetic dose is appreciably lower than doses used in the treatment of psychosis.

The type and dose of the drug selected depends on several factors: (1) the severity of agitation or anxiety (2) pre-existing diseases or conditions (if any), and (3) the age of the patient. For example, a more potent phenothiazine such as chlorpromazine (Thorazine) might be used in the treatment of a severely disturbed patient whereas one of the less potent drugs might be used for maintenance therapy. The more potent phenothiazines might also be given in lower doses for maintenance therapy. Once anxiety and/or agitation are lessened the patient may become more amenable to psychotherapy.

MISCELLANEOUS MAJOR TRANQUILIZERS
chlorprothixene (Taractan)
haloperidol (Haldol)
thiothixene (Navane)

There is a miscellaneous group of drugs also classified as major tranquilizers. These drugs have the same uses as other major tranquilizers. Chlorprothixene and thiothixene are chemically related to the phenothiazines.

THE MINOR TRANQUILIZERS

These drugs are most frequently employed in the treatment of neuroses, psychosomatic conditions, and mild forms of anxiety and tension. Some uses of these

---

THE MINOR TRANQUILIZERS
benzodiazepine group
    chlorazepate (Tranxene)
    chlordiazepoxide (Librium)
    diazepam (Valium)
    oxazepam (Serax)
propanediol group
    meprobamate (Miltown)
diphenylmethane group
    hydroxyzine (Atarax, Vistaril)
miscellaneous group
    chlormezanone (Trancopal)

---

drugs are in menopausal symptoms, preoperative anxiety states, and anxiety due to organic disease states. Sometimes these drugs are used in combination with other drugs in the treatment of diseases or conditions that may give rise to anxiety. For example, a minor tranquilizer might be administered along with female hormones in the treatment of menopausal symptoms. Or, these drugs might be used to treat hypertension, along with antihypertensive and/or diuretic agents.

Chlordiazepoxide (Librium) and diazepam (Valium) may be used in acute alcoholic withdrawal. Diazepam

also has skeletal muscle relaxing properties and has been useful in the treatment of musculoskeletal disorders such as chronic low back pain. The patient with a musculoskeletal disorder may also exhibit some anxiety—due to constant pain—and the drug may have a twofold effect, that is, muscle relaxation and sedation.

Originally barbiturates were used when it became necessary to control certain forms of anxiety, but these drugs have a sedative effect and cause varying degrees of drowsiness. In most patients the minor tranquilizers appear to cause less drowsiness as well as have less addiction potential.

Lithium (Lithane), while not classed as a tranquilizer, is a drug with a specific use, namely in the treatment of manic episodes of manic-depressive psychosis. This drug has the ability to calm the patient and control the acute symptoms. Drug effect may be noted in several days, and in some instances the patient can be discharged and returned to the home environment continuing therapy with the drug.

THE ANTIDEPRESSANTS

Depression is something that happens to all at one time or another; however, depression requires treat-

---

ANTIDEPRESSANT AGENTS
monoamine oxidase inhibitors
    phenelzine sulfate (Nardil)
    tranylcypromine (Parnate)
other agents
    amitriptyline (Elavil)
    desipramine (Norpramin)
    imipramine (Tofrānil)
    nortriptyline (Aventyl)
    protriptyline (Vivactil)

---

ment whenever it is severe, lasts for prolonged periods, or has no apparent cause. It would not be unusual to be depressed over the loss of a loved one or a serious illness, but a depression that is severe *and* prolonged may require treatment with drugs and psychotherapy.

There are two types of antidepressant agents: monoamine oxidase inhibitors and those agents that are not monoamine oxidase inhibitors. The latter group appears to be more commonly used because of the potential toxicity of the former group.

There is also a combination of an antidepressant drug *and* a tranquilizer. This combination is used in treating manic-depressive states where the patient's mood swings in cycles from the manic state to the depressive state, thus keeping the patient midway between these two states. Triavil is an example of the combination of perphenazine (Trilafon), a tranquilizer, and amitriptyline (Elavil), an antidepressant. This drug is available in several combination doses which allow the drug to be tailored to the patient's response.

Another drug, doxepin (Sinequan) is a single drug rather than a combination, and is also used to treat mixed anxiety and depression, depressive states, and anxiety states.

Psychotherapeutic agents are only adjuncts in the treatment of mental disorders. They do not cure the illness, they only help manage the patient and his symptoms and make him more amenable to therapy. Not all drugs will be of value in treating any one patient and a trial-and-error method may have to be used until the right drug and dose are found to produce a desired response.

General Drug Action

THE TRANQUILIZERS

THE MAJOR TRANQUILIZERS

The phenothiazines appear to affect the hypothalamus and other subcortical sites responsible for emotional reactions to stimuli from the environment. Some drugs of the piperazine subgroup (prochlorperazine—Compazine; perphenazine—Trilafon) also have greater antiemetic activity because of a depressant effect on the CTZ (*c*hemoreceptor *t*rigger *z*one). The piperazines also appear somewhat more selective in their effect on subcortical sites, accounting for less sedation while still lessening anxiety.

The psychotherapeutic action of the rauwolfia alkaloids is unclear. Large doses are usually required to produce beneficial effects, and the side effects produced by these large doses reduces their usefulness in psychotherapeutic disorders.

Chlorprothixene (Taractan) and thiothixene (Navane) have a mode of action basically the same as the phenothiazines. Haloperidol's (Haldol) mode of action is unknown although it is thought to also act like the phenothiazines on subcortical areas of the brain.

THE MINOR TRANQUILIZERS

The minor tranquilizers have a depressant effect on the subcortical levels of the central nervous system. These agents also have a variety of other effects such as skeletal muscle relaxing qualities. Their central nervous system effects appear to be less potent (when used in normal doses) than the major tranquilizers.

LITHIUM

The exact mode of action of lithium is unknown, but it appears to effect norepinephrine metabolism in the brain. Serum lithium levels must be determined routinely since the drug is highly toxic.

THE ANTIDEPRESSANTS

The monoamine oxidase inhibitors (MAO inhibitors) inhibit the action of monoamine oxidase, which is an enzyme partly responsible for the inactivation of norepinephrine. Thus, there is an increase in norepinephrine levels in the brain and other organs of the body. Increased levels of this neurohormone may account for the antidepressant ability of these agents.

The action of antidepressants that are nonmonoamine oxidase inhibitors is not clearly understood. It is thought that these agents may either prolong or potentiate the activity of norepinephrine.

Side Effects of Psychotherapeutic Agents

THE TRANQUILIZERS

THE MAJOR TRANQUILIZERS

Use of the rauwolfia alkaloids results in many side effects, especially with higher doses. Nasal congestion and dry mouth are experienced by almost all using the drug—regardless of the dose. Depression may occur, especially if the patient is on maintenance therapy.

The phenothiazines are capable of causing a wide variety of side effects as shown in Table 28-1.

Nervous system side effects may appear early or after prolonged use. Postural hypotension may be transient and disappear after several weeks of use. Patients should be cautioned against arising from a sitting or lying position suddenly. However, since the patient may be in an agitated state, this warning may go unheeded. The parkinsonism is reversible if the drug is discontinued, but occasionally the physician may wish to continue therapy at dose levels capable of creating this syndrome and use *anti*parkinsonism agents rather than stop the medication. If parkinsonism is severe, another major tranquilizer may be prescribed.

Muscle dystonia and tardive dyskinesia are other series of side effects that may be frightening. Carpopedal spasm (spasm of the hands and feet), rigidity of back and neck muscles, swallowing difficulties, rolling back of the eyes, and convulsions are signs of muscle dystonia. Rhythmical and involuntary movements of the tongue, face, mouth, jaw, and extremities are symptoms of tardive dyskinesia. A protruding tongue, puffing of the cheeks, puckering of the mouth, and chewing movements may also be seen.

Hematological side effects can also occur with agranulocytosis, eosinophilia, leukopenia, hemolytic anemia, thrombocytopenic purpura, and pancytopenia reported as possible changes in the blood picture. A decrease in the white blood cells can result in signs of susceptibility to infections, e.g., fever, sore throat, malaise, sores in the mouth.

Adverse behavioral effects are also a risk of phenothiazine therapy. An exacerbation of the psychosis, confusion, motor restlessness, catatonic-like states, and lethargy may be seen. The patient may appear weak and complain of weakness in the arms and legs. Just the reverse can occur and the patient may be restless, unable to sit still, pace constantly, and have a constant movement of the hands.

These drugs also have the ability to *potentiate* the effects of other drugs such as alcohol, barbiturates, narcotics, analgesics, and antihistamines. If it is necessary to use narcotics and the like, the dose of these agents must be lower than the one normally used.

Not all these side effects may appear with any one phenothiazine, yet because the drugs of this group are chemically similar, all the phenothiazines are thought to be potentially capable of these side effects.

The side effects of chlorprothixene (Taractan), haloperidol (Haldol), and thiothixene (Navane) are essentially the same as the phenothiazines. Extrapyramidal symptoms (parkinsonism, tardive dyskinesia, muscle dystonia) appear to occur frequently during the administration of haloperidol (Haldol).

Sudden deaths have been seen during the use of the phenothiazines or related compounds. In some cases death has resulted from cardiac arrest or asphyxia. Other cases have shown no specific cause of death. Because of the possibility of cardiac arrest, it is important to be familiar with cardiopulmonary resuscitation (CPR) techniques.

THE MINOR TRANQUILIZERS

These drugs have a wide variety of side effects, which are listed in Table 28-1. Drowsiness appears with the use of these drugs, especially early in therapy. Depression may also occur and could precipitate suicide attempts.

Drug dependence, both physical and psychological, has been known to occur with the use of some of these agents, namely chlordiazepoxide (Librium), chlorazepate (Tranxene), diazepam (Valium), and meprobamate (Miltown). *At no time should the tranquilizers* (both major and minor) *be suddenly discontinued* after prolonged usage. These agents are also subject to abuse by outpatients who may elect to increase the dose when (and if) tolerance develops. Close medical supervision regarding the number of tablets used in a given length of time is necessary to prevent drug abuse.

LITHIUM

Early in therapy, patients receiving lithium may notice drowsiness, polyuria, and mild nausea. Occasionally these symptoms may persist throughout ther-

---

LITHIUM INTOXICATION

early signs
diarrhea, vomiting, drowsiness, muscle weakness, lack of muscle coordination

later signs
ataxia, giddiness, tinnitus, polyuria, blurred vision

toxic reactions
tremor, muscle hyperexcitability, ataxia, blackout spells, vertigo, seizures, slurred speech, incontinence, restlessness, stupor, coma, cardiac arrhythmias, hypotension, circulatory collapse, anorexia, nausea, vomiting, diarrhea, dry mouth, blurred vision, fatigue, lethargy, weight loss, albuminuria, oliguria, polyuria

---

apy. The dose of lithium is regulated according to serum lithium levels. When serum levels are monitored, the incidence of toxic effects is minimal, yet a patient may take an overdose resulting in signs of lithium intoxication. Toxic effects can also occur when the dose of lithium reaches therapeutic levels; consequently the early signs of lithium intoxication may occur when the patient appears to be obtaining optimum effects from the drug. When the early signs of toxicity appear, the drug dose is either reduced or the drug stopped for 24 hours, after which time therapy is resumed at a lower dose.

THE ANTIDEPRESSANTS

MAO INHIBITORS

The MAO inhibitors are potent drugs capable of causing serious side effects. Hypertensive crisis has occurred when foods containing tyramine have been eaten. Foods such as aged cheeses, sour cream, beer, sherry and chianti wine, chicken livers, pickled herring, canned figs, chocolate, raisins, and soy sauce are examples of foods containing this enzyme. Other drugs may also interact with MAO inhibitors producing serious side effects; therefore the patient must be warned *not* to take *any* preparations unless prescribed by the physician. OTC (over the counter) preparations such as those for colds and hay fever must also be avoided. If the patient is unable to observe these restrictions, and many are, other antidepressants must be used.

Overstimulation—e.g., symptoms of anxiety, insomnia and so forth—may be apparent in some patients, and dose adjustment may reduce these side effects.

SYMPTOMS OF HYPERTENSIVE CRISIS	
bradycardia	palpitations
chest pain	stiff or sore neck
dilated pupils	sweating
nausea	tachycardia
occipital headache	vomiting

OTHER ANTIDEPRESSANTS

The non-MAO inhibitors also have a wide variety of side effects; however, they appear to be less toxic than the MAO inhibitors and therefore are used more frequently in the treatment of depressive states. Side effects of these drugs are shown in Table 28-1.

Some of these symptoms—for example, weakness or dizziness—may be vague, and if the patient complains of these problems, it may be difficult to determine if these are drug side effects or complaints that might be part of the patient's mental illness.

Triavil, a combination of perphenazine (Trilafon) and amitriptyline (Elavil) used for treating anxiety *and* depression, has side effects relevant to both drugs. Doxepin (Sinequan) is a single drug also used for anxiety and depression, and anticholinergic side effects (dry mouth, blurred vision, etc.), tachycardia, hypotension, gastrointestinal disturbances, paresthesias, and weight gain may occur during use.

Clinical Considerations

Psychotherapeutic agents may be administered in the general hospital situation as well as in areas involved in the treatment of mental illness. The nurse plays a very important role in the administration of these drugs in both the psychiatric and nonpsychiatric setting for several reasons: (1) patient response to medication, almost always the result of a *24-hour per day* observation, is made by nursing personnel and (2) astute and accurate observation of side effects is most important in the patient who has a mental illness. Some patients may be unable to verbally state that they are having problems because they cannot communicate or are unaware of physical changes. For example, their illness may prevent them from relating to the physician or nurse that they have a rash that itches or are constipated or have a headache. It is the nurse then, who must *closely* observe these patients for *any physical or mental changes*. Observation of patient activities may also lead one to suspect the occurrence of side effects; for instance, a patient who holds his forehead may have a headache and the patient who scratches himself may have urticaria.

Patient response to medication should be noted throughout the day *and* night. Daily activities—eating, occupational therapy, interactions with others—should be closely observed. The depressed patient who cries at 10 A.M. may still be depressed at 6 P.M. or be the reverse and show signs of anxiety and restlessness. All activity and patient responses are important as drug therapy may be changed or adjusted according to changes (or lack of changes) seen. It is also important to stay with the patient when medications are taken. If there is any doubt as to whether the patient is swallowing the drug or possibly vomiting (self-induced) immediately after the drug is taken, the physician should be told as other routes of administration may be necessary.

In the hospital situation it is important to be aware of the potential hazards associated with the use of the major tranquilizers, lithium, and antidepressant agents. The first step in recognizing side effects is knowing *what they are*. Listing the side effects of these agents on cards which can be posted in the medicine room will remind personnel. The second step is to take routine precautions for each type of drug.

PHENOTHIAZINES

PRECAUTIONS
1. avoid exposure to sunlight (due to photosensitivity reactions)
2. vital signs monitored, especially during the early phase of therapy (hypotension, cardiac irregularities)
3. bed patients—assist in and out of bed or chair slowly (postural hypotension)
4. parenteral form of these drugs—give *deep* I.M. and keep the patient flat one-half hour after administration (postural hypotension)
5. inspect skin for redness, rash, color changes, pigmentations daily
6. those with history of seizures—watch for convulsions, keep airway handy (but not necessarily in the patient's room)
7. supervise routine activities if excessive drowsiness is apparent
8. suicide risk if patient appears depressed; suicide precautions may be necessary

ANTIDEPRESSANTS

PRECAUTIONS FOR MAO INHIBITORS

1. strict dietary control, no food brought from the outside unless approved by the physician, dietitian, or nurse in charge (hypertensive crisis)
2. vital signs monitored frequently, especially early in therapy
3. report any incidence or suspicion of a headache immediately (may be first sign of hypertensive crisis)
4. bed patients—assist in and out of bed or chair (postural hypotension)
5. those with history of seizures—watch for convulsions, airway available
6. watch for signs of a swing from depression to a manic state or manic to depressive state
7. supervise patient in daily activities if drowsiness is apparent

PRECAUTIONS FOR NON-MAO INHIBITORS

1. monitor vital signs frequently, especially early in therapy
2. avoid exposure to sunlight
3. supervise patient in daily activities if drowsiness is apparent
4. those with history of seizures—watch for convulsions, have airway available
5. note aggravation of psychosis, especially a shift to a manic state
6. suicide risk, especially if patient becomes depressed

ANTIDEPRESSANT ANTIANXIETY AGENT

PRECAUTIONS FOR DOXEPIN (SINEQUAN)

1. monitor vital signs, especially early in therapy
2. supervise routine activities if drowsiness is apparent
3. note aggravation of psychosis
4. suicide risk, especially if depression is apparent

MINOR TRANQUILIZERS

PRECAUTIONS

1. supervise daily activities, especially if drowsiness is noted
2. physical and psychological dependence can occur. If the patient asks for different medication or wishes to have more medication, this must be reported

LITHIUM

PRECAUTIONS

1. normal diet, fluid up to 3000 ml. per day is important. See that the patient has water available. Encourage the patient to use salt liberally on food
2. serum lithium levels (as ordered)—be sure the laboratory test has been done on the days specified

In certain patients additional precautions may be necessary due to age, pre-existing disease, severity of illness, and specific physician orders.

Discharge Teaching

Many patients may be treated on an outpatient basis, and thorough instruction of the patient and/or family may be necessary. Although each type of drug and physician preferences vary, there are some common areas which should be presented.

1. take only the prescribed number of tablets or capsules; *do not* increase or decrease the dose without first contacting the physician
2. keep these (and all) medications out of the reach of children
3. keep all office or clinic appointments, including the appointments for laboratory tests (when ordered)
4. report *any* unusual effects or physical changes to the physician who will then decide what to do; side effects (the ones told to the patient or family) must also be reported
5. if drowsiness occurs, do not drive, operate heavy machinery, or engage in any task that may be potentially hazardous

Drug dependence has been reported after prolonged use of some of the minor tranquilizers. Abrupt stopping of the drug may precipitate drug withdrawal symptoms and extreme anxiety. When these drugs are to be discontinued, gradual tapering of the dose is recommended.

The major tranquilizers, lithium, and antidepressants should also not be abruptly discontinued as acute psychotic episodes may occur. References should be consulted regarding changes from one agent to another, as well as the dose schedules recommended by the manufacturers during the change.

Table 28-1.
PSYCHOTHERAPEUTIC AGENTS

GENERIC NAME	TRADE NAME	USES	SIDE EFFECTS	DOSE RANGES
MAJOR TRANQUILIZERS				
RAUWOLFIA ALKALOIDS				
rauwolfia serpentina	Raudixin	agitated psychotic states (also used as antihypertensive)	gastrointestinal disturbances, angina-like symptoms, arrhythmias, drowsiness, depression, nervousness, anxiety, nightmares, nasal congestion, pruritus, rash, dry mouth, headache, dyspnea, purpura, decreased libido, weight gain, dysuria	200-400 mg. daily orally (in some cases doses may be higher)
reserpine	Rau-Sed Serpasil	same as rauwolfia serpentina	same as rauwolfia serpentina	0.1-1 mg. daily orally

Generic Name	Trade Name	Uses	Side Effects	Dose Ranges
PHENOTHIAZINES acetophenazine	Tindal	management of manifestations of psychotic disorders	*cardiovascular and hematological:* cardiac arrest, hematological disorders, tachycardia; *gastrointestinal and related:* dry mouth, nausea and vomiting, diarrhea, constipation, nasal congestion, jaundice; *nervous:* postural hypotension, pseudoparkinsonism, motor restlessness, dystonia, cerebral edema, tardive dyskinesia, faintness, adverse behavioral changes, drowsiness, blurred vision, dizziness, hyper- or hypotension; *other:* itching, urticaria, photosensitivity reactions, skin pigmentation, breast enlargement (both sexes), change in libido, amenorrhea, glycosuria, hypo- or hyperglycemia	40-600 mg. daily in divided doses orally
butaperazine	Repoise	same as acetophenazine	same as acetophenazine	5-10 mg. T.I.D. orally; increased until maximum effect obtained. Total daily dose over 100 mg. not recommended. Maintenance is usually ¼-½ dose required during acute phase

Table 28-1. (*Continued*)

Generic Name	Trade Name	Uses	Side Effects	Dose Ranges
chlorpromazine	Thorazine	same as acetophenazine plus use as antiemetic, treatment of hiccups, alcohol withdrawal	same as acetophenazine	30-1000 mg. daily in divided doses orally. I.M., I.V. use 25-50 mg. per dose
fluphenazine	Permitil	same as acetophenazine	same as acetophenazine	0.5-20 mg. daily in divided doses orally; average daily dose: 3 mg.
perphenazine	Trilafon	antiemetic, management of neurosis	same as acetophenazine	2-16 mg. B.I.D. to Q.I.D. in divided doses orally; 5-10 mg. I.M. per dose
piperacetazine	Quide	same as acetophenazine	same as acetophenazine	20-160 mg. daily in divided doses orally; 2-4 mg. I.M. per dose
prochlorperazine	Compazine	same as perphenazine	same as acetophenazine	15-150 mg. daily in divided doses orally; 5-20 mg. I.M. per dose
thioridazine	Mellaril	same as acetophenazine plus alcohol withdrawal, intractable pain, senility, psychoneuroses	same as acetophenazine	150-800 mg. daily in divided doses orally
trifluoperazine	Stelazine	same as acetophenazine plus control of anxiety, tension, agitation seen in neuroses or associated with somatic conditions	same as acetophenazine	2-40 mg. daily in 2 divided doses orally; 1-10 mg. I.M.
triflupromazine	Vesprin	same as acetophenazine	same as acetophenazine	100-150 mg. daily in divided doses orally; 60-150 mg. daily in divided doses I.M. Maintenance outpatient dose 30-150 mg. daily orally

Generic Name	Trade Name	Uses	Side Effects	Dose Ranges
MISCELLANEOUS AGENTS				
chlorprothixene	Taractan	same as acetophenazine	same as acetophenazine	75-600 mg. daily in divided doses orally; 25-50 mg. I.M. per dose
haloperidol	Haldol	same as acetophenazine	same as acetophenazine	0.5-5 mg. B.I.D., T.I.D. orally; 3-5 mg. I.M. per dose
thiothixene	Navane	same as acetophenazine	same as acetophenazine	20-60 mg. daily in divided doses orally; 8-20 mg. daily in divided doses I.M.
MINOR TRANQUILIZERS				
chlorazepate	Tranxene	anxiety of anxiety neuroses, psychoneuroses in which anxiety symptoms are prominent	drowsiness, dizziness, nervousness, blurred vision, dry mouth, rash, headache, mental confusion, diplopia, depression, slurred speech, gastrointestinal distress; drug dependence may occur	15-60 mg. daily in divided doses orally
chlordiazepoxide	Librium	anxiety, tension, alcohol withdrawal	drowsiness, ataxia, rash, confusion, edema, nausea, constipation, extrapyramidal symptoms, physical and psychological dependence	5-25 mg. T.I.D., Q.I.D. orally; in severe anxiety or preoperatively 50-100 mg. I.M., I.V.
chlormezanone	Trancopal	anxiety and tension	rash, dizziness, flushing, edema, nausea, inability to void, weakness, depression, jaundice, drowsiness	100-200 mg. T.I.D., Q.I.D. orally

Table 28-1. (*Continued*)

Generic Name	Trade Name	Uses	Side Effects	Dose Ranges
diazepam	Valium	same as chlorazepate plus acute alcohol withdrawal, skeletal muscle spasm, preoperatively for surgery and endoscopic procedures	drowsiness, fatigue, ataxia, depression, constipation, hypotension, diplopia, rash, nausea, confusion, vertigo, acute hyperexcitability, urinary retention, jaundice, slurred speech; drug dependence may occur	2-10 mg. B.I.D. to Q.I.D. orally; 2-15 mg. per dose I.M., I.V.
hydroxyzine	Vistaril	anxiety, tension, psychomotor agitation	drowsiness, dry mouth, involuntary motor activity in higher doses	75-400 mg. daily in divided doses orally; 25-100 mg. per dose I.M.
meprobamate	Miltown	same as chlorazepate	physical and psychological dependence, drowsiness, ataxia, dizziness, headache, weakness, paresthesias, euphoria, nausea, vomiting, diarrhea, tachycardia, rash, urticaria, hematological changes	1200-2400 mg. daily in divided doses orally
oxazepam	Serax	same as chlormezanone	hypotension, vertigo, headache, excitement, rash, nausea, edema, lethargy, tremor, slurred speech	10-30 mg. T.I.D., Q.I.D. orally

Generic Name	Trade Name	Uses	Side Effects	Dose Ranges
OTHER				
lithium	Lithane	control of manic episodes in manic-depressive psychosis	drowsiness, fine tremors, polyuria, thirst, nausea, diarrhea, vomiting, muscle weakness; see text for signs of drug toxicity	600 mg. T.I.D. average dose; regulated according to serum levels
ANTIDEPRESSANTS				
MAO INHIBITORS				
phenelzine	Nardil	moderate to severe depressive states	hypertensive crisis, dizziness, dry mouth, constipation, postural hypotension, weakness, edema, gastrointestinal disturbances, overstimulation	initially: 15 mg. T.I.D. orally; maintenance: 15 mg. daily to Q.I.D.
tranylcypromine	Parnate	same as phenelzine	hypertensive crisis, overstimulation, restlessness, insomnia, weakness, dry mouth, nausea, diarrhea, constipation, tachycardia, palpitation, anorexia, edema, headache, rash, hepatitis	initially: 10 mg. A.M. and P.M. orally; maintenance: 10-30 mg. daily in divided doses

255

Table 28-1. (*Continued*)

Generic Name	Trade Name	Uses	Side Effects	Dose Ranges
OTHER ANTIDEPRESSANTS				
amitriptyline	Elavil	depression	*allergic reactions:* edema (of face, tongue), photosensitivity, rash, urticaria; *cardiovascular:* cardiac arrhythmias, hypo- or hypertension, tachycardia; *CNS-neuromuscular:* anxiety, ataxia, blurred vision, confusion, delusions, disorientation, drowsiness, dizziness, fatigue, hallucinations, restlessness, insomnia, nightmares, tremors, paresthesias, seizures, tinnitus, weakness; *endocrine:* breast enlargement (both sexes), change in libido, testicular swelling; *gastrointestinal:* anorexia, nausea and vomiting, stomatitis, peculiar taste, jaundice, diarrhea, swelling of the parotid, black tongue, constipation, dry mouth; *other:* alopecia, urinary retention or frequency, bone marrow depression	initially: 25 mg. T.I.D. and up to 300 mg. per day orally; maintenance: 40-100 mg. daily orally
desipramine	Norpramin	same as amitriptyline	same as amitriptyline	50 mg. T.I.D. and up to 200 mg. daily orally

GENERIC NAME	TRADE NAME	USES	SIDE EFFECTS	DOSE RANGES
imipramine	Tofrānil	same as amitriptyline	same as amitriptyline	initially: 100 mg. per day and up to 300 mg. daily orally; maintenance: 50-150 mg. per day in divided doses
nortriptyline	Aventyl	same as amitriptyline	same as amitriptyline	25 mg. T.I.D., Q.I.D.; daily dose ranges: 30-100 mg. orally
protriptyline	Vivactil	same as amitriptyline	same as amitriptyline	15-60 mg. per day in 3-4 divided doses orally

ANTIDEPRESSANT ANTIANXIETY AGENTS

GENERIC NAME	TRADE NAME	USES	SIDE EFFECTS	DOSE RANGES
doxepin	Sinequan	anxiety and/or depressive reactions, mixed anxiety/depression, involutional depression, manic-depressive reactions	dry mouth, blurred vision, constipation, drowsiness, tachycardia, hypotension, gastrointestinal distress, extrapyramidal symptoms, weight gain, edema, paresthesias, flushing, photophobia, decreased libido, rash, itching	25 mg. T.I.D. and up to 300 mg. daily orally
perphenazine plus amitriptyline	Etrafon Triavil	moderate to severe anxiety and/or agitation and depressed mood, depression when anxiety and/or agitation are severe, depression and anxiety associated with physical diseases	side effects of perphenazine and amitriptyline	available in dose combinations

NOTE: Doses of psychotherapeutic agents are adjusted upward and downward according to patient response. In some instances doses higher or lower than those stated may be used.

Histamine and Antihistamines

Histamine is a substance present in various tissues of the body—liver, lungs, intestines, and skin. The highest concentration of histamine is found in basophils (a type of white blood cell) and mast cells, which are found in the capillaries. On occasion, histamine may be used as a drug.

Antihistamines are drugs used to combat the effects of histamine on body organs and structures.

Actions and Uses of Histamine and Antihistamines

HISTAMINE

Histamine when liberated by body cells affects the vascular system resulting in dilatation of blood vessels and smooth muscles and increased secretions from exocrine glands of the stomach and respiratory tract. Injecting histamine under the skin (intradermally) produces a "triple response": A red flush appears in the center (where the drug was injected). Immediately around the red area is a flare or diffuse redness. There is a localized edema and the center red area is raised. This *flush, flare,* and *wheal* (the raised area) is the "triple response" of histamine. Any chem-

Chapter **22**

Histamine and Antihistamines, Antitussives and Mucolytics

ical or physical injury to the skin can result in a release of histamine.

Histamine is used as a diagnostic agent in gastric analysis. The injection of histamine stimulates gastric secretion of hydrochloric acid. Absence of hydrochloric acid (achlorhydria) in the gastric contents may be an indication of conditions such as pernicious anemia, gastric ulcer, chronic gastritis, and gastric carcinoma.

ANTIHISTAMINES

Antihistamines appear to be *competitors* for *receptor sites*, thereby preventing histamine from occupying these receptor sites and producing a histamine reponse.

Antihistamines are used for relief of the symptoms of seasonal allergies. Small doses of antihistamines are included in some O.T.C. preparations advertised as useful for the relief of colds and symptoms of seasonal allergies. Antihistamines are also employed for the relief of allergies due to environmental factors such as house dust and animals. They may also be used to treat the symptoms of drug allergies, especially skin manifestations. Some antihistamines are of value in treating or preventing motion sickness, nausea, and vomiting, but these drugs do not work equally well in all patients. Occasionally, an antihistamine may be used as a sedative or hypnotic for an elderly patient who cannot tolerate barbiturate/nonbarbiturate sedative/hypnotics. One antihistamine, promethazine (Phenergan), is used for the relief of the symptoms of allergy and motion sickness and is also of value as a sedative, particularly for the elderly. This drug also potentiates the action of central nervous system depressants. Promethazine, when combined with a narcotic,

allows for a reduction in the dose of the narcotic. This may be of value when (1) the patient cannot tolerate the depressing effect of a narcotic yet requires an analgesic for moderate to severe pain and (2) narcotic doses are being tapered in those who have received these agents for a long period of time and show some signs of psychological or physical addiction.

Side Effects of Histamine and Antihistamines

HISTAMINE

The side effects of histamine, when used medically, are due to drug overdose. This does not necessarily mean that the wrong dose was ordered or given, since some patients are more *sensitive* to histamine than others. Headache, nausea, vomiting, epigastric burning, flushing of the skin, and hypo- or hypertension may occur after the injection of histamine. If the hypotensive episode approaches a shock-like state, epinephrine may be ordered to counteract vasodilatation—the cause of the hypotension.

ANTIHISTAMINES

Most antihistamines are capable of causing some degree of drowsiness. Other commonly seen side effects are dry mouth, dizziness, lethargy, muscle weakness, and gastrointestinal disturbances. Antihistamines with atropine-like (or cholinergic blocking) side effects should be given with caution to those with bronchial asthma. Rare side effects include hypersensitivity reactions, hematological changes, nervousness, and anxiety.

Clinical Considerations

When histamine is used as a diagnostic agent, it is important to remain with the patient during and after administration of the drug. The blood pressure is taken prior to the gastric analysis—preferably one-half to one hour before, lest anxiety just immediately before the procedure raise the blood pressure and cause a false reading. Epinephrine should be readily available, in case it is needed. Histamine should be given with great caution to those with a history of allergies, and an allergy history should be obtained *before* the drug is given. If there is any question regarding allergies, the physician should be notified before the test is begun.

Discharge Teaching

Patients should be warned of the drowsiness that may occur when antihistamines are prescribed and should be cautioned against operating machinery, driving, or engaging in any task that may be hazardous. Drowsiness may disappear with continued use but if it interferes with normal daily activities, the drug may have to be discontinued and another tried. Patients should also be warned that these agents can potentiate the action of alcohol and other central nervous system depressants. Those taking antihistamines should make this fact known if they are prescribed medications by other physicians. In fact, it is a good policy to always tell patients that if another physician prescribes a medication, they must be very sure they tell the physician they are receiving other medications.

On rare occasions some antihistamines may produce signs of a *histamine reaction.* Anaphylactic shock, hypotension, rash, urticaria, and other manifestations of drug allergy are signs of a histamine reaction to these agents.

Antitussive and Mucolytic Agents

An **antitussive** agent is one used to relieve coughing. **Mucolytic** agents are used to reduce the thickness and tenacity of sputum, thereby facilitating the removal of sputum from the trachea and bronchi.

Types, Uses, and Actions of Antitussive and Mucolytic Agents

ANTITUSSIVES

Some antitussive agents act on the central nervous system and *depress* the cough reflex center of the medulla. Included in this group are narcotics such as codeine and morphine and non-narcotics such as dextromethorphan (a common ingredient of O.T.C. cough medications) and carbetapentane. Other antitussives act on peripheral structures. These agents may soothe the throat thereby temporarily decreasing local irritation; have expectorant action; or inhibit the cough reflex by anesthetizing stretch receptors in the lungs.

Drugs with expectorant action stimulate secretion of mucous glands in the bronchi which then aids in liquefying thick mucus obstructing the small branches of the bronchi (bronchioles). An example of an expectorant drug is ammonium chloride, which is usually found in combination with other antitussive agents.

Glycyrrhiza is an example of an agent that soothes the lining of the throat and thereby decreases local irritation. Benzonatate (Tessalon) has both peripheral and central action. This antitussive not only depresses the cough reflex center but also is believed to anesthetize stretch receptors in the lungs. This may account for the drug's ability to relieve symptoms of tightness in the chest.

The physician chooses an antitussive that will best suit the needs of the patient. A drug that acts centrally and depresses the cough reflex would be contraindicated in those with chronic respiratory disease such as asthma or emphysema. These agents might stop excessive coughing but would not help the patient raise mucus. Since the lungs are already diseased and may have lost their elasticity these patients already have difficulty raising mucus from the deeper respiratory passages. Centrally acting drugs also may decrease lung volume and those with chronic respiratory disease may already have a decreased lung volume. Obviously, indiscriminate use of O.T.C. antitussives by those with chronic lung disease can be more of a hindrance than a help.

Many antitussive agents contain several drugs, namely, an antitussive, an expectorant, and flavoring which makes the compound more palatable. Other drugs may also be added, for example, antihistamines.

MUCOLYTICS

Mucolytic agents are administered by nebulization or are instilled (carefully!) into the trachea. This is called an intratracheal instillation. In most instances the latter technique is performed by a physician. Acetylcysteine (Mucomyst) is an example of a muco-lytic agent that reduces the viscosity (thickness) of pulmonary secretions. Pancreatic dornase (Dornavac), an enzyme with mucolytic activity, is also administered by nebulization.

Side Effects of Antitussive and Mucolytic Agents

Some antitussive agents may produce gastric distress, especially when doses are exceeded. Some compound preparations contain antihistamines or antihistamine-related drugs and therefore are capable of causing drowsiness, sedation, and dryness of the mouth. Usually antitussives are well-tolerated, except in those individuals who occasionally show sensitivity or idiosyncrasy to the one or more agents of the preparation. Mucolytic agents have a low incidence of side effects when used as directed.

Clinical Considerations

Antitussive agents may be prescribed for the hospital patient who has a mild upper respiratory infection and/or cough due to respiratory disease. Sometimes the patient will ask for a "cough medicine" and finds it hard to believe that it cannot be given without a physician's order. The patient's rebuttal to the nurse's refusal to dispense an antitussive may refer to the fact that prescriptions aren't needed for cough medicines, therefore why can't one be given? This is a good opening for patient education! First, some antitussive preparations are available *only* by prescription. Second, the indiscriminate use of nonprescription antitussives by those with chronic lung disease, asthma, etc. can do more harm than good.

The cough mechanism is nature's method of cleaning out the respiratory passages. If the small bronchioles become plugged with mucus, oxygen and carbon dioxide cannot be exchanged adequately. If many of these structures become plugged for any length of time, a small (or even large) part of the lung can collapse. This is called atelectasis.

Those using O.T.C. antitussive agents for a chronic cough should be encouraged to see their physician. The cause of the cough should be determined and proper treatment instituted. While the cause of the cough may be minor and easily treated, coughing can also be a sign of a more serious disease such as lung cancer.

The patient who has an order for an antitussive preparation may also need additional measures to aid in the raising of sputum and to help cough. Depending on the degree of illness, the patient may need assistance in assuming a sitting position, and the postoperative patient may need support of the surgical incision. Abdominal incisions can be supported with a pillow or hand, and the patient can be shown how to use either of these methods.

A low humidity in the hospital room may also cause irritation of the nose, throat, and trachea. A bedside humidifier may be ordered, but if one is unavailable, frequent sips of water may relieve minor throat irritation due to a dry atmosphere.

Table 29-1.
HISTAMINE AND ANTIHISTAMINES

GENERIC NAME	TRADE NAME	USES	SIDE EFFECTS	DOSE RANGES
histamine phosphate U.S.P.		diagnostic for achlorhydria	headache, urticaria, hypo- or hypertension, nausea, vomiting, epigastric burning, flushing, dyspnea, syncope, circulatory collapse	300-500 mcg. of histamine base S.C.
ANTIHISTAMINES				
brompheniramine	Dimetane	symptomatic treatment of allergic rhinitis, vasomotor rhinitis, allergic conjunctivitis, allergic skin manifestations; also to lessen severity to allergic reactions to blood or plasma; in anaphylactic shock (along with other agents)	drowsiness, dry mouth, thickening of bronchial secretions, fatigue, restlessness, anorexia, blurred vision, headache, epigastric distress, vertigo, tinnitus, nasal congestion, hematological changes, difficulty in urination	4-8 mg. T.I.D., Q.I.D. orally; 5-20 mg. per dose I.M., S.C.; 10 mg. I.V.

Table 29-1. (*Continued*)

GENERIC NAME	TRADE NAME	USES	SIDE EFFECTS	DOSE RANGES
chlorpheni-ramine	Chlor-Trimeton	same as brompheniramine	drowsiness, restlessness, nervousness, dry mouth, anorexia, nausea, headache, polyuria, transitory hypotension with parenteral use	2-4 mg. T.I.D., Q.I.D. orally; 5-20 mg. I.M., S.C.; 10-20 mg. I.V.
cyclizine	Marezine	prevention and treatment of motion sickness, postoperative nausea and vomiting	drowsiness	50 mg. per dose and repeated q4-6h p.r.n. I.M., orally; 100-mg. suppository
dimenhy-drinate	Dramamine	prevention and treatment of motion sickness	drowsiness	50-100 mg. per dose and repeated q4h p.r.n. I.M., orally; I.V. use, same dose but must be diluted before administration
diphenhy-dramine	Benadryl	same as brompheniramine plus treatment of motion sickness, parkinsonism (including drug-induced)	same as brompheniramine	50 mg. T.I.D., Q.I.D. orally; 10-50 mg. I.V., I.M.; CHILD: 12.5-25 mg. T.I.D., Q.I.D. orally; 5 mg./Kg./day in 4 divided doses I.M., I.V.
meclizine	Bonine	same as dimenhydrinate	drowsiness	25-50 mg. per dose
promethazine	Phenergan	same as brompheniramine plus pre- and postoperative sedation, control of nausea and vomiting associated with anesthesia or surgery, adjunct to analgesics to control pain, also sedation, motion sickness	sedation, dry mouth, mild hypo- or hypertension, blurred vision	12.5-50 mg. per dose orally, I.M., rectal suppositories

Generic Name	Trade Name	Uses	Side Effects	Dose Ranges
trimeprazine	Temaril	pruritic symptoms of urticaria and other dermatitis	see side effects of phenothiazines, Chapter 28	10-40 mg. per day in divided doses, orally; CHILD: 1.25-2.5 mg. per dose
triprolidine	Actidil	symptomatic treatment of allergic rhinitis, conjunctivitis, rash	drowsiness	2.5 mg. B.I.D., T.I.D. orally; CHILD: 1.25 mg. B.I.D., T.I.D.
triprolidine and pseudo-ephedrine	Actifed	symptomatic relief of allergic and vasomotor rhinitis	drowsiness	1 tablet T.I.D.; CHILD: ½ tablet T.I.D.

Table 29-2.
ANTITUSSIVE AGENTS

The following are examples of the many antitussive preparations available:

Benylin expectorant —contains antihistamine diphenhydramine (Benadryl) which has antitussive action, and expectorants

Coryban-D cough syrup —contains a centrally acting antitussive (dextromethorphan), an antihistamine, vitamin C, expectorants, and an analgesic (acetaminophen)

Robitussin —contains an expectorant. Also available as Robitussin A-C (expectorant plus codeine plus a centrally acting antitussive); Robitussin D-M (expectorant plus dextromethorphan)

Tessalon (benzonatate) capsules—this drug has both centrally and peripherally acting antitussive activity

The gastrointestinal tract is subject to more diseases and disorders than any other system of the body. Some disorders, such as constipation, may be self-treated (although this can be dangerous in some instances); other disorders such as a peptic ulcer may require a variety of agents in the medical management of the disease.

Types, Uses, and Actions of Gastrointestinal Agents

ANTACIDS

Antacids counteract the hydrochloric acid found in the stomach. Excess hydrochloric acid can produce gastric distress which can be treated with an antacid. The medical management of a peptic ulcer includes the use of these products to aid in the healing of the ulcer as well as relieve the pain and/or discomfort associated with peptic ulcer. Other uses of antacids are in gastritis, food indiscretions, gastric distress and discomfort with vague causes.

There are two types of antacids: *systemic antacids* and *nonsystemic antacids*. A systemic antacid, for example, sodium bicarbonate (baking soda) neutralizes the hydrochloric acid of the stomach. After leaving the stomach, the systemic antacid is absorbed into

Chapter **30**

Agents Used in the Management of Gastrointestinal Disorders

the bloodstream through the blood vessels of the duodenum. This is followed by an alteration of electrolyte balance (e.g., too much alkali) and the kidney excretes the excess alkali. There are several problems here. One, the action of bicarbonate in the stomach produces a gas—carbon dioxide. The patient may feel relieved by the belching of gas, but there is also the danger of perforation of the stomach wall in those with peptic ulcers or conditions which may cause a weakening of this area. Second, excessive use of this type of antacid can result in systemic alkalosis, an excess of alkali in the body. This is more of a danger in those patients with impaired kidney function since it is the kidney that aids in the maintenance of electrolyte balance by excreting excess bicarbonate ions. The third problem is acid rebound. The presence of a strong alkali prompts the gastric cells to secrete *more* acid in an attempt to neutralize the alkali.

A nonsystemic antacid is an alkali that is not readily absorbed and forms relatively insoluble compounds after combining with the hydrochloric acid of the stomach. These products are more often prescribed than the systemic antacids because of the dangers of the latter products.

Various alkali can be employed as nonsystemic antacids. Some products, for example, Amphojel (aluminum hydroxide gel) contain one antacid; others, such as Maalox (magnesium and aluminum hydroxides) contain more than one antacid. Some of these alkali are also included as buffering agents in aspirin products such as Bufferin and Ascriptin.

The nonsystemic antacids buffer the gastric secretions to a pH that prevents the digestive action of pepsin affecting the stomach and duodenal lining.

DIGESTANTS

Digestants are agents that aid in the digestion of food when certain diseases or conditions prevent or hinder this process. Digestants are *not* intended to be used when there is a normal production of digestive enzymes. Achlorhydria (insufficient or absent hydrochloric acid), deficiency of bile and bile salts due to *partial* biliary tract obstruction or liver disease, and absence or deficiency of pancreatic enzymes due to pancreatitis or surgical removal of the pancreas or pancreatic duct are indications for the use of digestants. Hydrochloric acid, bile salts, and digestive enzymes are agents prescribed for those with deficiency states.

Hydrochloric acid is administered for achlorhydria. When it is given as a liquid a glass straw must be used, with the tip of the straw well behind the teeth. Hydrochloric acid can damage tooth enamel and this method of administration will reduce the possibility of erosion. The capsule form—glutamic acid hydrochloride (Acidulin)—is often preferred as there is no danger of the drug coming in contact with the teeth. Use of

---

NONSYSTEMIC ANTACIDS

aluminum hydroxide
aluminum phosphate
magaldrate
magnesium carbonate
magnesium hydroxide
magnesium oxide
magnesium trisilicate
milk of magnesia (magnesia magna, an aqueous
    suspension of magnesium hydroxide)

this agent in achlorhydria provides hydrochloric acid which is necessary for (1) the digestion of protein (2) activation of hepatic and pancreatic secretions (3) neutralization of the bicarbonate contained in intestinal secretions, and (4) the conversion of pepsinogen to active pepsin.

Bile salts aid in fat digestion and absorption by emulsifying (breaking up) fats, which are then acted on by pancreatic lipase. Bile salts are used as replacement therapy for those with biliary tract obstruction, fistulas, or deficiences. These drugs, in tablet form, are usually taken after meals. Bile salts are contraindicated in those with *complete* biliary obstruction as they also increase the flow of bile from the liver (this is called a choleretic activity) and may produce or increase jaundice.

The *digestive enzymes* are pepsin and pancreatic enzymes. Pepsin may be administered with hydrochloric acid, although a total lack of pepsin is rare—even in patients with achlorhydria. Also, pancreatic enzymes are capable of protein digestion and therefore supplemental therapy rarely appears necessary.

Pancreatic enzymes may be given to patients with pancreatitis, surgical removal of the pancreas, or cystic fibrosis. These tablets are usually taken before or with meals depending on the manufacturer's recommendations. The coating, or lack of a coating, or the capsule form dictates how the drug is taken.

EMETICS AND ANTIEMETICS

Emetics are drugs capable of causing vomiting. Drugs in this class are used only occasionally, as gastric lavage is the preferred method of emptying the stomach of its contents. Apomorphine is an emetic that has a direct effect on the CTZ (chemoreceptor trigger zone) of the medulla and may be used in cases of poisoning or drug overdose. The danger in the use of an emetic is in the aspiration of vomitus, especially if the patient is semiconscious or irrational. Ipecac syrup is also an emetic that may be kept in the household for use in cases of accidental poisoning and drug ingestion. The induction of vomiting carries hazards, especially in the hands of nonmedical personnel; therefore emergency first aid, a call to the poison center, and getting the patient to the hospital as soon as possible are probably more advantageous than the indiscriminate use of ipecac. An emetic must *never* be administered if (1) the agent swallowed is a caustic substance—for example, lye (2) the patient is unconscious, semiconscious, extremely restless, hyperventilating, or unable to swallow, or (3) the substance is a petroleum product—kerosene, gasoline, cleaning fluid, paint thinner, or fuel oil.

Antiemetics are used to treat nausea and vomiting, which may be due to a wide variety of reasons—drugs, food poisoning, dietary indiscretions, and anxiety are some causes.

These drugs make the chemoreceptor trigger zone of the medulla less sensitive to nerve impulses passing through this center to the vomiting center. These impulses may arise from the inner ear (motion sickness) or the stomach. The exact mode of action of some of these preparations is unknown.

Locally acting agents may also be used in the treatment of nausea and vomiting. Over-the-counter preparations such as Alka-Seltzer and Pepto-Bismol may have limited value in the relief of gastric distress or mild nausea, but severe cases require a centrally acting agent.

CATHARTICS AND LAXATIVES

The terms **cathartic** and **laxative** are used interchangeably. In some cases the term laxative denotes a product that is less harsh and produces a soft, formed stool with minimal abdominal cramping.

Cathartics are given to empty the bowel of fecal contents and gas. There are different types of cathartics: stimulant cathartics, saline cathartics, bulk-forming cathartics, and emollient (softening) cathartics.

STIMULANT CATHARTICS

aloe

bisacodyl (Dulcolax)

cascara sagrada

castor oil

danthron (Dorbane)

phenolphthalein

senna

Stimulant cathartics increase peristalsis, rapidly propelling the fecal mass through the intestine, resulting in one or more liquid stools. Castor oil acts in the small intestine and when taken internally splits into glycerol and ricinoleic acid. It is the ricinoleic acid that increases peristalsis. The other stimulant cathartics principally work in the large intestine.

Saline cathartics are rapid acting and usually produce loose, watery stools within several hours. The effect is produced by an increase in the amount of water in the large intestine. Epsom salts, citrate of magnesia, and sodium phosphate and sodium biphosphate (Fleet Brand Enema and Phospho-Soda) are examples of saline cathartics.

This type of cathartic is usually administered in the morning or afternoon because of the rapid effect—usually in one or two hours. Saline cathartics are utilized when a complete emptying of the intestinal tract is desired—X-rays of the intestine, following administration of an anthelmintic for certain types of helminths, and ridding the intestinal tract of poisons. The extremely salty taste of these products is unpleasant for some individuals. Some products are flavored and/or effervesced, making them more palatable.

Saline cathartics may be given by enema, and as in the case of Fleet Brand, come packaged in an enema administration form, eliminating the need for enema administration equipment.

The *bulk-forming cathartics* increase in size when combined with water. Like the saline cathartics, they stimulate nerve endings of the large colon, thereby increasing peristalsis. They also may form a jelly-like mass which helps soften the stool and allows for easy passage through the large colon. Methylcellulose, psyllium, plantago seed, and bran are examples of this type of cathartic.

The *emollient cathartics* soften the fecal mass thereby allowing easy passage through the intestine. There are two types of emollient cathartics: oils, such as mineral oil and glycerin suppositories, and surface active agents. Mineral oil, an indigestible product, is taken orally and softens the fecal mass by means of its lubricating properties. Other oils (cottonseed oil, olive oil) can be used in oil retention enemas to soften the fecal mass in the lower colon and rectum. Medically, these latter products are not used orally as cathartics. Glycerin suppositories also have lubricating properties and act in the same manner.

Surface active agents, for example, dioctyl sodium sulfosuccinate (Colace) lower surface tension, thereby allowing water to enter into and soften the fecal mass. This results in a soft, semiformed stool with minimal if any abdominal cramping. This action is similar to the action of detergents on grease.

Surface active agents are also available in combination with other cathartics—usually ones that produce mild peristalsis. An example is Peri-Colace, a combination of dioctyl sodium sulfosuccinate and casanthranol, a mild stimulant.

ANTIDIARRHEAL AGENTS

Diarrhea is a symptom rather than a disease. Treatment will depend on the cause, if known. Diarrhea, for example, may be a symptom of food or drug allergy, emotional stress, poor eating habits, constipation, partial intestinal obstruction, or other intestinal pathology.

There are two types of antidiarrheal agents: locally acting agents and systemic agents. Locally acting agents such as kaolin and pectin have adsorbent and soothing action. Kaolin attracts chemicals, bacteria, and toxins to its surface. Pectin has water-adsorbing qualities.

Systemic agents, the opiates and cholinergic blocking agents, usually are more effective than locally acting agents. One side effect of the opiates is constipation, due to the drugs' ability to slow peristalsis. This drug action is utilized in the treatment of diarrhea. Paregoric (camphorated tincture of opium) is the most commonly used opiate since morphine and other narcotics are too potent when used for this purpose. Paregoric is used for infants and adults and like all opiates it has addiction potential. Lomotil is a combination of a chemical related to meperidine—diphenoxylate—and a cholinergic blocking agent—atropine. This drug may also be habit-forming.

Cholinergic blocking agents block the action of the parasympathetic nervous system on the gastrointestinal tract, thereby slowing peristalsis. These drugs may be combined with phenobarbital or other drugs with sedative action. Other combinations are the inclusion of one or more cholinergic blocking agents and locally acting agents. An example of this combination is Donnagel, which contains hyoscyamine, atropine, and hyoscine (cholinergic blocking agents) and kaolin and pectin.

OTHER ANTIDIARRHEAL AGENTS

If diarrhea is due to a reduction of normal intestinal flora, as may be seen during antibiotic therapy, Bacid capsules (*Lactobacillus acidophilus*), Lactinex (*Lactobacillus acidophilus* and *Lactobacillus bulgaricus*) or buttermilk may be used to enhance regrowth of intestinal flora. These agents do not directly stop diarrhea but may eliminate the cause.

Diarrhea due to infection of the gastrointestinal tract may be treated with antibiotics, antifungals, or sulfonamides specific for the infectious microorganism. Systemic-acting agents may be given concurrently.

Side Effects of Gastrointestinal Agents

ANTACIDS

Aluminum hydroxide antacids may be constipating, and magnesium hydroxide antacids may cause diarrhea —especially when they are used in larger doses or continuously. Some commercial preparations combine magnesium and aluminum hydroxides in an effort to eliminate these problems.

One danger of antacid overuse is the possibility of disguising more serious gastrointestinal disorders, especially when these drugs are used continuously without medical advice.

Misuse of sodium bicarbonate or commercial products that "fizz" (effervescent products) in the presence of a peptic ulcer can result in perforation of the stomach wall—a serious emergency requiring immediate surgical intervention. Sodium bicarbonate overuse can also result in alkalosis and, in those with cardiac disease, hypernatremia (excess sodium). While the occasional use of both products by healthy individuals apparently is safe, overuse can be dangerous.

DIGESTANTS

Hydrochloric acid, if administered in liquid form, must be given with a glass straw with the tip of the straw well behind the front teeth. This product can damage tooth enamel if allowed to come in contact with the teeth or remain in the mouth. Administration should be followed with water.

Other digestants have few side effects; however, if a product contains additional cholinergic blocking agents, the side effects of these agents may be seen.

EMETICS

Emetics are to be used with caution as aspiration of the vomitus may occur, especially if the patient is unresponsive or extremely restless. Usually gastric lavage is the preferred method of emptying the stomach of its contents.

ANTIEMETICS

The side effects of systemic antiemetics vary with the type of drug used. Many of these agents may cause varying degrees of drowsiness. Some antiemetics may

---

SYSTEMIC ANTIEMETICS
dimenhydrinate (Dramamine)
hydroxyzine (Vistaril)
meclizine (Antivert)
*perphenazine (Trilafon)
*prochlorperazine (Compazine)
promethazine (Phenergan)
*thiethylperazine (Torecan)
* drugs with phenothiazine side effect potential

---

be phenothiazines or phenothiazine-related drugs; and therefore the side effects pertinent to this group of drugs must be considered during administration. See Chapter 28 for the action and side effects of the phenothiazines.

CATHARTICS AND LAXATIVES

Stimulant cathartics rapidly propel the fecal mass through the intestine which can result in excessive water and electrolyte loss, especially in debilitated individuals, children, and the aged. Saline cathartics also pose the same danger.

The use of saline cathartics, even in enema form, may be contraindicated in those with cardiac disease, as there is some absorption of sodium, even with the enema form. Many cardiologists prefer the use of stool-softening agents, as there is less intense action and results are more comparable to a normal soft stool. Some stool softeners contain sodium, and their use may be avoided in those with severe cardiac disease. Other surface active agents such as Surfak (dioctyl *calcium* sulfosuccinate) contain no sodium and may be preferred. The amount of sodium absorbed during the use of products containing sodium may vary and may or may not be significant in a particular patient.

The bulk-forming agents have no known toxic effects, but there are several possible dangers in the use of these products. If the patient has an undiagnosed intestinal obstruction due to tumors, an impacted fecal mass, adhesions, etc., these agents may compound the problem and possibly create a total intestinal obstruction. Also, sufficient water *must* be taken along with these agents, followed by extra water within the next two hours, or else the gelatinous mass can become impacted in the esophagus, stomach, or intestine.

Mineral oil, an emollient cathartic, is relatively inexpensive and is often used by older individuals who suffer from chronic constipation. There are several dangers associated with the chronic use of mineral oil. One: mineral oil hinders the absorption of the fat-soluble vitamins A, D, K, and E. A vitamin deficiency may result after prolonged use. Lack of vitamin K, which is essential in the manufacture of prothrombin (see Chapter 11) may result in a prolongation of the clotting time. When taken in large amounts, mineral oil may leak past the anal sphincter. If a patient has had recent rectal surgery, the leakage may retard healing. In other patients rectal leakage can cause embarrassment, stain clothing, irritate the skin, and lead to skin breakdown.

Surface active agents are apparently nontoxic when used as directed, but occasionally diarrhea may be seen even with normal doses.

The continued use of *any* cathartic—no matter how mild—can result in the loss of the defecation reflex and a decrease in (normal) peristalsis when use is discontinued. This is sometimes referred to as the laxative habit.

Another danger is the masking of a change in bowel habits. Constipation could be a sign of serious intestinal pathology, such as cancer of the bowel; usage of a cathartic may prevent the individual from seeking medical advice until it is too late.

ANTIDIARRHEALS

When used as directed, the nonopiate antidiarrheal agents have few side effects. Those containing cholinergic blocking agents may exhibit the side effects of those drugs (see Chapter 5). The opiate products, such as paregoric, or Lomotil may be habit-forming if use is prolonged. Like the cathartics, these products can also mask serious intestinal pathology, and continued diarrhea warrants examination by a physician.

Clinical Considerations

Antacids are often prescribed for patients being treated medically for peptic ulcers or conditions such as gastritis, gastric distress, or gastric hyperacidity.

Patients with a peptic ulcer may receive these drugs several times per day or as often as every two to four hours, alternating the antacid with milk or milk and cream. In some cases the physician may order the antacid left at the bedside. There are several nursing implications here; the nurse is responsible for seeing that (1) there is always a supply of antacid at the bedside (2) the patient fully understands *how much* of the antacid is to be taken each time and *how often* it is to be taken (3) an ample supply of measuring glasses is available (4) the patient is shown how to measure the dose and (5) the patient has a watch or clock. It is also important that the patient understands the importance of the antacid in the treatment of ulcers, as this may motivate him to take the drug as ordered—both in the hospital and after discharge. If milk or milk and cream is also included in the treatment, these products should be kept in thermal containers to prevent souring.

Antacids taken before, with, or after some drugs—tetracyclines for example—can interfere with drug action. Consequently antacids are not to be given to patients without a specific order from the physician.

Stimulant cathartics, in suppository form, may be used in a bowel retraining program. Those who have no control over bowel function—the para- or quadraplegic, stroke, or geriatric patient—may respond to this method of bowel stimulation. After physician approval, three things are necessary: (1) a well-balanced diet (2) plenty of liquids (2000+ ml. per day), and (3) cooperation of nursing personnel. The suppository is inserted at the *same time* each morning. Within 15-60 minutes the patient will have the urge to defecate,

at which time he is taken to the bathroom or placed on a portable commode. If the patient is unable to tell if he has to defecate, due to paralysis or other pathology, he can be placed on his side (or on a bedpan, *providing defecation will occur soon*) and the bedding protected with waterproof pads. This procedure should continue for one or two weeks, after which time the patient may have established a routine evacuation. The use of the suppository can then be discontinued and reinstituted when necessary for future retraining sessions. Variations of this program may be necessary to suit a particular patient.

The average adult dose of paregoric is 4-5 ml., and the drug must be measured accurately as overdose will result in signs of opiate poisoning. If the order is written in the apothecaries' system—℥ ī ——(4 ml.)—this should not be confused with—℥ ī ——which is 30 ml.

Overdose of antidiarrheal agents can lead to constipation; therefore these drugs should be given only if the stool is loose and watery. A soft, semiformed stool does not ordinarily require medication and the drug should be discontinued. Some O.T.C. antidiarrheal agents contain cholinergic blocking drugs and are contraindicated in those with glaucoma or enlarged prostate. Although these warnings are printed on the label or container, they may be ignored.

Discharge Teaching

The nurse can perform an educational service as to the use and misuse of nonprescription gastrointestinal agents. There are some who will ignore admonitions regarding the hidden dangers of these products, but if only one person seeks medical advice, it is well worth the effort.

The continued use of cathartics, mild or otherwise, should be discouraged, as laxative dependence with a loss of bowel tone can occur. Consistent use of mineral oil is definitely to be avoided as it hinders absorption of fat-soluble vitamins. Unfortunately, advertisements lead some to believe that "regularity" is a must and "irregularity" leads to a poor disposition or other personality changes.

There is a definite danger in the misuse of antacids without prior approval of a physician, as their use may be masking a more serious disease such as ulcers, stomach cancer, or gallbladder disease. People should be encouraged to consult a physician if they frequently use antacids for "stomach problems."

Table 30-1.
GASTROINTESTINAL AGENTS

GENERIC NAME (OR CONSTITUENTS)	TRADE NAME	DOSE RANGES
ANTACIDS		
aluminum hydroxide gel	Amphojel	1-2 teaspoonfuls or 1 tablet 5 or 6 times daily
aluminum hydroxide, magnesium hydroxide	WinGel	2-4 teaspoonfuls, tablets as required
aluminum hydroxide, milk of magnesia	Aludrox	1-2 teaspoonfuls or 1-2 tablets as required
calcium carbonate, magnesium carbonate, magnesium trisilicate	Dicarbosil	1-4 tablets Q.I.D.
magaldrate	Riopan	1-2 teaspoonfuls, tablets Q.I.D.
magnesium hydroxide, aluminum hydroxide	Maalox (No. 1 tablets, No. 2 tablets, suspension)	No. 1 tablets: 2-4 tablets Q.I.D. No. 2 tablets: 1-2 tablets Q.I.D. suspension: 2-4 teaspoonfuls Q.I.D.

Table 30-1. (*Continued*)

GENERIC NAME (OR CONSTITUENTS)	TRADE NAME	DOSE RANGES
magnesium trisilicate, aluminum hydroxide	Gelusil	2 or more tablets, teaspoonfuls Q.I.D.
magnesium trisilicate, aluminum hydroxide, magnesium hydroxide	Gelusil-M	1-2 tablets, teaspoonfuls as required

ANTACIDS WITH ANTIFLATULANTS

aluminum hydroxide, magnesium carbonate, magnesium hydroxide, simethicone (liquid does not contain magnesium carbonate)	Silain-Gel	2 tablets, teaspoonfuls as required
aluminum hydroxide, magnesium hydroxide, simethicone	Mylanta	1-2 tablets, teaspoonfuls Q.I.D.
dicyclomine (Bentyl), aluminum hydroxide, magnesium hydroxide	Kolantyl	1-4 wafers, teaspoonfuls or 1-2 tablets as required

CATHARTICS AND LAXATIVES

aloe—an ingredient in some O.T.C. preparations		varies
bisacodyl	Dulcolax	2-6 tablets; CHILD: 1-2 tablets; suppository: ADULT—1, CHILD—½
cascara sagrada		aromatic fluid extract: 2-12 ml., fluid extract: 0.6-2 ml., tablets: 300 mg.

GENERIC NAME (OR CONSTITUENTS)	TRADE NAME	DOSE RANGES
castor oil (oleum ricini)		15-60 ml.; CHILD: 4-15 ml.
danthron, d-calcium pantothenate	Modane	1 tablet or 1-2 teaspoonfuls; CHILD: ¼-1 teaspoonful
danthron, dioctyl calcium sulfosuccinate	Doxidan	1-2 capsules daily
dioctyl calcium sulfosuccinate	Surfak	same as Doxidan
dioctyl sodium sulfosuccinate	Colace	50-200 mg.; CHILD: 10-120 mg.
dioctyl sodium sulfo-succinate, casanthranol	Peri-Colace	1-2 capsules or tablespoonfuls; CHILD: 1-3 teaspoonfuls
glycerin—suppository or liquid		1 suppository as needed. 60 ml. with 30 ml. of 50% solution magnesium sulfate and 90 ml. of water as enema
milk of magnesia		15-30 ml.
mineral oil		15-30 ml.
mineral oil, phenol-phthalein	Agoral	½-1 tablespoonful h.s.; CHILD: ½-2 teaspoonfuls
psyllium	Metamucil	1 rounded teaspoonful stirred into water
senna concentrate, dioctyl sodium sulfosuccinate	Gentlax S	1-2 tablets; CHILD: 1 tablet

Table 30-1. (*Continued*)

Generic Name (or constituents)	Trade Name	Dose Ranges
sodium biphosphate, sodium phosphate (available as enema or oral liquid)	Fleet Brand (enema) Fleet Brand Phospho-Soda (oral liquid)	enema: 1 unit; oral preparation: 2-4 tablespoonfuls with water
DIGESTANTS		
dehydrocholic acid	Decholin	1-2 tablets T.I.D.
glutamic acid hydrochloride	Acidulin	1-3 Pulvules T.I.D. a.c.
glutamic acid hydrochloride, pepsin	Muripsin	1-2 tablets with meals
hydrochloric acid		2-8 ml. diluted—sipped during meal. USE GLASS STRAW
lipase, amylase, protease, bile constituents, hemicellulose	Festal	1-2 tablets T.I.D. with meals
ox bile extract		300 mg. with water T.I.D.
pancreatic enzymes	Cotazym	1-3 capsules a.c.
pancreatin, pepsin, bile salts	Entozyme	2 tablets p.c.
EMETICS		
apomorphine U.S.P.		5-10 mg. S.C.; INFANT: 1 mg. S.C.
ipecac U.S.P.		8-15 ml. ipecac syrup; 0.5-1 ml. ipecac fluid extract

GENERIC NAME (OR CONSTITUENTS)	TRADE NAME	USES	SIDE EFFECTS	DOSE RANGES
ANTIEMETICS*				
chlorpromazine	Thorazine	systemic antiemetic (also psychotherapeutic agent)	side effects of phenothiazines—see Chapter 28; hypotension is most common side effect when used as antiemetic	10-25 mg. q4-6h p.r.n.; 25-50 mg. q3-4h I.M.; rectal: 100 mg. suppository q6-8h p.r.n.
dimenhydrinate	Dramamine	vertigo, nausea and vomiting of motion sickness	drowsiness	50-100 mg. q4h orally; 50 mg. I.M., I.V.; 100 mg. as suppository; CHILD: 25-50 mg. T.I.D. orally
hydroxyzine	Vistaril	systemic antiemetic (also psychotherapeutic agent)	drowsiness, dry mouth	25-100 mg. I.M., orally
levulose, dextrose, orthophosphoric acid	Emetrol	locally acting antiemetic		1-2 tablespoonfuls at 15-minute intervals until vomiting stops; CHILD: 1-2 teaspoonfuls
meclizine	Antivert	nausea, vomiting, dizziness of motion sickness	drowsiness, dry mouth	25-50 mg. daily, orally
perphenazine	Trilafon	severe nausea, vomiting	side effects of phenothiazines	8-24 mg. daily in divided doses. 1 Repetab B.I.D. orally; 5-10 mg. I.M.
prochlorperazine	Compazine	severe nausea, vomiting	side effects of phenothiazines	5-10 mg. T.I.D., Q.I.D.; Spansule: 10 mg. q12h; suppository: 25 mg. B.I.D.; 5-10 mg. I.M. q3-4h; 5-10 mg. I.V.
promethazine	Phenergan	motion sickness, prevention and control of nausea and vomiting associated with certain surgeries and anesthetic agents	drowsiness, dry mouth, blurred vision	12.5-25 mg. I.M., rectally, orally

279

Table 30-1. (*Continued*)

Generic Name (or constituents)	Trade Name	Uses	Side Effects	Dose Ranges
thiethylperazine	Torecan	nausea, vomiting, vertigo	side effects of phenothiazines	10-30 mg. daily I.M. suppository, orally
trimethobenzamide	Tigan	nausea, vomiting	drowsiness, hypersensitivity reactions, hypotension, Parkinson-like syndrome	250 mg. T.I.D., Q.I.D. orally; 200 mg. T.I.D., Q.I.D., I.M. or suppository; CHILD: 100-200 mg. T.I.D., Q.I.D. orally; suppository, I.M. not recommended
Antidiarrheal Agents				
diphenoxylate, atropine	Lomotil	diarrhea	cholinergic blocking agent side effects (see Chapter 5), nausea, vomiting, sedation, headache, hypersensitivity reactions	2 tablets Q.I.D.; 10 ml. Q.I.D.
kaolin, pectin, hyoscyamine, atropine, hyoscine	Donnagel	diarrhea	cholinergic blocking agent side effects	1-2 tablespoonfuls after each loose stool
Lactobacillus acidophilus	Bacid	restoration of normal intestinal flora		2 capsules B.I.D., Q.I.D.
Lactobacillus acidophilus, Lactobacillus bulgaricus	Lactinex	same as Bacid		4 tablets T.I.D., Q.I.D.
mepenzolate	Cantil	irritable bowel syndrome	cholinergic blocking agent side effects	1-2 tablets T.I.D. with meals and h.s.
paregoric (camphorated tincture of opium)		diarrhea	opiate side effects—see Chapter 6	5-10 ml. per dose

*NOTE: Drugs with phenothiazine side effects may not cause these side effects in the lower doses used to control nausea and vomiting. However, since some phenothiazine side effects may be noted even in lower doses, they should be kept in mind.

At one time poisoning with heavy metals, which had been major components of some drugs, was a concern in medical practice. With the advent of newer agents, metal poisoning due to drugs is rarely seen. Poisoning with heavy metals may be seen in children who eat or chew on furniture, plaster chips, or other objects that have been covered with a lead-based paint. Adults working in industry may also come in contact with heavy metals, for example, as air pollutants, and may develop heavy metal poisoning.

Types and Uses of Heavy Metals and Heavy Metal Antagonists

Arsenic is no longer used in medicine, although it has historical interest in that it was the first effective agent used to treat syphilis. Arsenic is found in weed killers and insecticides. Poisoning with arsenic is treated with *dimercaprol* (BAL—British Anti-Lewisite), which is also used in gold and mercury poisoning.

Silver as silver nitrate or silver protein is a heavy metal used as a topical antiseptic agent. Silver nitrate is sometimes used in the treatment of extensive burns. In some states one or two drops of 1% ophthalmic silver nitrate is instilled into the eyes of all new-

Chapter

31

Heavy Metals and Heavy Metal Antagonists

born infants immediately after delivery, for the prevention of gonorrheal conjunctivitis. Children born of mothers with active gonorrhea (which may be without symptoms in the female) may come in contact with the microorganism during passage through the birth canal. Since the microorganism does not survive on the skin but on mucous membranes, the conjunctiva may become infected. If untreated, blindness may result.

Mild silver protein may be used in bladder irrigation or as an antiseptic on the mucous membranes of the nose, mouth, or throat. Toughened silver nitrate may be used as a mild caustic on wounds, scar tissue, and granulation tissue.

Gold is sometimes employed in the treatment of rheumatoid arthritis (aurothioglucose—Solganal) and although toxic effects can occur, dimercaprol may be given at the first sign of a severe reaction.

Calcium disodium edetate (calcium disodium Versenate) is used in the treatment of lead poisoning in both children and adults. In some large cities, lead poisoning detection centers have been set up to detect and treat this condition. The oral form of the drug is used for follow-up therapy or to treat asymptomatic patients with laboratory evidence of lead poisoning. The intramuscular route is painful, and procaine 0.5% may be added to the solution to minimize discomfort.

Penicillamine (Cuprimine) is used to treat poisoning by copper or to remove copper in Wilson's disease (a degenerative liver disease).

Side Effects of Heavy Metals and Heavy Metal Antagonists

Poisoning by silver is rare, since it is poorly absorbed through the skin or mucous membrane. The drug does stain the skin, and permanent discoloration of clothing, furniture, and bedding will occur if the solution comes in contact with these objects. Staining of the skin is not permanent and will wear (but not wash) off.

The use of gold can result in toxic reactions. Lesions of the mucous membranes, dermatitis, diarrhea, abdominal cramps, and blood dyscrasias may be seen. This drug must be administered by the *deep* intramuscular route. Periodic blood counts are usually ordered to monitor hematological changes, should they occur.

The side effects of dimercaprol (BAL) are nausea, vomiting, paresthesias, pain at the site of injection, burning sensation of the mouth, lips, and throat, a constricting sensation in the chest, and hypertension. Sterile abscesses may be seen at injection sites.

Calcium disodium edetate (calcium disodium Versenate) is a potentially toxic drug with the possibility of renal damage occurring during therapy. Daily urinalysis is recommended to monitor kidney function. Since severe lead poisoning can, in itself, cause proteinuria and hematuria, daily monitoring of these findings must also be made and compared with any changes that may occur during therapy. Ordinarily, the patient who begins therapy and has proteinuria and hematuria will begin to show an improvement in these findings *unless* the drug is beginning to show toxic side effects. Then, the findings will appear unchanged or worse than those seen before institution of therapy. Other renal studies may also be ordered. Changes in renal function may necessitate stopping therapy.

Penicillamine (Cuprimine) is relatively nontoxic although occasionally rash and easy bruising may be seen. Should these occur, the physician must be notified.

Clinical Considerations

When silver nitrate is used as a local antiseptic, care must be taken to avoid contact of the liquid with areas other than those being treated. The patient's personal belongings (clothes, rings, watch, etc.) should be protected if near the area treated. Hospital equipment, furniture, and walls should also be protected when possible, since staining is permanent. In burn treatment centers using silver nitrate, it is almost impossible not to stain bedding and furniture as large areas of the body are being treated with the silver nitrate solution.

In applying the ophthalmic solution to the eyes of newborn infants, the solution must be applied onto the conjunctiva. Care is necessary that the solution does not run down the infant's face, and although the grayish stain is not permanent, it may be nonetheless distressing to the parents. In addition, care should be taken to avoid contact of the tip of the applicator with the infant's cornea.

Good oral care is essential when gold is used in the treatment of rheumatoid arthritis, since lesions of the mucous membranes of the mouth and throat may occur. Frequent rinses with mouth wash, warm water, or dilute hydrogen peroxide will keep the mouth free of food particles. Since rheumatoid arthritis is a crippling disease and the hands are frequently affected, the patient may need assistance with oral care. Daily inspection of the oral cavity with the aid of a tongue blade and flashlight will be necessary. Should oral lesions (whitish spots or red ulcerations) become apparent, they must be reported to the physician.

Lead poisoning is a definite problem, especially in areas of older homes. Those who live in these areas should be encouraged to have their children tested for lead poisoning at local clinics or health departments. Lead poisoning can result in mental retardation, if untreated; therefore early detection and prompt treatment are of great importance. Magazines, newspapers, and television have done much to bring this problem to the attention of the public, but health professionals must also make an effort to encourage families to avail themselves of the services offered by these detection centers.

Discharge Teaching

When calcium disodium edetate is administered orally for the treatment of lead poisoning, it may be necessary to explain dose schedules to the family. The importance of taking the drug as ordered plus return visits to the clinic must be *stressed*. The teaching of families usually must be a team approach with physicians, nurses and other health personnel explaining the problems that can occur if therapy is *not* instituted promptly or if dose schedules are not followed.

Table 31-1.
HEAVY METALS AND HEAVY METAL ANTAGONISTS

GENERIC NAME	TRADE NAME	USES	SIDE EFFECTS	DOSE RANGES
HEAVY METALS				
aurothioglucose	Solganal	rheumatoid arthritis	lesions of mucous membranes, dermatitis, diarrhea, abdominal cramps, blood dyscrasias	initially 10 mg., then 25 mg. × 2, then 50 mg. I.M.; doses given weekly
silver nitrate solution, 1% ophthalmic		prevention of gonorrhea of conjunctiva in newborn		1-2 drops, each eye
silver nitrate solution		treatment of burns, antiseptic for mucous membranes, caustic for wounds, scar tissue, granulation tissue	staining of skin	applied topically
HEAVY METAL ANTAGONISTS				
calcium disodium edetate	calcium disodium Versenate	lead poisoning	renal toxicity, pain at site of injection	ADULTS: 4 Grams daily in divided doses orally; 1 Gram in 250-500 ml. of isotonic sodium chloride solution B.I.D. × 5 days I.V.; CHILD: up to 1 Gram per 30 lbs. of body weight per day in divided doses I.M.
dimercaprol U.S.P. (BAL)		arsenic, gold poisoning	nausea, vomiting, paresthesias, pain at injection site, burning sensation of lips, mouth, throat, constricting sensation of chest, hypertension	2.5-5 mg./Kg. q4h × 2 days I.M.; then 2 injections on third day; then daily × 5 days
penicillamine	Cuprimine	copper poisoning, removal of excess copper in Wilson's disease	occasionally rash, easy bruising	250 mg. Q.I.D. orally

Vitamins

A **vitamin** is a substance needed for normal growth and function. The exact role of some vitamins in human nutrition remains unclear. Most vitamins must be obtained from outside sources, namely food, as the body does not manufacture them. The vitamins manufactured by the body are vitamin D, which is produced upon the exposure of the skin to sunlight, and vitamin K, synthesized by intestinal bacteria.

Types, Uses, and Actions of Vitamins

Vitamins are divided into two main groups: the *water-soluble vitamins,* which are vitamin C and the B-complex group, and *fat-soluble vitamins,* vitamins A, D, E, and K.

THE WATER-SOLUBLE VITAMINS

Vitamin C (ascorbic acid) is found in citrus fruits and some vegetables. A deficiency of this vitamin results in scurvy, a condition well known to sailors who were deprived of fruit and vegetables on long sea voyages. In the early nineteenth century the British navy began to issue limes and lemons to their crews. This move led to the almost complete disappearance of scurvy among their sailors, who were then nicknamed "limeys."

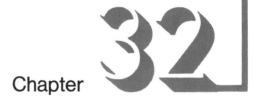

Chapter **32**

Vitamins and Drugs Used in the Treatment of Anemias

The signs of scurvy are swollen, red, bleeding gums, a loosening of the teeth, hemorrhage of the skin, joints, and muscles due to capillary fragility, fatigue, pallor, and anemia. In most instances a normal diet provides sufficient vitamin C but additional vitamin C may be required by:

1. those with a decreased or inadequate food intake
2. pregnancy
3. surgical patients—particularly patients who have had major surgery
4. infants and growing children

There is no absolute proof that this vitamin is of value in the prevention of colds.

Vitamin C is concerned with the development of teeth, bone, blood vessels, and collagen and is involved with carbohydrate metabolism. It appears to aid in wound healing; thus it may be prescribed postoperatively either by the oral or intravenous route.

The B-complex group includes:

1. thiamine (B_1)
2. riboflavin (B_2)
3. pyridoxine (B_6)
4. niacin
5. pantothenic acid

Thiamine (B_1) is found in meats and whole cereal grains. Deficiency results in beriberi, a disease characterized by neurological and cardiovascular symptoms: muscular weakness, anorexia, peripheral neuritis, cardiac arrhythmias, and edema of the lower extremities. Poor nutritional states, as might be seen in alcoholics or those with severe diet inadequacies, give rise to a thiamine deficiency. In the hospital, postoperative patients may be given B-complex—sometimes along with vitamin C—when dietary intake is limited. Other patients, such as the chronically ill, the elderly, and the chronic alcoholic also may be given thiamine or B-complex, which includes all of the B vitamin group. This vitamin is thought to play an important role in carbohydrate metabolism.

Riboflavin (B_2) is found in milk, eggs, meat, green vegetables and whole cereal grains. Deficiency of this vitamin rarely exists alone. Characteristic lesions of the cornea, tearing, burning and itching of the eyes, inflammation of oral mucous membranes, and cracks or fissures at the corner of the mouth may be seen if a riboflavin deficiency (along with other vitamin deficiencies) occurs. Riboflavin is found in body cells and appears to be active in cellular respiration.

Pyridoxine (B_6) is found in many of the foods containing thiamine. Like riboflavin, pyridoxine deficiency rarely exists alone. This vitamin is usually included in most B-complex preparations administered for vitamin deficiencies. Pyridoxine plays an important role in amino acid and fatty acid metabolism.

Niacin (nicotinic acid) is found in lean meat, fish, beans, peas, and liver. Deficiency results in pellagra. This vitamin is important in oxidation-reduction reactions in body cells. Niacin and riboflavin deficiencies are most likely to exist together, hence the treatment of niacin deficiency includes niacin *and* riboflavin and usually thiamine. Niacin deficiency is not uncommon in poverty areas where cost factors limit the purchase of foods containing niacin and other B-complex vitamins.

Pantothenic acid is present in many foods and deficiency is relatively rare. This vitamin plays an important role in carbohydrate and fatty acid metabolism, the formation of acetylcholine (a neurohormone), and the synthesis and degradation of sterols and steroid hormones.

THE FAT-SOLUBLE VITAMINS

These vitamins, unlike the water-soluble vitamins, are stored in body muscle and fat and in the liver. Absorption of the fat-soluble vitamins requires the presence of fat and bile salts in the digestive tract. Since these vitamins are stored in the body, deficiencies develop more slowly.

Vitamin A is found in eggs, liver, and the fat of milk. *Carotene*, which is found in green vegetables and carrots, is the substance the body is able to convert into vitamin A. Deficiency of this vitamin results in night blindness (inability to see in dim light), dry skin, and diarrhea. Kidney stones may also develop as the loss and clumping of epithelial cells that line the urinary tract provide a starting point for stone formation.

Vitamin A deficiency may occur in those with a *prolonged* inadequate dietary intake, for example, the terminally ill patient who eats very little food. Also prone to deficiency are those with biliary disease, hepatic disease, chronic digestive disorders that interfere with the absorption of fats (and therefore the fat-soluble vitamins), and prolonged use of a mineral oil cathartic. Vitamin A is essential for growth, the normal development of bones and teeth, and the maintenance of epithelial tissues.

Vitamin D deficiency in children causes rickets—a softening and bending of the bones, especially the bones of the legs. Adults develop osteomalacia—a softening of bone due to either a lack of vitamin D or a loss of calcium from the bone. This vitamin is found in small amounts in milk and egg yolk, but the chief source of vitamin D is obtained by exposure to sunlight. Ultraviolet rays change sterols in the skin to vitamin D. Other sources are milk and other foods that are artificially enriched with vitamin D. This vitamin is necessary for the absorption of calcium from the digestive tract and the deposition of phosphorus and calcium in the bones and teeth.

Vitamin E is found in wheat germ oils, green and leafy vegetables, milk fat, and eggs. There has been a great deal of controversy about this vitamin; however, there is no absolute proof that a deficiency causes a specific problem, or that taking the vitamin will be of therapeutic value.

Vitamin K is found in fats, wheat, rye, alfalfa, and other foods. Deficiency is rare as this vitamin is found in a wide variety of foods and is also synthesized by intestinal bacteria. Deficiency can occur if there is an alteration of intestinal flora (as might be seen during antibiotic therapy), biliary disease, and severe prolonged diarrhea. Vitamin K is used by the liver in the manufacture of *prothrombin*, a necessary element in blood coagulation. Signs of deficiency are manifested by bleeding tendencies; however, bleeding tendencies can have a cause other than a vitamin K deficiency.

This vitamin may be administered to those with a vitamin K deficiency (which is relatively rare), severe and prolonged diarrhea as might be seen in those with ulcerative colitis, to patients with biliary tract disease including hepatitis, cirrhosis, and biliary obstruction, and to newborn infants. Newborns normally have a deficiency of vitamin K for a few days after birth, after which time they are able to synthesize this vitamin in their intestinal tract.

Other compounds which do not appear to be related to any group of vitamins are biotin, inositol, and para-aminobenzoic acid (PABA). Since these substances are found in many foods and deficiencies do not appear to exist, they are not used as singular substances in the treatment of vitamin deficiencies. They may be included in some multivitamin preparations.

Side Effects of Vitamins

There appear to be no side effects associated with the use of the water-soluble vitamins with the exception of niacin, which may cause a flushing and feeling of warmth. This is a normal reaction when niacin is given in larger doses.

Overdose of vitamin A results in hypervitaminosis A, with skin and bone lesions, jaundice, alopecia and lethargy—an extremely toxic condition. Because of the dangers of hypervitaminosis A, preparations of the larger doses require a prescription.

Hypervitaminosis D will result in a *loss* of calcium from the bones, calcium deposits in soft tissues, and increased blood serum levels of calcium (hypercalcemia). There is no known toxic effect from overdoses of vitamins E and K.

Clinical Considerations

On occasion health professionals may be asked to recommend a "good vitamin preparation." Obviously, there are several problems here. If the individual "feels tired" or has some other vague complaint, it may *not* be due to a lack of vitamins but may indicate other problems, diseases, or conditions which require medical investigation. Those who eat a well-balanced diet rarely are in need of a vitamin supplement. Pregnancy, certain disease states, and infants and children may require vitamin supplements, especially during the early growth years, but these are best prescribed by a physician as each condition may require a different balance of vitamins and minerals.

Secondly, vitamins are overpriced, since the individual may be taking a product that is actually not needed. In dollars and cents, the preparation may be worth the price paid—when it is in the bottle—but may be of little value once taken. Some vitamin preparations may contain substances—such as biotin—which have no known deficiency states, and the cost of the preparation must then outweigh its value. Advertising claims as to the importance of some vitamin preparations are at best questionable.

Drugs Used in the Treatment of Anemias

Anemia is a decrease in the number of red blood cells *or* a decrease in the amount of hemoglobin in red blood cells or *both* a decrease in the number of red blood cells and hemoglobin. *Iron*, which is essential for the manufacture of hemoglobin, is widely distributed in the body. Iron is also found in a wide variety of foods—meats, egg yolks, and green vegetables. The body stores iron and uses it over and over; therefore there is usually little need for supplemental iron therapy *except* in the treatment of an iron deficiency anemia.

If an iron deficiency anemia is diagnosed, it then becomes necessary to find the *cause* of the anemia. Some causes of an iron deficiency anemia are bleeding (which may or may not be obvious), inadequate dietary intake of iron over a period of time, and pregnancy. The symptoms of this type of anemia include pallor, weakness, fatigue, headache, and anorexia.

Iron may be administered by the oral or parenteral route, although the oral route is preferred. Parenteral routes are used when: (1) the patient cannot take oral preparations (2) oral iron would not be absorbed from the intestine (3) a rapid replacement of iron is necessary, and (4) the patient has an inflammatory gastrointestinal disorder such as ulcerative colitis. Examples of iron preparations are shown in Table 32-1.

Iron may also be found in multivitamin preparations or in mixtures of iron and B-complex or other vitamins and/or mineral combinations.

Deficiency of vitamin B_{12} is rare as the vitamin is found in meats, milk, eggs, and cheese. The body also stores this vitamin, using approximately 30 *micro*grams per month. A deficiency may be seen in those who (1) are strict vegetarians (2) have had a total gastrectomy or subtotal gastric resection (3) have intestinal diseases such as ulcerative colitis, and (4) have gastric carcinomas. Removal of all or part of the stomach involves loss of the cells that secrete the *intrinsic factor,* which is necessary for the absorption of vitamin B_{12} in the intestine. Deficiency, for any reason, will not result for several years because of the body's ability to store this vitamin.

Vitamin B_{12} is used in the treatment of pernicious anemia (a lack of the intrinsic factor) and megaloblastic anemias due to fish tapeworm, gastric carcinomas, gastrectomy, and nutritional deficiencies. This vitamin is also used in the Schilling test (vitamin B_{12} absorption test). The value of this vitamin in treating *anything but a true vitamin B_{12} deficiency is unfounded.* Massive doses—for example, 1000 mcg. daily—are also unnecessary except in the initial treatment of pernicious anemia.

Folic acid, or pteroylglutamic acid, is a B-complex vitamin used in the treatment of megaloblastic and macrocytic anemias resulting from folate deficiency. Folate deficiency may occur as a result of a nutritional deficiency and may also be seen in those undergoing renal dialysis, administration of folic acid antagonist drugs such as methotrexate, and during the long-term administration of drugs such as diphenylhydantoin (Dilantin) and barbiturates, and in those who consume large amounts of alcohol. Folic acid may also be used in the treatment of pernicious anemia as a substitute for liver extract. It is not used in place of vitamin B_{12}, but may be used in conjunction with this vitamin.

Liver extract is occasionally used to treat pernicious anemia and other macrocytic anemias. The action of liver extract lies in its vitamin B_{12} content. Because some patients develop allergic reactions to liver extract, vitamin B_{12} is usually preferred.

Side Effects of Drugs Used in the Treatment of Anemias

Iron, given orally, may cause nausea, vomiting, epigastric distress, abdominal cramping, diarrhea and/or constipation. Usually the stool will appear black, which is to be expected and should cause no alarm. If side effects do develop, the iron preparation may be discontinued for several days and resumed at lower doses.

Iron preparations that are enteric-coated appear to cause less gastric irritation than the uncoated forms. Side effects also may be minimized by taking the drug immediately after meals. Oral iron is contraindicated in patients with ulcerative colitis and peptic ulcer.

Injectable iron—iron dextran (Imferon) and iron sorbitex (Jectofer)—is used only when oral therapy is not possible, as fatal anaphylactic reactions have occurred following administration. Iron dextran can be given by the intramuscular or intravenous route whereas iron sorbitex is given only by the intramuscular route. Both drugs produce pain and/or discomfort at injection sites when given intramuscularly. Doses are computed according to the patient's weight and hemoglobin. A recommended test dose of 0.5 ml. on the first day of therapy is advised.

There appear to be no side effects with vitamin B_{12} and folic acid.

Clinical Considerations

Patients should be encouraged to take oral iron preparations immediately after meals, as this appears to minimize gastrointestinal side effects. Additionally, the black color to the stool should be explained to the patient, lest this cause undue alarm.

Patients should also be advised to keep iron preparations away from children, as acute iron toxicity and poisoning can occur if the tablets are ingested. Vomiting, tarry stools, vomiting of blood, weak and rapid pulse, hypotension, and coma can occur soon after ingestion of toxic doses. The child may appear to recover, yet 24 hours later a second set of symptoms—cyanosis, shock, pulmonary edema, coma, and death—may be seen.

Intramuscular injections of iron sorbitex (Jectofer) and iron dextran (Imferon) are given by the "Z-track" technique. Injection is made only in the upper outer quadrant of the buttock. The needle should be two to three inches long and 19 or 20 gauge.

Table 32-1.

VITAMINS AND DRUGS USED IN THE TREATMENT OF ANEMIAS

GENERIC NAME	TRADE NAME	USES	SIDE EFFECTS	DOSE RANGES
VITAMINS vitamin A		vitamin A deficiencies	hypervitaminosis A with anorexia, alopecia, dry skin, pruritus, enlarged liver, irritability	INFANT: 4,500 units; CHILD: 9,000 units; ADULT: 12,000 units daily; in some cases higher doses may be used
vitamin B complex	many trade names	vitamin B deficiencies		recommended therapeutic doses: *Thiamine* (B_1): 5-90 mg. daily in single or divided doses orally; up to 50 mg. B.I.D. I.M. *Riboflavin* (B_2): 2-10 mg. daily S.C., orally *Pyridoxine* (B_6): 25-200 mg. daily I.V., I.M., orally *Niacin:* 10-20 mg. daily I.V., I.M., orally
vitamin C (ascorbic acid)		scurvy, vitamin C deficiency		25-200 mg. or more daily I.M., I.V., orally
vitamin D		vitamin D deficiency	overdose: loss of calcium from bones, calcium deposits in soft tissues, hypercalcemia	average dose: 400 units daily (higher doses may be necessary in some cases)
vitamin E		unknown		unknown; preparations are available for oral use
menadiol sodium diphosphate (a vitamin K analog)	Synkayvite	prothrombin deficiency states		5-10 mg. daily I.M., I.V., S.C., orally
menadione sodium bisulfite	Hykinone	same as menadiol		0.5-2 mg. daily I.M., I.V., S.C., orally

Table 32-1. (Continued)

GENERIC NAME	TRADE NAME	USES	SIDE EFFECTS	DOSE RANGES
phytonadione (vitamin K_1)	Konakion	same as menadiol		1-20 mg. daily I.M.

Drugs Used for Anemias

GENERIC NAME	TRADE NAME	USES	SIDE EFFECTS	DOSE RANGES
ferrocholinate	Ferrolip	iron deficiency anemias	rare	50 mg. T.I.D. orally
ferrous fumarate	Ircon	same as ferrocholinate	gastrointestinal distress, diarrhea	200 mg. T.I.D., Q.I.D. orally
ferrous gluconate	Fergon	same as ferrocholinate	same as ferrous fumarate	320-640 mg. T.I.D. orally
ferrous sulfate	Feosol	same as ferrocholinate	same as ferrous fumarate	200 mg. T.I.D., Q.I.D. orally
folic acid	Folvite	megaloblastic and macrocytic anemias, pernicious anemia, folate deficiency		250 mcg.-1 mg. daily orally; in some instances doses may be higher
iron dextran	Imferon	iron deficiency anemia	arthralgia, muscle aching, anaphylactoid reactions, rash, itching, headache, nausea, pain at site of injection	dose calculated by formula using patient's weight and hemoglobin; I.M. using "Z-track" technique. Test dose of 0.5 ml. should be given on first day. Also I.V.
iron sorbitex	Jectofer	same as iron dextran	nausea, vomiting, chest pain, hypotension, cardiac arrhythmias, headache, anaphylactoid reactions, pain at site of injection	same as iron dextran but I.M. use only, use "Z-track" technique
vitamin B_{12} (cyanocobalamin)	Rubramin	pernicious anemia; occasionally used for peripheral neuritis and other neuropathies, vitamin B_{12} deficiency		7-30 mcg. and up to 1 mg. (1000 mcg.) I.M. per dose

In 1798 Edward Jenner, a British physician, introduced a vaccination process for smallpox. Since the time of Jenner, the spread of many diseases has been controlled and contained; vaccines have almost completely eradicated some diseases.

Active and Passive Immunity

When an infection occurs, the body will begin to build an **immunity** to the disease.

There are three types of immunity: (1) actively acquired immunity, (2) artificially acquired active immunity, and (3) passive immunity.

An **antigen** is an invading virus, bacteria, or foreign protein. An **antibody** is a protein substance, manufactured by lymphoid tissue and the reticuloendothelial system, that provides immunity to a disease. A *specific disease*, such as mumps or smallpox, has *specific antibodies*. Once manufactured by these specialized tissues, antibodies circulate in the blood serum. When an antigen enters the body, specific antibodies neutralize the specific invading antigen.

Antibody-producing tissues cannot distinguish between a live antigen that is capable of causing disease *or* an attenuated (weakened) or killed antigen. It is therefore pos-

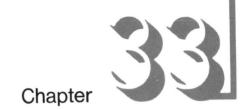

Chapter **33**   **293**

Immunological Agents

sible to create an acquired active immunity with either killed or attenuated antigen. A *live* antigen results in a *naturally* acquired active immunity, whereas a killed or attenuated antigen results in an *artificially* acquired active immunity (see chart on facing page).

A **vaccine** is a preparation containing an attenuated or a killed infectious agent.

A **toxin** is a substance produced by some bacteria such as the *Clostridium tetani* (the microorganism causing tetanus). A toxin is also capable of stimulating the lymphoid tissues and reticuloendothelial system into producing antibodies. Toxins, which are usually powerful substances, can be attenuated or weakened.

vides immediate immunity. Passive immunity lasts only for a short time. Development of an active immunity takes *time,* sometimes a few weeks to a few months, but immunity lasts for a long time and in some cases a lifetime.

With artificial immunity, a *booster* injection is sometimes necessary to keep the level (titer) of antibodies adequate to ward off disease. If the antibody titer drops too low, the individual, if exposed, could develop the disease. The booster dose, usually smaller than that given originally, is injected at an appropriate time after primary immunization.

Most vaccines administered give artificially acquired

EXPOSURE TO AN ANTIGEN (bacteria, virus, foreign protein)	=	ANTIBODY FORMATION
EXPOSURE TO A TOXIN	=	ANTITOXIN FORMATION

They are then called **toxoids,** which are also capable of stimulating the body to produce antibodies. Both toxins and toxoids are also antigens.

An **antitoxin** is formed after exposure to a toxin, just as an antibody is formed after exposure to an antigen. An antitoxin is an antibody, but these two terms are used to differentiate antibodies formed on exposure to toxins from those formed on exposure to bacteria, virus, or any foreign protein.

Passive immunity, or the receiving of antibodies manufactured by another human or by an animal, pro-

active immunity. Use of attenuated or killed microorganisms is safer than the administration of live microorganisms. In cases where immunity must be produced immediately, passive immunity techniques are employed.

Skin testing may be employed to determine if there is a sufficient amount of circulating antibodies against some microorganisms. The *Schick test* is performed as a diagnostic for diphtheria antibodies, and the *Dick test* for scarlet fever antibodies. If no localized reaction is seen after an intradermal injection, it is pre-

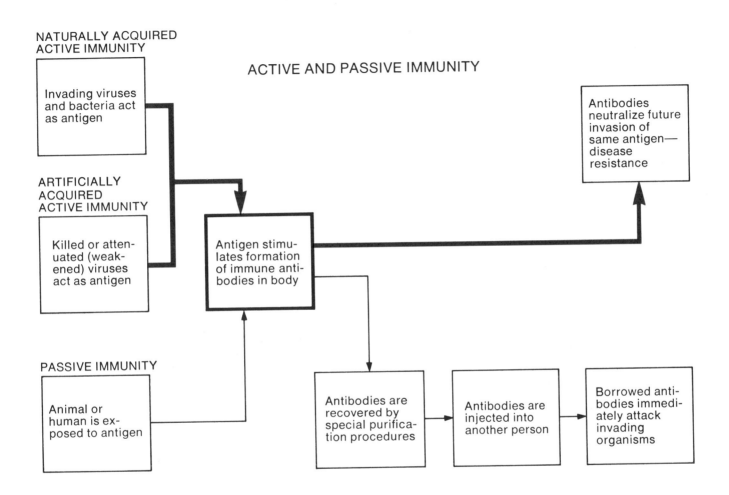

NATURALLY ACQUIRED
ACTIVE IMMUNITY

Invading viruses
and bacteria act
as antigen

ACTIVE AND PASSIVE IMMUNITY

ARTIFICIALLY
ACQUIRED
ACTIVE IMMUNITY

Killed or atten-
uated (weak-
ened) viruses
act as antigen

Antigen stimu-
lates formation
of immune anti-
bodies in body

Antibodies
neutralize future
invasion of
same antigen—
disease
resistance

PASSIVE IMMUNITY

Animal or
human is ex-
posed to antigen

Antibodies are
recovered by
special purifica-
tion procedures

Antibodies are
injected into
another person

Borrowed anti-
bodies immedi-
ately attack
invading
organisms

295

sumed the individual has a sufficient number of circulating antibodies. The Schick test is read 4 days after injection and the Dick test 1 day after injection. Other examples of skin tests are tuberculosis testing—Tine, PPD, Mantoux—and skin tests for blastomycosis and histoplasmosis.

Vaccines and doses are listed in Table 33-1.

Clinical Considerations

Parents should be encouraged to have infants and young children receive the vaccinations and immunizations suggested by their pediatrician or family physician. Those without a family physician should be given information regarding public health, city, or hospital clinics or physicians near their place of residence. Infectious diseases can be crippling or even fatal, and in some instances could have been prevented or lessened through an immunization program.

Those traveling outside the country should be encouraged to contact their physician and/or local health department regarding what precautions (if any) are to be taken and the immunizations (if any) that are required. Travelers should follow suggestions offered by the health department regarding health hazards of a particular country. Immunizations should be obtained *well in advance* of departure, as some vaccines require several weeks to produce adequate immunity.

Table 33-1.
VACCINES AND IMMUNIZATIONS

Vaccine	Type of Immunity	Dose Range	Route	Use and Comments
BCG vaccine (bacillus Calmette Guérin)	active	Intradermal: 0.1 ml. Multipuncture: 1 gt.	Intradermal or multipuncture method	Used only in those with negative tuberculin skin test. Skin test is administered 2-3 months after, to determine success of vaccination. USE: to provide active immunity to tuberculosis
botulism antitoxin	passive	Therapeutic: 10,000 U of bivalent types A and B	I.M., I.V.	Hypersensitivity test should be done prior to use. USE: treatment of botulism

Vaccine	Type of Immunity	Dose Range	Route	Use and Comments
cholera vaccine	active	0.5 ml. followed by 0.5-1 ml. 7-10 days later. Third dose of 1 ml. 7-10 days after second dose	S.C.	Immunity develops about 10 days after last injection and lasts 4-6 months. A stimulating dose of 1 ml. may be given every 6 months as needed. USE: to provide active immunity to cholera
diphtheria toxoid	active	0.5-1 ml. per dose. See comments	S.C.	Hypersensitivity test should be done prior to use. Precipitated and absorbed types require 2 doses, plain toxoid 3 doses, 3-4 weeks between each dose. USE: to provide active immunity to diphtheria
influenza vaccine	active	0.5-1 ml.	S.C.	Vaccines have been developed for various strains. Consult manufacturers' package inserts for doses. USE: to provide immunity to influenza. Period of immunity usually brief
measles virus vaccine, live, attenuated (Attenuvax)	active	0.5 ml.	S.C.	Some brands contain streptomycin, penicillin, neomycin. Immunity lasts 4+ years. May produce symptoms of measles (noncommunicable form). Immune globulin may be given at same time to reduce symptoms. Allergy to included drugs prevents use

Table 33-1. (Continued)

VACCINE	TYPE OF IMMUNITY	DOSE RANGE	ROUTE	USE AND COMMENTS
mumps vaccine, attenuated	active	1 vial	S.C. (use syringe provided by manufacturer)	USE: to provide immunity to mumps. Length of immunity 1-2+ years. Revaccinate about 1 month for antibody development
pertussis vaccine (whooping cough)	active	3 doses of 0.5-1 ml. 4-6 weeks apart	S.C., I.M.	USE: to provide immunity against pertussis. Does not always prevent an attack but may lessen severity
poliomyelitis vaccine, live oral poliovirus vaccine	active	MONOVALENT TYPE: each type administered separately at 4-6 week intervals and fourth reinforcing dose 8-12 months later. TRIVALENT TYPE: 3 dose series. Second dose 6-8 weeks after first. Third dose 8-12 months after second. Fourth dose may be given if vaccine administered to an infant. Ages of infant schedule: 8 weeks, 16 weeks, 32 weeks, 15-18 months	oral	USE: provides active immunization against poliomyelitis caused by types 1, 2, 3 poliovirus. Preferably given from November to May when interference enteroviruses are at a minimum (Enteroviruses may prevent multiplication of virus in G.I. tract which is necessary for development of immunity.) This is also called the Sabin vaccine
poliomyelitis vaccine	active	3 doses of 1 ml. each; second dose 4-6 weeks after first, third dose 7 months after second	I.M., S.C.	USE: to provide active immunity against poliomyelitis. Also called the Salk vaccine
rabies vaccine	active	1 dose daily × 14 days or 21 days	S.C. in abdomen, lower back, lateral aspect of thighs	USE: to promote immunity to rabies in those exposed or thought to be exposed. Booster given 10-20 days after initial series.

Vaccine	Type of Immunity	Dose Range	Route	Use and Comments
Rocky Mountain spotted fever vaccine	active	1 ml. × 3, 7-10 days apart	S.C.	USE: to promote immunity to Rocky Mountain spotted fever
smallpox vaccine	active	contents of 1 container	multiple skin puncture method	Clean skin first with acetone. World Health Organization defines 2 types of reactions. MAJOR REACTION: vesicular, pustular lesion or palpable induration. All other reactions are EQUIVOCAL REACTIONS and require repeat vaccination
tetanus toxoid	active	0.5-1 ml. according to label instructions × 3 at 3-4 week intervals	S.C.	USE: to provide active immunity to tetanus
tetanus antitoxin	passive	Therapeutic: 10,000-200,000 U I.V., 10,000-20,000 U injected into tissues. Prophylactic: 1,500-3,000 U S.C.	S.C., I.V., I.M.	HYPERSENSITIVITY TEST FOR HORSE SERUM BEFORE ADMINISTRATION. Known sensitivity to horse serum: DO NOT DO SKIN TEST OR GIVE ANTITOXIN
typhoid vaccine	active	0.5 ml. × 3 at 7-28 day intervals	S.C.	USE: to provide active immunization against typhoid
typhus vaccine	active	1 ml. × 2 at 7-10 day intervals	S.C.	USE: to provide active immunity against louse-borne typhus
yellow fever vaccine	active	0.5 ml.	S.C.	Available only through U.S. Public Health Service facilities and clinics approved by the Federal government

Table 33-1. (*Continued*)

Vaccine	Type of Immunity	Dose Range	Route	Use and Comments
COMBINED VACCINES				
diphtheria, tetanus toxoid, pertussis vaccine (D.P.T.)	active	0.5 ml. 4-6 weeks apart. Reinforcing dose 1 year later	S.C.	One vaccine for 3 disease immunities
tetanus and gas gangrene antitoxins	passive	1 vial repeated every 5-7 days as indicated	I.M., S.C.	HYPERSENSITIVITY TEST BEFORE ADMINISTRATION
typhoid and paratyphoid vaccines	active	0.5 ml. × 3 at 7-10 day intervals	S.C.	Combined vaccine may be given to those traveling to areas where both diseases are prevalent or to those living, working in, or in contact with both diseases.

Antiseptics and Disinfectants

Aseptic surgical technique was introduced by Lister although the use of antiseptics goes back to ancient civilizations. An **antiseptic** is an agent that stops, slows, or prevents the growth of microorganisms. A **disinfectant** is an agent that destroys microorganisms. The most important aspect of an antiseptic or disinfectant is its *effectiveness*.

Types, Uses, and Actions of Antiseptics and Disinfectants

ACIDS

Boric acid is a mild antiseptic and as a weak solution may be used as a wash, irrigation fluid, gargle, or eye solution. It is also available as an ointment or dusting powder. The liquid preparations are also used in the form of wet dressings or soaks. Continual application of full strength boric acid powder or solution to large denuded areas can cause toxic reactions and death due to the absorption of the boric acid. The effectiveness of boric acid is questionable.

Methenamine mandelate (Mandelamine) is a salt of mandelic acid and methenamine. This oral drug is rapidly absorbed, and excreted in the urine. Methenamine, in the pres-

Chapter

34

Antiseptics, Disinfectants, and Other Locally Acting Agents

ence of *acid* urine, breaks down into ammonia and formaldehyde—the latter of which is bactericidal. Mandelic acid acidifies the urine and also has bacterial action. This drug is effective only in acid urine; therefore it is essential that foods capable of making the urine alkaline be avoided *or* an acid-forming agent such as ammonium chloride be administered. Methenamine mandelate is used in the treatment of urinary tract infections, usually along with other antibiotic agents. It is especially useful for long-term therapy because of the low incidence of side effects and because bacterial resistance to formaldehyde does not appear to occur.

Nalidixic acid (NegGram) is also used for urinary tract infections. This drug is excreted primarily in the urine and appears to inhibit the synthesis of DNA. Nalidixic acid is used to treat infections due to susceptible gram-negative bacteria.

ALCOHOL

Two forms of alcohol may be used as surface antiseptics—ethyl alcohol, usually as 70% solution, and isopropyl alcohol, full strength. Both alcohols are used to cleanse the skin prior to venipuncture and parenteral injections.

DYES

Dyes are used as antiseptics and diagnostic agents. One dye, phenazopyridine hydrochloride (Pyridium) is an azo dye taken orally. This agent has urinary analgesic action and provides a soothing effect on bladder mucosa (innermost lining). It is used, often in conjunction with urinary antibiotics, to treat bladder infections. Burning, frequency, and urgency often accompany a bladder infection. The action of phenazopyridine helps to relieve these symptoms. Being a dye, this drug will color the urine a reddish-orange. A combination of phenazopyridine and methenamine mandelate (Azo-Mandelamine) is also used to treat urinary tract infections, the methenamine providing antiseptic activity and the phenazopyridine analgesic activity.

Gentian violet is used topically to treat vaginal infections caused by *Candida albicans* (see Chapter 18). Gentian violet as well as other dyes may also be used as a skin-marking agent during radiation therapy.

Fluorescein, sulfobromophthalein (Bromsulphalein—B.S.P.), and phenolsulfonphthalein (P.S.P.) dyes are used as diagnostic agents. Fluorescein is placed in the eye for detection of foreign objects and corneal ulcers. Sulfobromophthalein (B.S.P.) is used as a diagnostic test of liver function, and phenolsulfonphthalein (P.S.P.) for kidney function.

FURANS

Three furan derivatives possess antibacterial activity: nitrofurantoin (Furadantin), nitrofurazone (Furacin), and furazolidone (Furoxone). Nitrofurantoin macrocrystals (Macrodantin) and nitrofurantoin (Furadantin) are essentially the same except for the size of the drug crystals, and are both used in the treatment of urinary tract infections due to susceptible organisms. Nitrofurazone (Furacin) is available as a powder, ointment, cream, solution, and as a gauze impregnated with the drug. Nitrofurazone is used in the treatment of second- and third-degree burns and skin grafts. The prepackaged sterile gauze dressing may be applied to burned areas, skin grafts, and large abraded areas. This drug is also available as urethral inserts, for use before and after urethral instrumentation. Furazolidone (Furoxone) is used in the treatment of diarrhea caused by bacteria or protozoa. The furan derivatives exert antibacterial activity against susceptible organisms.

HALOGENS

A halogen is any element that combines with hydrogen to form an acid or metal to form a salt. Iodine, bromine, chlorine, and fluorine are halogens. Iodine, as tincture of iodine (2% iodine and 2% sodium iodide diluted with alcohol) is a topical antiseptic. Iodine solution contains the same ingredients as tincture of iodine except that water is the diluent rather than alcohol. The former agent is less irritating when applied to cuts or abraded areas. Povidone-iodine (Betadine) is another form of iodine which is an iodophor—the combination of iodine and an agent that makes the iodine more soluble in water. The mechanism of action of iodine is unknown, but it does exert antibacterial action against many types of bacteria, fungi, and viruses, when applied topically.

HEAVY METALS AND THEIR SALTS

Mercury compounds used topically as antiseptics include merbromin (Mercurochrome), thimerosal (Merthiolate), ammoniated mercury ointment, and nitromersol (Metaphen). At best, mercurial compounds appear to be only fair antiseptics and have largely been replaced by more effective agents.

Silver nitrate is used both as an antiseptic and as a caustic agent for the removal of excess granulation tissue. See Chapter 31 for the action, uses, and side effects of silver compounds.

Zinc oxide is used as a paste, powder, or ointment. This agent has a toughening action on the skin. It may be applied over bony prominences to prevent skin breakdown and around colostomy and ileostomy stomas and draining fistulas in an effort to prevent skin breakdown caused by draining fecal matter.

OXIDIZING AGENTS

An oxidizing agent releases free oxygen which in turn is germicidal. The germicidal effect of oxygen varies, but oxygen is especially effective against anaerobic organisms. Three oxidizing agents are hydrogen peroxide, potassium permanganate, and zinc peroxide. Hydrogen peroxide rapidly gives off oxygen (as seen by its foaming effect) and is useful in cleansing wounds and removing mucus and food particles from the oral cavity. It may also be used in the treatment of Vincent's infection. Hydrogen peroxide can also be used on inanimate objects and may be used to remove mucus and purulent material from instruments and objects such as tracheostomy tubes. When used to cleanse wounds or rid the oral cavity of food and/or debris it should be diluted as one part hydrogen peroxide to two or four parts water—that is, 1:2 or 1:4.

Potassium permanganate ($KMnO_4$), a deep purple crystal that is soluble in water, is used in varying strengths. This preparation is applied topically, as well as employed as a bladder irrigant and vaginal douche. Solutions stronger than 1:5000 may be irritating to the tissues, therefore a 1:5000 or 1:10,000 strength is usually used in the bladder or vagina. Like hydrogen peroxide, free oxygen is liberated on contact. When the potassium permanganate solution turns brown, it has lost its oxygen.

Phenol (carbolic acid) is rarely used today except perhaps in areas where other disinfectants are unobtainable. Phenol is irritating to the tissues. Cresol is a derivative of phenol and is used to disinfect inanimate objects such as eating utensils, bedpans, basins, and sinks. Resorcinol is both bactericidal and antifungal and is used topically in the treatment of ringworm, fungus, eczema, and other skin disorders. Hexylresorcinol is an anthelmintic and is discussed more fully in Chapter 20. Hexachlorophene is a chlorinated phenol and has been used as a preparation for reducing the bacterial flora present on the skin. Due to its possible toxic effects if absorbed systemically, use has been curtailed.

SURFACE-ACTIVE AGENTS

Surface-active agents are those which change surface tension, aiding in the removal of dirt and bacteria. Some of these agents may also be bactericidal against some organisms. Benzalkonium chloride (Zephiran) is used as a (1) topical antiseptic for cuts, wounds, and lacerations (2) bladder irrigant (3) wet dressing for wounds and skin ulcers, and (4) disinfectant for utensils and instruments.

Side Effects of Antiseptics and Disinfectants

Boric acid use can cause toxic effects when applied full strength over large areas of the body. The solution should *not* be left on the patient's bedside stand (especially in pediatric units) unless colored with a vegetable dye. Taken internally this agent can be poisonous.

If left in the patient's room, it is best placed in an area other than the bedside stand, kept tightly capped, and labeled "DO NOT DRINK."

Methenamine mandelate (Mandelamine) and phenazopyridine hydrochloride (Pyridium) have few side effects. Occasionally a patient may experience gastrointestinal side effects.

The use of nalidixic acid (NegGram) for *more than* two weeks necessitates periodic blood counts and renal and liver function tests. This drug is capable of causing side effects, notably central nervous system and gastrointestinal in nature. False-positive reactions for glucose may be obtained if Clinitest Reagent tablets, Benedict's, or Fehling's solutions are used to test the urine for glucose. Use of Tes-Tape and Clinistix Reagent Strips will *not* result in false-positive reactions. Urine samples sent to the laboratory should be labeled to show the patient is receiving this drug.

Nitrofurantoin (Furadantin) and nitrofurantoin macrocrystals (Macrodantin) have the same side effects. Both agents are capable of causing gastrointestinal distress, which may be helped by a reduction in dose or administration of these drugs with food. It is recommended that both drugs be *given with food or milk* to minimize gastric distress. Macrodantin appears to be less irritating to the stomach for some patients. Hypersensitivity reactions can also occur.

Furazolidone (Furoxone) may cause gastrointestinal disturbances and hypersensitivity reactions. This drug is also capable of *monoamine oxidase inhibition* (see Chapter 28), especially if used in doses larger than recommended. The manufacturer also warns of the use of this drug in certain ethnic groups—Mediterranean,

Negro, and Near East origins—as hemolysis of red cells can occur. Occasionally patients may exhibit an Antabuse (disulfiram)-like reaction if alcohol is taken while on this medication. An Antabuse-alcohol reaction produces severe vomiting, throbbing headache, sweating, thirst, hypotension, blurred vision, mental confusion, tachycardia, respiratory difficulty, and chest pain. Patients receiving furazolidone (Furoxone) should be cautioned to avoid alcoholic beverages during therapy.

Potassium permanganate ($KMnO_4$) can be irritating to tissues, especially mucous membranes. Care must be taken that the correct concentrations are used when the drug is employed as a vaginal douche or bladder irrigant. This drug can also stain clothing, skin, and inanimate objects.

Clinical Considerations

Topical antiseptics such as iodine, silver nitrate, and dyes stain the skin and clothing and therefore care must be executed during their use. Watches and rings should be removed if these solutions are used on or near the hands, wrists, or arms. The patient's personal clothing should also be protected.

B.S.P. dye is given only by the intravenous route. If the drug extravasates into surrounding tissues, the arm should be immediately elevated and ice packs applied, as cellular destruction can result. This drug is given with extreme caution to those with an allergic history, asthmatics, or those who have had a prior occurrence of this drug extravasating into tissues, as anaphylactoid reactions have been known to occur.

Patients receiving phenazopyridine (Pyridium) should be told about the change in the color of their urine. As minor as this may seem, failure to mention this can create unnecessary anxiety in patients, since they may have no way of knowing if a drug or some other event is causing the urine to change color.

Sterile technique must be employed when Furacin gauze or ointment is applied to burned or abraded areas. The gauze can be handled with sterile gloves or forceps and should be applied according to the directions of the physician—that is, single layers, multiple layers, spread thinly, etc. Burn treatment centers usually have policies regarding the routine applications of this agent, but when it is applied in the emergency room or general hospital unit, first check to see if specific directions have been written.

Other Locally Acting Agents

Absorbable hemostatics are agents used to control bleeding. They are capable of being absorbed and therefore need not be removed from the area after bleeding has been controlled. This makes them useful for insertion into body cavities or deep wounds.

Enzymes are agents used to absorb fluid, blood, or purulent accumulations. Some are used topically whereas others are injectable solutions.

Types and Uses of Locally Acting Agents

Absorbable gelatin sponge (Gelfoam), oxidized cellulose (Oxcel), and thrombin are examples of absorbable hemostatic agents used to control capillary bleeding and oozing. Absorbable gelatin sponge and oxidized cellulose—which resembles gauze—may be left in surgical wounds or body cavities. Absorption will take place in approximately four to six weeks if gelatin sponge is used and in as little as two days and as long as six or more weeks with oxidized cellulose. The gelatin sponge should be moistened with isotonic normal saline immediately prior to use. Oxidized cellulose does not require moistening. Both products may be used in the control of bleeding in surgery as well as the control of superficial bleeding.

Thrombin, which comes from bovine plasma, is used only topically to control capillary bleeding. It is available as a powder and may be sprinkled on the area or may be dissolved in isotonic normal saline and then applied.

Enzymes have a rather limited use in medicine mainly because they have very specific actions and therefore specific uses. Enzymes are substances (complex proteins) that act as catalysts; that is, they induce a chemical change without themselves being changed. An example of a body enzyme is ptyalin. This enzyme, present in saliva, acts on starch. The end product is dextrin and maltose. Further down the digestive tract another enzyme, amylase, also performs the same task.

Hyaluronidase (Wydase) is an enzyme used to aid in the absorption of fluids. It is principally used to encourage absorption of fluids given by hypodermoclysis. Hypodermoclysis is used when veins are unavailable for the administration of intravenous fluids. As this method of administration causes subcutaneous swelling and pain, the enzyme is either added to the intravenous solution *or* injected subcutaneously at the site used (usually the thigh) prior to starting the infusion. Hyaluronidase can also be used to aid in the diffusion of local anesthetics, especially nerve block anesthesias. This drug must *not* be injected into infected areas, as it will aid in the spread of infection to surrounding tissues.

Streptokinase-streptodornase (Varidase) is used to remove clotted blood or purulent material in such conditions as empyema, hematomas, hemothorax, osteomyelitis, and infected wounds. This enzyme combination may be applied topically in the form of wet dressings or injected directly into a body cavity or wound. Used orally, in the form of buccal tablets, it is used in the treatment of edema due to an injury or infection.

Pancreatic dornase (Dornavac) is an enzyme administered by aerosol inhalation or as an irrigating solution. It is used to reduce the thickness and tenacity of sputum in diseases or conditions such as bronchiectasis, atelectasis, emphysema, chronic bronchial asthma, and pulmonary abscesses. This drug can be administered in conjunction with antibiotics, antihistamines, and adrenergic drugs.

Chymoral—a combination of chymotrypsin and trypsin—may be used for treatment of inflammation and edema after an episiotomy.

Side Effects of Locally Acting Agents

Occasionally gastrointestinal distress is noted with the use of the *oral* enzymes. Other side effects appear to be relatively rare.

Clinical Considerations

Patients receiving oral enzymes for localized inflammatory conditions and edema should be observed for any increase or decrease in symptoms. A decrease in symptoms may mean that the drug is effective, whereas an increase in symptoms may indicate a more serious event such as a spread of infection or bleeding or the development of an abscess. When agents are used topically and applied to open wounds or ulcers the area must be inspected for changes, that is, the color of drainage (if any), the wound edges, appearance of granulation tissue, etc. Again, any change must be made known to the physician, especially those changes involving the appearance or spread of infection.

If pancreatic dornase (Dornavac) is used in aerosol form, the general appearance of the patient's sputum *before* and *after* treatment will be of value in determining drug efficacy.

Table 34-1.
ANTISEPTICS, DISINFECTANTS, AND OTHER LOCALLY ACTING AGENTS

GENERIC NAME	TRADE NAME	USES	SIDE EFFECTS	DOSE RANGES
furazolidone	Furoxone	bacterial or protozoan diarrheas and enteritis caused by susceptible organisms	gastrointestinal distress, MAO inhibition (see Chapter 28), hypersensitivity reactions, Antabuse-like reaction to alcohol	100 mg. Q.I.D. orally; CHILD: 25-50 mg. Q.I.D.
methenamine mandelate	Mandelamine	recurring urinary tract infections	dysuria, gastrointestinal distress, rash	1 Gram Q.I.D. orally; CHILD over 5: ½ the adult dose
nalidixic acid	NegGram	urinary tract infections caused by susceptible organisms	drowsiness, weakness, headache, dizziness, vertigo, nausea, vomiting, diarrhea, abdominal pain, rash, urticaria, arthralgia, photosensitivity reactions, angioedema, false-positive urine test (sugar) with Benedict's, Fehling's, Clinitest	1 Gram Q.I.D. orally initially; may be reduced to 2 Grams daily after initial treatment; CHILD: 25 mg./lb./day in 4 equally divided doses initially; may be reduced to 15 mg./lb./day

Table 34-1. (*Continued*)

Generic Name	Trade Name	Uses	Side Effects	Dose Ranges
nitrofurantoin, nitrofurantoin macrocrystals	Furadantin, Macrodantin	same as nalidixic acid	nausea, vomiting, rash, diarrhea, urticaria, pruritus, hypersensitivity reactions, headache, dizziness, muscle ache, malaise, nystagmus	50-100 mg. Q.I.D. with food; CHILD: 5-7 mg./Kg./day in 4 divided doses
nitrofurazone	Furacin	topical antibacterial for second- and third-degree burns, skin grafting, urethritis, prophylaxis before and after urological procedures, bacterial vaginitis and cervicitis, prophylaxis before and after cervicovaginal surgery and radiation therapy	rare, occasionally skin reactions	TOPICALLY: apply as directed. Urethral inserts, vaginal cream, and suppositories: 1-2 × day
phenazopyridine hydrochloride	Pyridium	symptomatic relief of pain, burning, urgency, frequency, and other discomforts of the bladder and urethra	gastrointestinal disturbance; will change color of urine	200 mg. T.I.D. p.c. orally
phenazopyridine hydrochloride, methenamine mandelate	Azo-Mandelamine	urinary tract infections and relief of symptoms of infection	side effects of both products	2 tablets Q.I.D.

The history of anesthesia dates back to antiquity when narcotics (as raw opium) and alcohol were used to quiet the patient during surgical procedures. Modern anesthesia began with the discovery of nitrous oxide gas by Priestley in 1776. In 1779, Davy suggested the use of this gas for surgical procedures, but it was not used for this purpose until 1844.

In 1846 Morton demonstrated the anesthetic properties of ether and in 1847 Simpson used chloroform to produce anesthesia. In this century many new and highly capable anesthetic agents, increasing patient safety and comfort, have been introduced.

Types and Uses of Anesthetic Agents

There are two general types of anesthetic agents: **general anesthetics** and **local anesthetics**.

GENERAL ANESTHETIC AGENTS

PREANESTHETICS

Before general anesthesia is administered, a **preanesthetic agent** is usually given. The general purpose of preanesthetic agents is to *prepare the patient for anesthesia*. The more specific purposes of these agents are:

Chapter 35

Anesthetic Agents

1. to decrease anxiety and apprehension immediately prior to surgery. Almost every patient has some degree of anxiety prior to surgery, especially in the few hours before. The patient who is calm and less apprehensive can be anesthetized more quickly, usually requires a smaller dose of the induction agent, may require less anesthesia during surgery, and may have a smoother recovery (wakening) from anesthesia. The preanesthetic agent, then, sedates the patient, thereby decreasing anxiety and apprehension

2. to dry secretions of the respiratory tract. Anesthetic gases are somewhat irritating to the lining of the respiratory tract, thereby increasing mucus secretions. The ability to cough and/or swallow is lost during general anesthesia and these secretions could pool in the lungs

3. to lessen the undesirable side effects of anesthesia—for example, nausea and vomiting.

The preanesthetic agent is usually chosen by the anesthesiologist and may consist of one or more drugs. (See Table 35-1.) The type of agent selected may be based on the patient's physical condition and/or disease or condition present, allergies (if any) to certain types of drugs, past history of anesthesia, type of surgery, type of anesthetic agents to be used, and the age, sex, and weight of the patient. The anesthesiologist may, for example, choose a tranquilizer that has both sedative *and* antiemetic properties and may combine this with a cholinergic blocking agent to dry secretions of the respiratory tract. In most hospitals an anesthesiologist will see the patient the day before surgery, although this might not be possible for emergency surgeries. The patient's physical status is evaluated and an explanation of how the patient will be anesthetized (geared to the patient's understanding) may be given at this time. At times patients will have many questions. Proper and adequate explanation of surgery and what will occur the morning or afternoon before surgery will often help to allay *some* of the apprehension experienced by the patient and/or family.

Table 35-1.
PREANESTHETIC AGENTS

GENERIC NAME	TRADE NAME
NARCOTICS	
meperidine	Demerol
morphine	
BARBITURATES	
pentobarbital	Nembutal
secobarbital	Seconal
TRANQUILIZERS	
chlorpromazine	Thorazine
hydroxyzine	Vistaril
perphenazine	Trilafon
prochlorperazine	Compazine
promethazine	Phenergan
triflupromazine	Vesprin
CHOLINERGIC BLOCKING AGENTS	
atropine	
scopolamine	

General surgical anesthesia is divided into four stages:

STAGE I—stage of analgesia
STAGE II—stage of delirium
STAGE III—stage of surgical anesthesia
STAGE IV—stage of respiratory paralysis

Induction is a part of Stage I anesthesia and begins with the administration of an anesthetic agent and lasts until consciousness is lost. With some *induction agents*, such as the short-acting barbiturates, this stage may last only 5-10 seconds.

Stage II, the stage of delirium, is also brief when modern anesthetic agents are used. During this stage the patient may move about and mumble incoherently. The muscles are somewhat rigid. The patient is unconscious and cannot feel pain, yet if surgery were attempted at this stage there would be a physical reaction to painful stimuli.

Stage III, the stage of surgical anesthesia, is divided into four planes (or substages). The anesthesiologist differentiates these planes by the character of the respirations, eye movements, certain reflexes, pupil size, etc. At Plane 2 or 3 the patient is usually ready for the surgical procedure.

SHORT-ACTING INTRAVENOUS
BARBITURATES
hexobarbital (Evipal)
methohexital (Brevital)
thiopental (Pentothal)

Stage IV, the stage of respiratory paralysis, is a rare and dangerous state. At this stage respiratory arrest and cessation of all vital signs may occur.

INTRAVENOUS ANESTHETICS

The short-acting barbiturates are usually used as induction anesthetics. They may also be used as the sole anesthetic agent for brief procedures such as the extraction of teeth. These agents have a rapid onset of action, in many instances a matter of a few seconds. Barbiturates are poor analgesic agents and if no other anesthetic agent is given, the patient may *physically* react to painful stimuli though he will not be consciously aware of the pain or remember the experience. Barbiturates are rapidly detoxified by the liver and because of this are contraindicated in those with liver disease. Hypotension follows an injection of these agents and consequently they cannot be used for patients in shock, as might be seen in an automobile accident victim needing emergency surgery.

GASEOUS ANESTHETICS

Nitrous oxide, once called "laughing gas," is the oldest gas anesthetic. It is nonflammable and almost odorless. Nitrous oxide is a weak anesthetic agent and can produce only upper Stage III anesthesia. The advantages of nitrous oxide are that it has a rapid induction, can be used in emergencies (when barbiturates cannot be used), recovery is rapid, minimal postoperative nausea is seen (as compared to other agents), and it has a relatively wide margin of safety. The disadvantages are poor muscle relaxation and minimal potency when used alone.

Cyclopropane was first used in 1933. This gaseous anesthetic has an ether-like odor and is highly flammable and explosive. The advantage of cyclopropane is that it can be used in those who are poor surgical risks, including patients in shock. The disadvantages are the development of cardiac arrhythmias, bronchospasm, and respiratory depression, the high incidence of postrecovery nausea and vomiting, and its explosive and inflammatory nature.

VOLATILE ANESTHETICS

These anesthetic agents are liquids at room temperature, but easily evaporate.

Ether has a characteristic and for most patients an unpleasant odor. Used alone, it is a slow induction agent causing extreme activity and restlessness during Stage II. Ether is rarely used alone and is usually combined with other anesthetic agents. The advantage of ether is that it is a versatile anesthetic that can be given in special situations, with simple equipment. There is also the advantage of the emergency administration of ether by nonanesthetist personnel. For example, it could be used for emergency surgery on a small ship and administered by a pharmacist's mate. Ether also stabilizes heart action, increases the heart rate and blood pressure, and dilates smooth muscle. The disadvantages of ether are its slow induction and recovery rate, the high incidence of postrecovery nausea and vomiting, its inflammatory and explosive nature, and the excitement occurring during induction.

Chloroform is a nonflammable volatile anesthetic. It is rarely used today, mainly because of its toxic effect on the liver. The advantages of chloroform are (1) it is a nonflammable agent and (2) it has rapid induction and emergence qualities. The disadvantages are (1) a high incidence of cardiac arrhythmias and (2) toxicity to the liver.

Fluothane (halothane) is a nonflammable volatile anesthetic that is usually used with other agents to maintain surgical anesthesia. It can be used alone for brief surgical procedures. Fluothane has a rapid induction and emergence. The advantages of this agent are (1) it is nonflammable (2) induction is rapid, and (3) emergence is rapid. The disadvantages are (1) poor relaxation and analgesia (2) cardiac arrhythmias may develop during use, and (3) rare instances of liver damage have been reported.

The liver damage produced by Fluothane appears to occur the *second* time the patient receives this particular anesthetic. Apparently, liver sensitivity develops in some patients, and when the anesthetic is repeated at a later time, liver damage results.

Penthrane (methoxyflurane) was first used about 1960. This agent produces good relaxation and analgesia in light surgical anesthesia. In low concentrations, Penthrane is nonflammable; however in high concentrations it is flammable. Induction and emergence is very slow, and ultra-short-acting barbiturates are usually used for induction. The advantages of Penthrane are (1) it is nonflammable (except in high concentrations) and (2) it is capable of producing good analgesia and muscle relaxation. The disadvantages are (1) the slow induction and emergence period and (2) rare occurrences of liver toxicity.

Vinethene (vinyl ether) is a volatile liquid similar to ether. It is given by the open drop method (i.e., the liquid is dropped on a face mask). Vinethene has a very rapid induction, and emergence is also rapid. It is usually used as a short-duration anesthetic. The advantages of this anesthetic agent are its rapid induction and emergence properties. The disadvantages are (1) it is a flammable agent and (2) it is liver toxic. Liver toxicity appears to occur if the anesthetic is used longer than one-half hour.

Trilene (trichloroethylene) has an odor similar to chloroform and a blue vegetable dye is added to the liquid to distinguish it from chloroform. This agent may be used as a "self-administered" anesthetic, by means of a hand-held inhaler mask. Induction and emergence are relatively short and analgesia can be produced without loss of consciousness.

NEUROLEPT ANALGESICS

Neurolept analgesics are agents that produce analgesia, or relief from pain, without a total loss of consciousness. Innovar, a neurolept analgesic agent, contains Sublimaze (fentanyl), which is a narcotic, and Inapsine (droperidol) a major tranquilizer. The effects of Innovar are shown in Table 35-2.

Sublimaze produces an effect in approximately 8-10 minutes after intramuscular injection and 2-3 minutes after intravenous injection. Inapsine produces sleepiness and detachment in approximately 5-10 minutes after intravenous administration.

The patient receiving this type of anesthesia will appear detached from his surroundings. There is no loss of consciousness but the patient will appear somnolent. Painful stimuli do not reach the higher nerve centers of the brain because of the selective action of

Table 35-2.
EFFECTS OF INNOVAR

EFFECTS OF SUBLIMAZE (FENTANYL) (A NARCOTIC)	EFFECTS OF INAPSINE (DROPERIDOL) (A MAJOR TRANQUILIZER)
CENTRAL NERVOUS SYSTEM	
potent analagesia	marked tranquilizing properties
weak emetic	potent antiemetic
	potentiates action of depressants
MUSCULAR	
skeletal muscle rigidity	
CARDIOVASCULAR	
bradycardia	peripheral dilatation
	mild transient hypotension
	alpha adrenergic blocking activity
	no myocardial depression
RESPIRATIONS	
marked depression	very little effect

these drugs on the thalamus, hypothalamus, and reticular formation.

The effects of Inapsine may last as long as 24 hours; however, the usual duration is 6-12 hours.

Innovar may be used as a preoperative medication, as an induction agent, and as an adjunct to general and spinal anesthesia. Inapsine (droperidol) and Sublimaze (fentanyl) can also be used separately rather than as the combined agent Innovar. Inapsine may be used as a preoperative medication and during induction of anesthesia. It also is an antianxiety, antiemetic, and tranquilizing agent that may be used during regional anesthesia. For example, the anesthesiologist may administer Inapsine during spinal (which is a regional) anesthesia. Sublimaze may be used preoperatively and postoperatively as well as during surgery whenever a potent analgesic agent is required.

DISSOCIATIVE ANESTHETICS

Ketamine (Ketalar) may be used for surgical and diagnostic procedures that do not require skeletal muscle relaxation, as an induction agent, or as an adjunct to other anesthetic agents.

Patients emerging from ketamine anesthesia may have vivid dreams, hallucinations, delirium, excitement, and irrational behavior. The patient may recall the

Table 35-3.
NEUROMUSCULAR BLOCKING AGENTS

GENERIC NAME	TRADE NAME
NONDEPOLARIZING	
benzoquinonium chloride	Mytolon
dimethyl tubocurarine chloride	Mecostrin
dimethyl tubocurarine iodide	Metubine
gallamine triethiodide	Flaxedil
tubocurarine chloride	Tubarine
DEPOLARIZING	
decamethonium bromide	Syncurine
succinylcholine chloride	Anectine

anesthetic as an unpleasant experience because of these psychotropic effects. Recurrences of these experiences have been recorded up to 24 hours after surgery. These reactions may be reduced if the patient is not disturbed and surrounding stimuli (noise, lights, etc.) are kept to a minimum. Cardiac arrhythmias, hypo- or hypertension, respiratory depression, nausea, emesis, and tonic and clonic movements resembling convulsive seizures may also occur.

NEUROMUSCULAR BLOCKING AGENTS

Neuromuscular blocking agents are used during anesthesia to relax skeletal muscles. General anesthetic agents are usually poor muscle relaxants; consequently other drugs must be used to facilitate surgical procedures—especially those of the abdomen.

The crude form of curare, although not used today, is the forerunner of neuromuscular blocking agents. South American Indians used curare-laden arrows to kill wild game. The curare paralyzed the victim's skeletal muscles, including the muscles of respiration. This resulted in death by asphyxia.

During anesthesia, neuromuscular blocking agents are given intravenously, and their effect is rapid. Respiratory support—by means of a respirator—must be given as the patient cannot breath on his own. Muscle relaxants do not have anesthetic properties.

There are two types of neuromuscular blocking agents: nondepolarizing (or curariform) and depolarizing. (See Table 35-3.) Nondepolarizing agents compete for acetylcholine at myoneural (nerve/muscle) junctions of skeletal muscle. The depolarizing agents occupy myoneural junctions and prolong depolarization by being unaffected by the action of acetylcholinesterase. (See also Chapter 4 for the action of acetylcholine and acetylcholinesterase in nerve impulse transmission.)

Neuromuscular blocking agents mainly affect skeletal muscles, first affecting muscles of the eyes, eyelids, and fingers and toes. Then the larger muscles of the arms, legs, and abdomen are affected and finally the diaphragm and intercostal muscles, with subsequent respiratory paralysis and apnea. The margin between the dose required to first show drug effects and the dose required for respiratory paralysis is very narrow; thus respiratory support is necessary.

Since large doses of gases or volatile anesthetic agents are necessary to produce muscle relaxation, use of these agents allows for lighter (i.e., less) anesthesia. Additionally, these agents can be used to facilitate the insertion of an endotracheal tube.

Antagonists used to stop the action of nondepolarizing neuromuscular blocking agents are cholinergic agents—edrophonium (Tensilon) and neostigmine (Prostigmin). These drugs are used when the anesthesiologist wishes to terminate the action of nondepolarizing agents. They are of *no value* for reversing the effects of the depolarizing agents, which because of the relatively short action do not require an antagonist.

LOCAL ANESTHETICS

A local anesthetic temporarily blocks pain sensations in a specific area. Except for cocaine, local anesthetics are synthetic preparations.

When a local anesthetic agent is injected into a specific part, sensory and autonomic fibers are first affected, followed by larger motor fibers. The higher the concentration of the drug the more rapid the onset of action. The duration of anesthesia is also prolonged when higher drug concentrations are utilized. The local anesthetic is injected around a nerve or nerve ending(s), the drug being concentrated in a small area.

Local anesthetics can be administered three ways:

1. They may be applied *topically* to the skin or mucous membranes. The anesthetic may be a liquid, ointment, cream, jelly, or powder. Some solutions may be applied as an aerosol spray. The topical method of administration gives minimal analgesia to small areas. This method may be used to relieve pain and itching as well as provide local analgesia to mucous membranes. Some examples of use are in sunburn, insect bites, and prior to urological examinations and minor surgical procedures of the mucous membranes of the eye, nose, and throat

2. *Infiltration* around nerve fibers provides analgesia to a small area but also affects deeper nerve fibers in subcutaneous tissues. Local anesthetics used for infiltration are available with epinephrine which will intensify the anesthetic effect and aid in the control of capillary bleeding, due to the vasoconstricting effects of epinephrine. Additionally, this effect prevents systemic ab-

sorption of the anesthetic agent, which could lead to serious drug reactions. Some examples of the use of this method of local anesthesia are in suturing of small wounds and lacerations, removal of superficial foreign bodies, removal of cysts, plantar warts, and moles, dentistry, and minor E.N.T. procedures

3. *Nerve block anesthesia* is the injection of a local anesthetic agent close to large nerve trunks or near nerve plexi. This method of local anesthesia may be used for surgery of the foot or hand. A more extensive nerve block is a spinal anesthetic. The local anesthetic agent is injected into the subarachnoid space of the spinal cord. There are different types of spinal anesthetics: high spinal anesthetics, low spinal anesthetics, caudal anesthetics, and saddle blocks.

LOCAL ANESTHETIC AGENTS

benzocaine
bupivacaine hydrochloride (Marcaine)
chloroprocaine hydrochloride (Nesacaine)
cocaine
cyclomethycaine (Surfacaine)
dibucaine hydrochloride (Nupercaine)
lidocaine (Xylocaine)
mepivacaine hydrochloride (Carbocaine)
prilocaine hydrochloride (Citanest)
procaine hydrochloride (Novocain)
tetracaine hydrochloride (Pontocaine)

Clinical Considerations

The physician may require assistance in the administration of local anesthetics. The required equipment should be obtained and placed on an accessible and sturdy table or Mayo stand. The patient must be placed in a position for the administration of the anesthetic. The physician will usually describe the desired position of the patient and/or the extremity involved. The patient may require physical restraint and/or support while the local anesthetic is administered. If the patient appears anxious, he should be reassured. If at all possible, the materials used for administration of the local anesthetic should be away from the patient's line of vision, as viewing of the preparations prior to administration, as well as the instruments used, creates unnecessary anxiety. Trays with the required equipment should be assembled away from the patient area, and brought to the area covered. If it is necessary to assemble the tray near the patient, it should be done out of the patient's line of vision—such as behind the head of the bed or cart.

When holding the bottle containing the local anesthetic while the physician withdraws the solution, make sure the label *faces* the physician so the drug and strength can be visibly checked. It is also advantageous to state the name and the strength at the time the physician fills the syringe. This double check (visual and auditory) may help eliminate any error of mistaken identity. After administration of a local anesthetic the patient should be observed for side effects, namely nausea, vomiting, pallor, hypotension, tachycardia, respiratory difficulty, and convulsions.

Diseases or injury to the musculoskeletal system may be major—requiring hospitalization or intensive and prolonged drug therapy—or minor—requiring no more than a mild analgesic such as aspirin.

A variety of drugs may be used to treat the many types of musculoskeletal disorders. These drugs may have a wide range of effects, from the relief of minor pain and discomfort to the delay of joint destruction and crippling of rheumatoid arthritis.

Types, Uses, and Actions of Agents Used in the Treatment of Musculoskeletal Disorders

The **salicylates** are used in the treatment of bone and joint diseases, for example, osteoarthritis, bursitis, and rheumatoid arthritis. Pain associated with muscle strains and minor musculoskeletal injuries such as sprains also respond to salicylate therapy.

Aspirin (acetylsalicylic acid) and sodium salicylate are two of the most commonly used agents of the salicylate group. Beside providing analgesia, both drugs are capable of relieving swelling, inflammation, stiffness, and fever. The anti-inflammatory action of the salicylates is not clearly understood, but those with rheumatic conditions often experience

Drugs Used in the Management of Musculoskeletal Disorders

relief with the use of these agents. This anti-inflammatory effect does not cure arthritis but *may* delay the crippling effects of this disease. The antipyretic effect of the salicylates also reduces the fever that may accompany some forms of arthritis. Chapter 7 discusses the action and effects of these drugs in more detail.

Phenylbutazone (Butazolidin) and **oxyphenbutazone** (Tandearil) are pyrazolone derivatives used in the treatment of rheumatoid arthritis, bursitis, and similar disorders. These agents are also used in the treatment of gout but appear to be of value only during acute attacks. The precise mechanism of action is not clearly understood. Although both drugs are analgesics, they are not used for the relief of minor pain because of their ability to cause serious side effects. Both drugs are usually used when the patient does not respond to less toxic agents. Sulfinpyrazone (Anturane) is related to phenylbutazone and is used in the prevention and treatment of gouty arthritis. It is a uricosuric agent—that is, it promotes the excretion of uric acid.

Colchicine is a drug that has been in use for several hundred years for the treatment of gout. This agent can be used for acute gout and as a prophylactic agent to prevent recurrent attacks. When a drug is given to prevent recurrent attacks of gout this is usually called interval therapy.

The exact mechanism of action of colchicine is unknown, although it appears to reduce the inflammation resulting from the deposit of urate crystals around joints. The drug itself has no analgesic properties, but its ability to relieve pain associated with gout appears to lie in its anti-inflammatory action.

Allopurinol (Zyloprim) is also an antigout agent. This drug interferes with the final steps of uric acid formation. Gout is a metabolic disease in which there is a defect in purine metabolism. This defect results in elevated uric acid blood levels and a deposit of uric acid (or urate) crystals in cartilage—especially around the joints. By inhibiting the formation of uric acid, allopurinol has the ability to prevent gout. It is of no value in the treatment of acute attacks and therefore is used as interval therapy.

Probenecid (Benemid) is an agent chemically related to the sulfonamides and is used in the treatment of gout and gouty arthritis. This drug is a uricosuric agent—that is, a compound capable of *promoting* or increasing the urinary excretion of uric acid. This agent also *inhibits* or delays the excretion of penicillin and amino-salicylic acid (PAS—an antitubercular agent) and therefore may be used to increase and prolong blood levels of these two drugs.

Indomethacin (Indocin) is an anti-inflammatory, antipyretic, and analgesic agent used in the treatment of severe rheumatoid arthritis, rheumatoid spondylitis, osteoarthritis of the hip, and gouty arthritis. This drug can cause severe adverse effects; therefore it is *not* employed as a simple analgesic agent. Use of this drug is recommended in those who do not respond to other agents.

Gold salts, aurothioglucose (Solganal) and gold sodium thiomalate (Myochrysine), are used in the treatment of active rheumatoid arthritis. The mechanism of action of the gold salts is not known.

Corticosteroids are widely used in the treatment of various musculoskeletal disorders. These drugs may be taken orally, parenterally, or injected in or near joints or bursae. Dexamethasone (Decadron) is an example of a corticosteroid used to treat various musculoskeletal disorders. As dexamethasone sodium phosphate, this drug can be injected into intra-articular spaces as well as given by the intramuscular or intravenous routes. The potent anti-inflammatory action of this drug makes it useful in treating conditions such as rheumatoid arthritis, bursitis, tenosynovitis, acute gouty arthritis, and ankylosing spondylitis. The various actions of corticosteroid agents are discussed in Chapter 21.

Skeletal muscle relaxants may also be used in the treatment of skeletal muscle disorders. These agents are centrally acting; that is, their site of action is the central nervous system rather than peripheral structures such as bones, muscles, or peripheral nerves. The precise mechanism of action is not clear, but some appear to depress various areas of the central nervous system—namely the thalamus, basal ganglia, brain stem, and spinal cord neurons.

Chlorphenesin (Maolate) appears to act on the brain stem and spinal cord and is used to reduce muscle spasm in such conditions as back sprains and bursitis. The effect of this drug is relatively brief. Carisoprodol (Soma) is a drug related to meprobamate (Miltown), a minor tranquilizer. The action and use of this drug are similar to chlorphenesin.

The beneficial effect of this group of drugs appears to vary. Some patients note decided relief, whereas others obtain only minimal relief.

Tranquilizers, especially diazepam (Valium) may also be used as muscle relaxants. Diazepam has been used in the treatment of muscle spasm and back strain. In some patients better results are obtained in the use of tranquilizers with muscle-relaxing properties than with the use of skeletal muscle relaxants. At times, other tranquilizers may be used to relieve the anxiety that might be associated with certain orthopedic conditions.

Side Effects of Drugs Used in Musculoskeletal Disorders

The side effects of salicylates, corticosteroids, tranquilizers and gold salts have been discussed in Chapters 7, 21, 28, and 31 respectively.

Phenylbutazone (Butazolidin) and oxyphenbutazone (Tandearil) are potentially toxic agents capable of creating serious and potentially fatal side effects. The side effects of these drugs are as follows:

ALLERGIC REACTIONS: anaphylactic reactions, arthralgia, fever, Stevens-Johnson syndrome, urticaria

CARDIOVASCULAR: hypertension

CENTRAL NERVOUS SYSTEM: agitation, confusion, lethargy

EYE/EAR: blurred vision, hearing loss

FLUID/ELECTROLYTE DISTURBANCES: edema, metabolic acidosis, respiratory alkalosis, sodium and chloride retention

GASTROINTESTINAL: diarrhea, gastritis, gastrointestinal bleeding, nausea and vomiting, ulceration of colon, ulcerative stomatitis

HEMOPOIETIC: agranulocytosis, aplastic and hemolytic anemia, leukemia, pancytopenia, thrombocytopenia

KIDNEY: oliguria and anuria, proteinuria and hematuria, renal failure, renal stones
LIVER: hepatitis
METABOLIC/ENDOCRINE: hyperglycemia, toxic goiter
SKIN: erythema nodosum, pruritus, rash

Gastrointestinal side effects may be minimized by giving these drugs with food. These drugs also potentiate the action of insulin and the oral hypoglycemic sulfonylureas—tolbutamide (Orinase), tolazamide (Tolinase), chlorpropamide (Diabinese), and acetohexamide (Dymelor)—therefore an adjustment in the dose of these drugs may be necessary. It is recommended that complete blood counts be taken every one to two weeks because of potentially serious hematological changes. Patients should also be warned to report *any* unusual symptoms immediately. This includes blurred vision, sore throat, weight gain, changes in the color of the stool or urine, and the appearance of skin or oral lesions. Appropriate references should be consulted if any symptom or patient complaint is noted.

Sulfinpyrazone (Anturane), though related to phenylbutazone, appears to be less toxic. Most side effects are related to the gastrointesinal tract. Taking the drug with meals may lessen these symptoms. This drug also potentiates the action of insulin and the oral hypoglycemic sulfonylurea agents. Salicylates *antagonize* the action of this drug and therefore should *not* be taken concurrently.

The side effects of colchicine are chiefly related to the gastrointestinal tract. When therapy for an acute attack of gout is initiated the drug is given every 1-2 hours *until* nausea, vomiting, or diarrhea occurs *or* until pain is relieved. The appearance of any of these effects indicates that therapy is to be terminated. The patient is then placed on a dose schedule ranging from daily to 1-4 times per week. Usually several days are allowed to elapse before instituting interval therapy. A uricosuric agent such as probenecid (Benemid) may also be administered concurrently during interval therapy. Gastrointestinal side effects may become *severe*; therefore it is important that therapy for acute attacks be stopped *immediately* when the pain is relieved *or* gastrointestinal side effects *first* appear.

The most common side effect of allopurinol (Zyloprim) is skin rash, which may be mild or take more severe forms such as exfoliative dermatitis, purpura, or the Stevens-Johnson syndrome. Gastrointestinal distress and drug idiosyncrasy consisting of fever, chills, joint pain, and leukopenia may also be seen.

Probenecid (Benemid) may cause gastrointestinal side effects, hypersensitivity reactions, sore gums, dizziness, and anemia. Use of salicylates is contraindicated because they antagonize the uricosuric effects of this drug. If a mild analgesic is necessary, acetaminophen (Tylenol) may be used.

Indomethacin (Indocin) is a potentially toxic drug capable of causing severe gastrointestinal reactions. Ulcerations of the esophagus, stomach, duodenum, and small intestine have been reported. Any sign of gastrointestinal bleeding warrants stopping the drug. Hepatic, hematological, cardiovascular, renal, and dermatological effects as well as hypersensitivity reactions may also be seen.

Side effects of the skeletal muscle relaxants include gastrointestinal distress, dizziness, lightheadedness and drowsiness. The side effects for each agent are listed in Table 36-1.

Clinical Considerations

Many patients with musculoskeletal diseases and disorders experience varying degrees of pain. For some, changes in the weather or dampness may bring on a general stiffness or soreness of the affected joints. The patient with rheumatoid arthritis may have severe joint damage and be unable to perform even the simplest of daily tasks. Each patient with a musculoskeletal disorder will require drug therapy that will provide optimum benefit. And though some disorders cannot be cured, the progression of disease and/or symptoms may be controlled with the use of one or more drugs. Patient care is planned according to the disease or condition the patient has and the drug therapy or other measures (for example, physiotherapy) instituted.

The patient with severe rheumatoid arthritis, for example, will first need an evaluation of physical limitations—that is, can the patient perform routine daily activities, ambulate (with or without assistance); is any special assistance required such as combing the hair, cutting food, etc. The amount of pain associated with these activities must also be evaluated so that personnel understand how much the patient can do for himself and what must be done for the patient.

Once therapy for any musculoskeletal disorder has been instituted, personnel must observe the patient for changes (if any) in the patient's status. The patient with acute gout, for example, may show marked improvement several hours after therapy is begun, whereas the patient with arthritis may not show any change for days or weeks.

Many of these patients may have had a musculoskeletal disorder for many months or even years. Pain may be almost constant with only occasional periods of relief. This tends to have an emotional impact, and many of these patients may be depressed or demanding, or show little desire to help themselves. For some, progress is very slow and improvement at best gradual.

Discharge Teaching

Once the physician is satisfied with the patient's progress and feels that therapy can be continued at home, the patient is discharged. Discharge teaching is tailored to suit the individual patient and should include the following points concerning drug therapy:

1. THE SALICYLATES—taking salicylates in large doses may result in salicylism (see Chapter 7). These signs may already have been experienced, but explanation might still be necessary. The patient should be encouraged to report any side effects to the physician, as dose adjustment may be necessary. Equally important is letting the physician know of any changes, particularly a flare-up of symptoms of the disorder
2. PYRAZOLONE DERIVATIVES: PHENYLBUTAZONE (Butazolidin), OXYPHENBUTAZONE (Tandearil)—as these

drugs are capable of causing serious side effects, patients should be encouraged to keep physician or clinic appointments. This can be impressed on the patient by a statement such as, "Your physician will probably want to see you at regular intervals. It is important that you keep these appointments as this is the way he will check on what the drug(s) is doing for you." The physician may not want all of the side effects explained to the patient, but patients should be told to contact their physician if *any* unusual symptoms occur—no matter how unimportant they may seem

3. COLCHICINE—when the patient is discharged, interval therapy for gout will be instituted. The patient should be told to contact the physician if gastrointestinal symptoms should occur or if any further symptoms of gout become apparent. If a uricosuric agent is concurrently prescribed, the patient must understand the dose schedule of both drugs. Colchicine may not be taken daily but only 1-4 times per week, whereas the uricosuric agent may be prescribed to be taken daily. Although prescription containers are labeled by the pharmacist, the patient should still have this information repeated

4. ALLOPURINOL (Zyloprim)—the most common side effect of this drug appears to be skin rash—which may be mild to severe. As in all patient teaching, the physician may or may not want this (or other) side effects specifically mentioned. If this is the case, state that *any* unusual changes or symptoms should be reported to the physician—as soon as they occur. It is important that the patient not decide what the cause or reason for any change is, but leave this decision to the physician

5. PROBENECID (Benemid)—since the use of salicylates antagonizes the uricosuric effects of this drug, the patient should be told that aspirin or any *aspirin-like product or O.T.C. medication containing aspirin* should be avoided. Since aspirin might be contained in some of the "cold" medications (and listed as acetylsalicylic acid and not aspirin), it is best if the patient not purchase *any* drugs without first consulting the physician. This warning also applies to any drug prescribed by another physician, even one prescribed *before* institution of therapy. If it is suspected that the patient may be taking other medications, suggest that the patient either show these medications to the physician or have his druggist check with the physician *before* any of these medications are taken

6. INDOMETHACIN (Indocin)—this drug is also capable of causing serious toxic effects. Here again, the physician may not want the patient to know all of the possible effects that might occur during therapy. Again, encourage the patient to contact his physician

should unusual symptoms occur. The physician also has good reason for not informing patients of the long list of side effects of some of the drugs administered. Even though numerous side effects are listed in references, it does not mean that these side effects will occur in any one particular patient

7. TRANQUILIZERS—these drugs are capable of causing drowsiness, especially during the early part of therapy. The patient should be told that this occurs in many individuals and is part of the drug's action. Operation of hazardous machinery or driving an automobile should be avoided if *any* drowsiness or lethargy is noted. Alcoholic beverages are to be avoided as they potentiate the action of these drugs

8. SKELETAL MUSCLE RELAXANTS—like tranquilizers, these agents may also cause drowsiness and the same warnings apply. Occasionally, muscle weakness may be noted and this should be reported to the physician

Table 36-1.

DRUGS USED IN THE MANAGEMENT OF MUSCULOSKELETAL DISORDERS

GENERIC NAME	TRADE NAME	USES	SIDE EFFECTS	DOSE RANGES
allopurinol	Zyloprim	treatment of: gout, hyperuricemia associated with blood dyscrasias, recurrent uric acid stone formation, uric acid nephropathy in patients receiving cancer chemotherapeutic agents capable of elevating serum uric acid levels	skin manifestations, nausea, vomiting, diarrhea, drug idiosyncrasy	200-800 mg. daily in single or divided doses orally
aspirin		rheumatoid arthritis, arthritis, minor muscle pain and aching, osteoarthritis and other arthritic conditions	see Chapter 7	up to 10 Grams per day orally; dose varies with reason for use; CHILD: varies according to weight
aurothioglucose	Solganal	rheumatoid arthritis	see Chapter 31	see Chapter 31

Table 36-1. (*Continued*)

Generic Name	Trade Name	Uses	Side Effects	Dose Ranges
carisoprodol	Soma	muscle relaxant for relief of skeletal muscle spasm and pain	drowsiness, vertigo, nausea, vomiting, tachycardia, postural hypotension, flushing, ataxia	350 mg. Q.I.D. orally
chlorphenesin	Maolate	same as carisoprodol	hematological reactions, drowsiness, dizziness, nausea, confusion	400-800 mg. T.I.D. orally
colchicine		treatment of gout—acute attacks and interval therapy	nausea, vomiting, diarrhea when full dosage reached; prolonged administration—bone marrow depression may be seen	at *immediate* onset of acute attack: 1-2 tablets (0.6-1.2 mg.) followed by 1 tablet q1-2h or 2 tablets q2h orally; interval therapy: 1 tablet 1-4 times per week
diazepam	Valium	relief of skeletal muscle spasm, spasticity of cerebral palsy, paraplegia, athetosis; also a minor tranquilizer	see Chapter 28	2-10 mg. B.I.D. to Q.I.D. orally; 5-10 mg. per dose I.M., I.V.
gold sodium thiomalate	Myochrysine	rheumatoid arthritis	same as aurothioglucose	initially: 10-15 mg.; then 25-50 mg. at weekly intervals I.M.
ibuprofen	Motrin	symptomatic treatment of rheumatoid arthritis, osteoarthritis	abdominal distress, heartburn, nausea, vomiting, constipation, diarrhea, skin rash	300-400 mg. T.I.D., Q.I.D., and up to 2400 mg. daily, p.o.
indomethacin	Indocin	moderate to severe rheumatoid arthritis, spondylitis and osteoarthritis of the hip	gastrointestinal ulcerations and bleeding, aggravation of epilepsy, Parkinson's, and psychiatric disturbances, toxic hepatitis, hematological reactions, tinnitus, hypersensitivity reactions, alopecia, edema, hypertension, headache, hematuria, hyperglycemia, glycosuria	50-200 mg. daily in 2-3 divided doses orally

Generic Name	Trade Name	Uses	Side Effects	Dose Ranges
methocarbamol	Robaxin	same as carisoprodol	dizziness, drowsiness, hypotension, gastrointestinal distress, pain at site of injection, urticaria, nasal congestion, mild muscular incoordination, bradycardia, blurred vision	1-1.5 Grams Q.I.D. orally; up to 3 ampuls per day I.M., I.V.
orphenadrine	Norflex	same as carisoprodol	dry mouth, blurred vision, mydriasis, nausea, vomiting, headache, tachycardia, dizziness, drowsiness	100 mg. B.I.D. orally; 60 mg. I.V., I.M. q12h
oxyphenbutazone	Tandearil	rheumatoid arthritis and spondylitis, psoriatic arthritis, osteoarthritis, gout, bursitis	see pages 319-320	100-600 mg. daily in 3-4 divided doses orally; in acute gouty arthritis 400 mg. initially, then 100 mg. q4h until inflammation subsides
phenylbutazone	Butazolidin	same as oxyphenbutazone	same as oxyphenbutazone	same as oxyphenbutazone
probenecid	Benemid	treatment of hyperuricemia of gout, maintenance of penicillin and aminosalicylic blood levels	headache, gastrointestinal distress, sore gums, anemia, dizziness, hypersensitivity reactions, flushing	gout: 0.5-2 Grams daily in divided doses orally; maintenance of penicillin and aminosalicylic acid blood levels: 2 Grams daily in divided doses
sodium salicylate		same as aspirin	same as aspirin	3-10 Grams per day in divided doses orally
sulfinpyrazone	Anturane	interval therapy in chronic gout	gastrointestinal distress, rash	200-400 mg. daily in 2 divided doses orally

This appendix is provided as a review of the basic mathematical principles necessary in using standard formulas taught in basic pharmacology courses. Also included are basic conversion tables and the formulas frequently used in the computation of drug doses.

Arithmetic Review

FRACTIONS

A fraction is often used to express a weight or volume in the apothecaries' system. A **proper fraction** may be defined as a part of a whole or any number less than a whole number. An **improper fraction** is a fraction having a numerator *the same as* or *larger than* the denominator.

PARTS OF A FRACTION		
PROPER FRACTION	$\dfrac{1}{2}$	← numerator ← denominator
IMPROPER FRACTION	$\dfrac{7}{6}$	← numerator ← denominator

It must be remembered that the numerator and the denominator of a fraction must be of like entities or terms, that is:

$$\frac{\text{grains}}{\text{grains}} \underset{\leftarrow}{\overset{\leftarrow}{\rightarrow}} \text{LIKE} \overset{\nearrow}{\underset{\searrow}{\rightarrow}} \frac{\text{ounces}}{\text{ounces}} \quad \text{NOT UNLIKE} \overset{\nearrow}{\underset{\searrow}{\rightarrow}} \frac{\text{grains}}{\text{ounces}}$$

MIXED NUMBERS AND IMPROPER FRACTIONS

It sometimes becomes necessary to change a mixed number (a whole number plus a proper fraction) to an improper fraction or to change an improper fraction to a mixed number.

To change a mixed number (example: 3 3/4) to an improper fraction:

1. multiply the denominator of the fraction by the whole number (4 × 3 = 12)

$$3\frac{3}{4}$$

2. add the numerator (12 + 3 = 15)

$$3\frac{3}{4}$$

3. place the sum over the denominator of the fraction

$$\frac{15}{4}$$

To change an improper fraction (example: 15/4) to a mixed number:

1. divide the denominator into the numerator; the quotient is the whole number

$$4\overline{)15} \\ \underline{12} \\ 3 \quad\to 3$$

2. place the remainder over the denominator of the improper fraction

$$3\frac{3}{4}$$

ADDING FRACTIONS WITH LIKE DENOMINATORS

When the denominators are the same, fractions are added by adding the numerators and placing the *sum* of the numerators over the denominator. If the answer is an improper fraction, as in the first example in the

---

ADDING FRACTIONS WITH
***LIKE* DENOMINATORS**

$$\frac{2}{3}$$

$$\frac{1}{3}$$ $$\frac{1}{8}$$

$$\frac{1}{3}$$ $$\frac{3}{8}$$

$$\frac{4}{3} \text{ or } 1\frac{1}{3}$$ $$\frac{4}{8} \text{ or } \frac{1}{2}$$

box, it may then be changed to a mixed number. In the second example, the answer is 4/8, which is reduced to 1/2. (Fractions should be reduced to the lowest possible terms.)

ADDING FRACTIONS WITH UNLIKE DENOMINATORS

Fractions with unlike denominators cannot be added until the denominators are converted to like numbers. First, the *lowest common denominator* is found. The lowest common denominator is the *lowest* number divisible by *all* the denominators. In the example shown in the box, the larger denominator is 4; however, 4 is not divisible by 3. The first number divisible by both denominators is 12; therefore 12 is the lowest common denominator. The next steps are:

1. divide the lowest common denominator by the denominators ($12 \div 3$ and $12 \div 4$)

$$\frac{2}{3} = \frac{}{12}$$

$$\frac{1}{4} = \frac{}{12}$$

2. multiply the quotient by the numerators (4×2, 3×1)

$$\frac{2}{3} = \frac{8}{12}$$

$$\frac{1}{4} = \frac{3}{12}$$

3. add the numerators

$$\frac{2}{3} = \frac{8}{12}$$

$$\frac{1}{4} = \frac{3}{12}$$

$$\frac{11}{12}$$

ADDING FRACTIONS WITH *UNLIKE* DENOMINATORS

$$\frac{2}{3} = \frac{8}{12}$$

$$\frac{1}{4} = \frac{3}{12}$$

$$\frac{11}{12}$$

COMPARISON OF FRACTIONS

When fractions with like denominators are compared, the fraction with the *largest* numerator is the largest fraction. Thus, 5/8 is larger than 3/8. When the denominators are not the same, for example the two fractions 2/3 and 1/10, the lowest common denominator must first be determined. The same procedure is followed as in the addition of fractions with unlike denominators. The fraction with the larger numerator, in this case 20/30, is the larger of the two fractions.

$$2 \times \frac{1}{2} = \frac{2}{2} = 1$$

$$4 \times \frac{2}{3} = \frac{8}{3} = 2\frac{2}{3}$$

$$2 \times \frac{3}{8} = \frac{6}{8} = \frac{3}{4}$$

COMPARISON OF FRACTIONS

$$\frac{2}{3} = \frac{20}{30}$$

$$\frac{1}{10} = \frac{3}{30}$$

In order to multiply mixed numbers, the mixed numbers are changed to improper fractions, which are then multiplied:

$$2\frac{1}{2} \times 3\frac{1}{4} = \frac{5}{2} \times \frac{13}{4} = \frac{65}{8} = 8\frac{1}{8}$$

$$3\frac{1}{3} \times 4\frac{1}{2} = \frac{10}{3} \times \frac{9}{2} = \frac{90}{6} = 15$$

MULTIPLYING FRACTIONS

When fractions are multiplied, the numerators are multiplied and the denominators are multiplied.

$$\frac{1}{8} \times \frac{1}{4} = \frac{1}{32}$$

$$\frac{1}{2} \times \frac{2}{3} = \frac{2}{6} = \frac{1}{3}$$

$$\frac{4}{5} \times \frac{3}{6} = \frac{12}{30} = \frac{2}{5}$$

When whole numbers are multiplied with fractions, the numerator is multiplied by the whole number, and the product is placed over the denominator. If necessary, the improper fraction is changed to a mixed number.

To multiply a whole number and a mixed number, both numbers are changed to improper fractions:

$$3 \times 2\frac{1}{2} = \frac{3}{1} \times \frac{5}{2} = \frac{15}{2} = 7\frac{1}{2}$$

$$2 \times 4\frac{1}{2} = \frac{2}{1} \times \frac{9}{2} = \frac{18}{2} = 9$$

Note that the whole number is converted to an improper fraction by placing the whole number over one. In the above examples 3 becomes 3/1 and 2 becomes 2/1.

DIVIDING FRACTIONS

When fractions are divided, the *second* fraction (the

divisor) is inverted (turned upside down). The fractions are then *multiplied*.

$$\frac{1}{8} \div \frac{1}{4} = \frac{1}{8} \times \frac{4}{1} = \frac{4}{8} = \frac{1}{2}$$

$$\frac{2}{3} \div \frac{5}{6} = \frac{2}{3} \times \frac{6}{5} = \frac{12}{15} = \frac{4}{5}$$

$$\frac{3}{4} \div \frac{1}{2} = \frac{3}{4} \times \frac{2}{1} = \frac{6}{4} = 1\frac{2}{4} = 1\frac{1}{2}$$

DIVIDING FRACTIONS WITH MIXED NUMBERS

Some problems of division may be expressed as fractions *and* mixed numbers or as two mixed numbers. When a mixed number and a fraction are divided, the mixed number is first changed to a fraction. When two mixed numbers are divided, both numbers are changed to fractions.

MIXED NUMBERS AND FRACTIONS

$$2\frac{1}{3} \div \frac{1}{4} = \frac{7}{3} \div \frac{1}{4} = \frac{7}{3} \times \frac{4}{1} = \frac{28}{3} = 9\frac{1}{3}$$

$$2\frac{1}{2} \div \frac{1}{2} = \frac{5}{2} \div \frac{1}{2} = \frac{5}{2} \times \frac{2}{1} = \frac{10}{2} = 5$$

MIXED NUMBERS

$$3\frac{3}{4} \div 1\frac{1}{2} = \frac{15}{4} \div \frac{3}{2} = \frac{15}{4} \times \frac{2}{3} = \frac{30}{12} = 2\frac{6}{12} = 2\frac{1}{2}$$

RATIOS

A ratio is a way of expressing a part of a whole or the relationship of one number to another. For example, a ratio written as 1:10 means 1 part to 10 parts, or 1 to 10. A ratio may also be written as a fraction; thus 1:10 can also be expressed as 1/10. Drug solutions may be expressed in ratios, for example 1:100 or 1:500. These ratios mean that there is 1 part of a drug in 100 parts of solution or 1 part of a drug in 500 parts of solution. A ratio is a way of expressing a part of a whole just as a fraction expresses a part of a whole.

PERCENT

The term *percent* (%) means parts per hundred. For example, 25% means 25/100, which can be further reduced to 1/4.

CHANGING A FRACTION TO A PERCENT

To change a fraction (example: 4/5) to a percent, divide the denominator into the numerator and multiply the quotient by 100.

$$4 \div 5 = 0.8; 0.8 \times 100 = 80\%$$

CHANGING A RATIO TO A PERCENT

To change a ratio to a percent, the ratio is expressed as a fraction; the first term of the ratio becomes the numerator and the second term the denominator. For example, 1:500 (ratio) changed to a fraction becomes 1/500. Then the fraction is changed to a percent.

The denominator is divided into the numerator, the quotient is multiplied by 100, and a percent sign (%) added.

$$1 \div 500 = 0.002; 0.002 \times 100 = 0.2\%$$

If the ratio is 1:10 (1/10):

$$1 \div 10 = 0.1; 0.1 \times 100 = 10\%$$

CHANGING A PERCENT TO A RATIO

To change a percent to a ratio, the percent becomes the numerator over a denominator of 100.

$$5\% = \frac{5}{100} = \frac{1}{20} \text{ or } 1{:}20$$

$$50\% = \frac{50}{100} = \frac{1}{2} \text{ or } 1{:}2$$

PROPORTIONS

A proportion is a method of expressing equality between two ratios. An example of two ratios expressed as a proportion is:

3 is to 4 as 9 is to 12

This may also be written as:

$$3 : 4 \text{ as } 9 : 12$$

or

$$3 : 4 : : 9 : 12$$

or

$$\frac{3}{4} = \frac{9}{12}$$

Proportions may be used to find an unknown quantity. The unknown quantity is assigned a letter, usually x, in the proportion. An example of a proportion with an unknown quantity is:

$$5 : 10 : : 10 : x$$

or

$$\frac{5}{10} = \frac{10}{x}$$

The first and last terms of the proportion are called the *extremes*. The second and third terms of the proportion are called the *means*.

$$\overbrace{5 : 10 : : 10 : x}^{\text{means}}$$
$$\underbrace{}_{\text{extremes}}$$

$$\begin{array}{cc} \text{extreme} & \\ \text{mean} & \end{array} \frac{5}{10} = \frac{10}{x} \begin{array}{c} \text{mean} \\ \text{extreme} \end{array}$$

In order to solve for x:

1. multiply the extremes and place the product to the left of the equal (=) sign

$$5 : 10 : : 10 : x$$
$$5x =$$

2. multiply the means and place the product to the right of the equal sign

$$5 : 10 : : 10 : x$$

$$5x = 100$$

3. solve for x

$$5x = 100$$

$$x = 20$$

To prove that the equation is correct, substitute the answer for x in the equation.

$$5 : 10 : : 10 : x$$

$$5 : 10 : : 10 : 20$$

Now multiply the means and extremes; if the numbers are the same on both sides of the equal sign, the problem has been solved correctly.

$$5 \times 20 = 10 \times 10$$

$$100 = 100$$

If the proportion has been set up as a fraction, cross multiply and solve for x:

1. 5 times $x = 5x$

$$\frac{5}{10} \searrow \frac{10}{x}$$

2. 10 times $10 = 100$

$$\frac{5}{10} \nearrow \frac{10}{x}$$

3. $5x = 100$

$$x = 20$$

To set up a proportion, it must be remembered that a sequence *must* be followed:

GRAINS is to GRAMS as GRAINS is to GRAMS
(GRAINS : GRAMS : : GRAINS : GRAMS)

or

$$\frac{\text{GRAINS}}{\text{GRAMS}} = \frac{\text{GRAINS}}{\text{GRAMS}}$$

DECIMALS

Decimals are used in the metric system. A **decimal** is a fraction in which the denominator is 10 or some power of 10. Thus 2/10 (read as two-tenths) is an example of a fraction with a denominator of 10. 1/100 (one one-hundredth) is a fraction with a denominator that is a power of 10.

A power (or multiple) of 10 is the number 1 followed by one or more zeros. Therefore 100, 1000, 10,000, and so on are powers of 10. Fractions whose *denominators* are 10 or a power of 10 are often expressed in decimal form.

There are three parts to a decimal:

1	**•**	**25**
number(s) to	d	number(s) to
the left of	e	the right of
the decimal	c	the decimal
point	i	point
	m	
	a	
	l	

A decimal may consist only of numbers to the *right* of the decimal point; this is called a *decimal fraction*. A decimal may also have numbers to the *left* and *right* of the decimal point; this is called a *mixed decimal fraction*. Both decimal fractions and mixed decimal fractions are commonly referred to as decimals. When there is *no* number to the left of the decimal, a zero may be written, for example 0.25. Although in general mathematics the zero may not be required, it should be used in the writing of drug doses in the metric system. Use of the zero lessens the chance of medication errors, especially when a drug dose is hurriedly written and the decimal point indistinct.

To read a decimal, the position of the number to the left or right of the decimal point will indicate how the decimal is to be expressed.

$$
\begin{array}{ccccc c ccccc}
\text{hundred thousands} & \text{ten thousands} & \text{thousands} & \text{hundreds} & \text{tens} & \textbf{DECIMAL POINT} & \text{tenths} & \text{hundredths} & \text{thousandths} & \text{ten thousandths} & \text{hundred thousandths} \\
0 & 0 & 0 & 0 & 0 & \bullet & 0 & 0 & 0 & 0 & 0
\end{array}
$$

To multiply a whole number by a decimal, move the decimal point of the product as many places to the *left* as there are places to the right of the decimal.

```
 500
 .05  ← there are two places to the right of the decimal
25.00. ← the decimal point is moved two places to the left
   ^
```

MULTIPLYING A DECIMAL BY A DECIMAL

To multiply a decimal by a decimal, move the decimal point of the product as many places to the left as there are places to the right in *both* decimals:

```
2.75 ← two places to the right of the decimal
0.5  ← plus one place to the right of the decimal equals
          three
1 375. ← move the decimal point three places to the left
   ^
```

DIVIDING DECIMALS

The divisor is a number which is divided into the dividend.

$$
\underset{\text{DIVIDEND}}{0.65} \div \underset{\text{DIVISOR}}{0.3} \qquad \underset{\text{DIVISOR DIVIDEND}}{0.3\overline{)0.65}}
$$

To divide decimals:

1. the divisor is changed to a whole number. In this example the decimal point is moved *one* place to the right

$$0.3_{\wedge}\overline{)0.65}$$

2. the decimal point in the dividend is moved the same number of places to the right

$$3. \overline{)0.6\wedge5}$$

3. the numbers are now divided

$$\begin{array}{r} 2.16 \\ 3\overline{)6.50} \end{array}$$

When only the dividend is a decimal, the decimal point is carried to the quotient in the same position:

$$\begin{array}{r} .375 \\ 2\overline{)0.750} \end{array}$$

When only the divisor is a decimal:

1. the divisor is changed to a whole number. In this example the decimal point is moved one place to the right

$$.3\wedge\overline{)66}$$

2. the decimal point in the dividend must also be moved one place to the right

$$3\overline{)66.0\wedge}$$

3. the numbers are now divided

$$\begin{array}{r} 220. \\ 3\overline{)660.} \end{array}$$

CHANGING A FRACTION TO A DECIMAL

To change a fraction to a decimal, divide the numerator by the denominator.

$$\frac{1}{5} = 5\overline{)1.0}^{\ \ .2}$$

$$\frac{3}{4} = 4\overline{)3.00}^{\ \ .75}$$

CHANGING A DECIMAL TO A FRACTION

To convert a decimal to a fraction:

1. remove the decimal point and make the resulting whole number the numerator

$$0.2 = \underline{2}$$

2. the denominator is stated as 10 or a power of 10. 0.2 is read as two-*tenths*; therefore in this example the denominator is 10

$$\frac{2}{10} = \frac{1}{5}$$

Other examples:

$$0.75 = \frac{75}{100} = \frac{3}{4}$$

$$0.5 = \frac{5}{10} = \frac{1}{2}$$

$$0.025 = \frac{25}{1000} = \frac{1}{40}$$

Note that all fractions are reduced to the lowest possible terms.

APPROXIMATE EQUIVALENTS

METRIC		APOTHECARIES'
WEIGHT		
1 milligram (mg.) (1000 micrograms [mcg.])	=	1/60 grain (gr.)
60 mg.	=	1 grain
1 Gram (Gm.) (1000 mg.)	=	15 grains
30 Gm.	=	1 ounce (oz.)
1 Kilogram (Kg.)	=	2.2 pounds (lb.) (avoirdupois)
VOLUME		
1 milliliter (ml.)	=	15 or 16 minims (♏)
4 ml.	=	1 fluid dram (fl ℨ)
30 ml.	=	1 fluid ounce (fl ℥)
500 ml.	=	1 pint (pt.)
1000 ml. (1 Liter)	=	1 quart (qt.)

Systems of Measurements:
The Apothecaries' and Metric Systems

The two systems of weights and measures used in pharmacology are the **apothecaries'** system and the **metric** system. Although both are presently used, the metric has largely replaced the apothecaries'.

The *Gram* is the unit of weight, the *Liter* the unit of volume, and the *meter* the unit of linear measurement in the metric system. In the apothecaries' system the *grain* is the unit of weight and the *minim* the unit of volume.

HOUSEHOLD MEASUREMENTS AND EQUIVALENTS

HOUSEHOLD	APOTHECARIES'	METRIC
1 teaspoonful	60 drops (gtt.) or 60 minims or 1 dram	4 or 5 ml.
1 tablespoonful	4 drams	15 or 16 ml.
2 tablespoonfuls	1 ounce	30 ml.

CONVERSION FROM METRIC TO APOTHECARIES' AND APOTHECARIES' TO METRIC

The above tables can be used to convert from one system to another. In some instances it may be necessary to convert within the same system. Some examples of the need for conversion are:

The physician's order reads: Seconal gr. īss
  (APOTHECARIES'—1½ grains)
The drug container reads: Seconal 0.1 Gram
  (METRIC)

The physician's order reads: Demerol 0.1 Gram
  (METRIC)
The drug container reads: Demerol 100 mg./ml.
  (METRIC)

In order to convert, it is necessary to know or have available some of the equivalents given in these tables.

Although several methods may be used to convert from one system to another or convert within a system, most conversions can be done by proportion.

EXAMPLE No. 1

Convert 120 *milligrams* to *grains* (metric to apothecaries').

Using proportion and known equivalents (60 mg. = 1 gr.):

$$1 \text{ gr.} : 60 \text{ mg.} : : x \text{ gr.} : 120 \text{ mg.}$$

or

$$\frac{1 \text{ gr.}}{60 \text{ mg.}} = \frac{x \text{ gr.}}{120 \text{ mg.}}$$
$$60x = 120$$
$$x = 2 \text{ grains}$$

Therefore 120 mg. is equal to 2 grains.

EXAMPLE No. 2

Convert 0.1 *Gram* to *milligrams* (conversion within the metric system).

$$1000 \text{ mg.} : 1 \text{ Gm.} : : x \text{ mg.} : 0.1 \text{ Gm.}$$

or

$$\frac{1000 \text{ mg.}}{1 \text{ Gm.}} = \frac{x \text{ mg.}}{0.1 \text{ Gm.}}$$

$$x = 100 \text{ mg.}$$

Therefore 0.1 Gm. is equal to 100 mg.

EXAMPLE No. 3

Convert *grains* 1/100 to *milligrams* (apothecaries' to metric).

$$60 \text{ mg.} : 1 \text{ gr.} : : x \text{ mg.} : 1/100 \text{ gr.}$$

or

$$\frac{60 \text{ mg.}}{1 \text{ gr.}} = \frac{x \text{ mg.}}{1/100 \text{ gr.}}$$

$$x = 60 \times \frac{1}{100} = \frac{60}{100} = \frac{3}{5} \text{ mg.}$$

Fractions are not used in the metric system; the fraction is converted to a *decimal* by dividing the denominator into the numerator:

$$5 \overline{)3.0} \quad \overset{.6}{}$$

Therefore gr. 1/100 is equal to 0.6 mg.

EXAMPLE No. 4

Convert 0.3 *milligram* to *grains* (metric to apothecaries').

$$1/60 \text{ gr.} : 1 \text{ mg.} : : x \text{ gr.} : 0.3 \text{ mg.}$$

or

$$\frac{1/60 \text{ gr.}}{1 \text{ mg.}} = \frac{x \text{ gr.}}{0.3 \text{ mg.}}$$

$$x = 1/60 \times 0.3 = \frac{0.3}{60} = \frac{3}{600} = \frac{1}{200}$$

Therefore 0.3 mg. is equal to 1/200 grains. Note that in this example the decimal was removed from the fraction.

If the equivalent 60 mg. = 1 grain is used in the above problem, the proportion would be:

$$60 \text{ mg. : } 1 \text{ gr. : : } 0.3 \text{ mg. : } x \text{ gr.}$$

or

$$\frac{60 \text{ mg.}}{1 \text{ gr.}} = \frac{0.3 \text{ mg.}}{x \text{ gr.}}$$

$$60x = 0.3$$
$$x = 0.005$$

Decimals are not used in the apothecaries' system; therefore this decimal is converted to a fraction. 0.005 is read as 5/1000 or 1/200.

EXAMPLE No. 5
Convert 30 *grains* to *Grams* (apothecaries' to metric).

$$15 \text{ gr. : } 1 \text{ Gm. : : } 30 \text{ gr. : } x \text{ Gm.}$$

or

$$\frac{15 \text{ gr.}}{1 \text{ Gm.}} = \frac{30 \text{ gr.}}{x \text{ Gm.}}$$

$$15x = 30$$
$$x = 2 \text{ Gm.}$$

Therefore 30 gr. is equal to 2 Gm.

Oral Dosages of Drugs

It is sometimes necessary to compute the oral dosage of drugs, as the dosage ordered by the physician may not be available in the strength ordered or may be expressed in a system (apothecaries' or metric) other than that stated on the drug container.

ORAL DOSAGES OF TABLETS AND CAPSULES

To find the correct dosage of a solid oral preparation, the following formula may be used:

$$\frac{\text{DOSE DESIRED}}{\text{DOSE ON HAND}} = \text{DOSE ADMINISTERED}$$

This formula may be abbreviated as:

$$\frac{\text{D (desired)}}{\text{H (have)}} = \text{X}$$

When the dose ordered by the physician (dose desired) is written in the *same* system as the dose on the drug container (dose on hand), these two figures can be substituted in the formula.

EXAMPLE
The physician orders ascorbic acid 100 mg.
The dose available is ascorbic acid 50 mg.

$$\frac{\text{D}}{\text{H}} = \text{X}$$

$$\frac{100 \text{ mg.}}{50 \text{ mg.}} = 2 \text{ tablets of ascorbic acid}$$

Note that the fraction in the above example denotes $\frac{milligrams}{milligrams}$. If the physician had ordered ascorbic acid 0.5 Gm. and the drug container was labeled ascorbic acid 250 mg., a conversion of *Grams* to *milligrams* or *milligrams* to *Grams* would be necessary *before* this formula could be used. Errors will be reduced if the entire dose is written, rather than just numbers:

$$\frac{100 \text{ mg.}}{50 \text{ mg.}} \text{ rather than } \frac{100}{50}$$

This will eliminate the possibility of using unlike terms in the fraction.

If the physician's order is written in the apothecaries' system and the drug container is labeled in the metric system, conversion is necessary.

EXAMPLE
The physician's order reads codeine sulfate gr. 1/4.
The drug container is labeled codeine sulfate 15 mg.

Grains must be converted to *milligrams* or *milligrams* converted to *grains*.

GRAINS TO MILLIGRAMS
$$60 \text{ mg.} : 1 \text{ gr.} : : x \text{ mg.} : 1/4 \text{ gr.}$$

or

$$\frac{60 \text{ mg.}}{1 \text{ gr.}} = \frac{x \text{ mg.}}{1/4 \text{ gr.}}$$

$$x = 60 \times \frac{1}{4}$$

$$x = 15 \text{ mg.}$$

MILLIGRAMS TO GRAINS
$$60 \text{ mg.} : 1 \text{ gr.} : : 15 \text{ mg.} : x \text{ gr.}$$

or

$$\frac{60 \text{ mg.}}{1 \text{ gr.}} = \frac{15 \text{ mg.}}{x \text{ gr.}}$$

$$60x = 15$$

$$x = \frac{1}{4} \text{ gr.}$$

The formula $\frac{D}{H} = X$ can now be used:

$$\frac{D}{H} = X$$

$$\frac{15 \text{ mg.}}{15 \text{ mg.}} = 1 \text{ tablet}$$

$$\frac{D}{H} = X$$

$$\frac{1/4 \text{ gr.}}{1/4 \text{ gr.}} = 1 \text{ tablet}$$

Knowing the most commonly used equivalents will sometimes eliminate the need for the use of formulas.

The physician's order reads codeine sulfate grains ī.
The drug container is labeled codeine sulfate 60 mg.

If the common equivalent 60 milligrams equals 1 grain is remembered, the need for further computation is eliminated.

ORAL DOSAGES OF LIQUIDS

Drugs in liquid form may be available in the clinical area or prepared by the pharmacist. In liquid preparations there is a specific amount of a drug in a specific volume of solution, for example 5 mg. per 5 ml. The physician usually orders the drug by weight, for example 5 mg., and indicates that a liquid is to be given by including words such as syrup, elixir, or solution along with the name of the drug.

EXAMPLES
Elixir of terpin hydrate; Erythromycin syrup.

The formula for computing the oral dosage of liquids is:

$$\frac{\text{DOSE DESIRED}}{\text{DOSE ON HAND}} \times \text{QUANTITY}$$
$$= \text{DOSE ADMINISTERED}$$

This can be abbreviated:

$$\frac{D}{H} \times Q = X$$

EXAMPLE
The physician's order reads codeine phosphate syrup gr. 1/3.
The drug container is labeled codeine phosphate syrup gr. 1/6 per 4 ml. (The 4 ml. is the quantity [amount] which contains 1/6 gr. of the drug.)

$$\frac{D}{H} \times Q = X \text{ (amount to be given)}$$

$$\frac{\text{gr. } 1/3}{\text{gr. } 1/6} \times 4 \text{ ml.} = x$$

$$\frac{1}{3} \div \frac{1}{6} = \frac{1}{3} \times \frac{6}{1} = \frac{6}{3} = 2$$

$$2 \times 4 \text{ ml.} = 8 \text{ ml.}$$

Therefore the amount administered is 8 ml.

Liquid forms of drugs may also be ordered in drops (gtt.) or in minims. With the former, a medicine dropper, which is usually supplied with the drug, is used. To measure a drug in minims, a measuring glass *calibrated in minims* must be used.

Parenteral Dosages of Drugs

Drugs for parenteral use must be in liquid form before they are administered. Parenteral drugs may be available:

1. as liquids in disposable cartridges or disposable syringes, which contain a specific

amount of a drug in a specific volume, for example Demerol 50 mg. per ml. After administration, the cartridge or syringe is discarded.

2. in ampuls or vials which contain a *dry* form of the drug or a *solution.* If the ampul or vial contains a dry form of the drug, a liquid (called the diluent) must be added before the drug is withdrawn from the container and administered.

3. as tablets manufactured for *parenteral use,* for example H.T. (hypo tablet) atropine sulfate.

LIQUID PREPARATIONS IN DISPOSABLE CARTRIDGES OR DISPOSABLE SYRINGES

These drugs may be available in one or more strengths. There may be instances when a particular dose is not available in a prepared strength, and it will be necessary to administer less than the amount in a syringe or cartridge.

EXAMPLE
The physician's order reads Valium 5 mg. I.M.
The drug on hand is Valium Tel-E-Ject 2 ml. = 10 mg.

$$\frac{D}{H} \times Q = X$$

$$\frac{5 \text{ mg.}}{10 \text{ mg.}} \times 2 \text{ ml} = x$$

$$x = \frac{1}{2} \times 2 = 1 \text{ ml. (dose administered)}$$

Since the syringe contains 2 ml., *1 ml. is discarded,* leaving 1 ml. in the syringe.

AMPULS AND VIALS

If the drug is a *liquid* in the ampul or vial, the desired amount is withdrawn from the vial. In some instances the entire amount is used; in others only part of the total amount is used. ALWAYS CHECK DRUG LABELS CAREFULLY. Some containers may be labeled in a manner different from others.

2 ml. = 0.25 mg.
2 ml. ampul

1 ml. = 5 mg.
2 ml. ampul

EXAMPLE
The physician's order reads H. atropine sulfate gr. 1/200.
The multidose vial reads H. atropine gr. 1/200. per ml.

1 ml. is withdrawn from the ampul.

On occasion the desired dose may not be available and computation may be necessary.

EXAMPLE

The physician's order reads H. atropine gr. 1/300. The multidose vial reads H. atropine gr. 1/200 per ml.

$$\frac{D}{H} \times Q = X$$

$$\frac{\text{gr. } 1/300}{\text{gr. } 1/200} \times 1 \text{ ml.} = x$$

$$\frac{1}{300} \div \frac{1}{200} = \frac{1}{300} \times \frac{200}{1} = \frac{2}{3}$$

$$\frac{2}{3} \times 1 \text{ ml. (15 minims)} = 10 \text{ minims}$$

When the dose is less than 1 ml., the milliliter amount can be converted to minims. The conversion factor of 15 minims per milliliter is used when the denominator of the fraction (in this example, 3) can be divided into 15. The conversion factor of 16 minims per milliliter is used when the denominator of the fraction can be divided into 16.

If the drug is in *powder or crystal form*, it must be reconstituted before use by the addition of a diluent. Sterile distilled water is a commonly used diluent, but in some cases the manufacturer may supply an ampul of another diluent. Before a drug is reconstituted, the label should be checked for instructions (if any) for dilution.

EXAMPLE OF DILUTION DIRECTIONS

Add 4 ml. of sterile distilled water to vial.

2.2 ml. = 0.5 Gram.

When no dilution directions are given, 1.0 to 1.5 ml. is usually added to single-dose vials. In multiple-dose vials 10 to 20⁺ ml. (depending on the size of the container) is added to the dry form of the drug. If there is any doubt regarding the dilution of a dry form of a drug and there are no manufacturer's suggestions for dilution, the hospital pharmacist should be consulted.

Once a diluent is added, the amount of solution to be administered is determined. In some cases, the entire amount is given; in others a part of the solution is given.

EXAMPLE

Buffered sodium penicillin G 5,000,000 units per vial. Diluted as per manufacturer's directions: add 23 ml., 18 ml., 8 ml., 3 ml. to provide 200,000 U, 250,000 U, 500,000 U, 1 million U per ml. respectively. There is a choice as to how much diluent will be added, according to the desired concentration per milliliter. If the physician orders 500,000 U to be administered, 8 ml. of diluent is added to the vial; *each* milliliter will contain 500,000 units. Once the dry powder or crystal has been reconstituted the bottle should be *clearly labeled* as to the amount of drug per milliliter and the date.

TABLETS

When *hypodermic* tablets are prepared for parenteral administration they may or may not be available in the dose desired. If available in the dose desired, the tablet is placed in the syringe and sterile diluent is drawn into the syringe, usually in the amount of 1.0 to 1.5 ml. The syringe is then gently rotated until the tablet is *completely* dissolved. If the dose desired is not available, the following formula may be used:

$$\frac{D}{H} = X \text{ (number of tablets used)}$$

EXAMPLE No. 1
H. morphine sulfate gr. 1/6 is ordered. The available strength is H.T. (hypo tablet) morphine sulfate gr. 1/4.

$$\frac{D}{H} = X$$

$$\frac{1/6}{1/4} = \frac{1}{6} \div \frac{1}{4} = \frac{1}{6} \times \frac{4}{1} = \frac{2}{3} \text{ tablet}$$

A small hypodermic tablet *cannot* be cut in half or thirds. The whole tablet is dissolved in 1 ml. (15 minims), and two-thirds of this amount, that is, 10 minims, is administered. (Two-thirds of the volume in the syringe equals two-thirds of a tablet.)

In the above sample problem, 15 minims was arbitrarily selected as the amount of solution in which to dissolve the hypodermic tablet. The final volume that is administered should be *no less than* 8 to 10 minims, as inaccuracy of the fractional dose may occur if less than 8 to 10 minims is administered. *This minimal amount applies to this type of drug administration only* (that is, the dissolving of hypodermic tablets in a diluent). In most instances, the maximum amount *administered* should be no more than 30 to 32 minims, as larger amounts cause discomfort at the site of injection.

In this problem other amounts can be used to dissolve the hypodermic tablet. Since the fractional amount is two-thirds of a tablet, the amount of diluent must be divisible by the denominator of the fraction, in this instance, 3.

EXAMPLE No. 2
H. atropine sulfate gr. 1/100 is ordered and H. atropine sulfate gr. 1/150 is available.

$$\frac{D}{H} = X$$

$$\frac{1/100}{1/150} = \frac{1}{100} \div \frac{1}{150} = \frac{1}{100} \times \frac{150}{1} = 1\frac{1}{2} \text{ tablets}$$

In this example two tablets are used, as one tablet cannot be broken in half. The amount of diluent can be arbitrarily chosen and the amount to be administered can be determined by using proportion.

$$2 \text{ tablets} : 32 \text{ minims} :: 1.5 \text{ tablets} : x \text{ minims}$$
(diluent)   (amount administered)

$$2x = 48$$
$$x = 24 \text{ minims}$$

Therefore two tablets are dissolved in 32 minims and 24 minims are administered. The 24 minims contain 1 1/2 tablets of the drug.

When more than one hypodermic tablet must be used, it is usually easier to use between 16 and 32 minims as a diluent. Some hypodermic preparations may be more difficult to dissolve in small amounts of solution.

Temperatures

Two scales are used in measuring temperatures, Fahrenheit and centigrade (also known as Celsius). On the Fahrenheit scale the freezing point is 32° F. and the boiling point of water is 212° F. On the centigrade scale 0° C. is the freezing point and 100° C. is the boiling point of water.

To convert from one scale to the other, the formula used is:

$$C : F - 32 :: 5 : 9$$

EXAMPLES

centigrade 30° = Fahrenheit ?°
$$C : F - 32 :: 5 : 9$$
$$30 : F - 32 :: 5 : 9$$
$$270 = 5 \text{ F} - 160$$
$$5 \text{ F} = 270 + 160 = 430$$
$$F = 86°$$

Fahrenheit 50° = centigrade ?°
$$C : F - 32 :: 5 : 9$$
$$C : 50 - 32 :: 5 : 9$$
$$9 \text{ C} = 5 \ (50 - 32)$$
$$9 \text{ C} = 90$$
$$C = 10°$$

Pediatric Dosages

The dosage of drugs given to children is usually lower than that given to adults. The dosage may be based on age, weight, or body surface area.

CLARK'S RULE

This formula uses the child's weight to determine a drug dose.

$$\frac{\text{weight of child in pounds}}{\text{average adult weight (150 lbs.)}} \times \text{adult dose} = \text{child dose}$$

EXAMPLE

The adult dose of Seconal is gr. 1 1/2; what is the dose given to a child weighing 50 pounds?

$$\frac{50}{150} \times 1\frac{1}{2} = x$$

$$\frac{1}{3} \times \frac{3}{2} = \frac{3}{6} = \frac{1}{2} \text{ grain}$$

YOUNG'S RULE

This formula is based on the child's age and is used when the child is more than one year of age and not more than twelve years of age.

$$\frac{\text{age}}{\text{age} + 12} \times \text{adult dose} = \text{child dose}$$

EXAMPLE

The adult dose of digitalis is 0.1 Gram (100 mg.); what is the dose given to a four-year-old child?

$$\frac{4}{4 + 12} = \frac{4}{16} = \frac{1}{4}; \frac{1}{4} \times 100 \text{ mg.} = 25 \text{ mg.}$$

FRIED'S RULE

This formula is used for infants.

$$\frac{\text{age in months}}{150} \times \text{adult dose} = \text{infant dose}$$

EXAMPLE

The average adult dose of aspirin is 10 grains; how much aspirin is given to a six-month-old infant?

$$\frac{6}{150} = \frac{1}{25}; \frac{1}{25} \times 10 \text{ grains} = \frac{2}{5} \text{ grain}$$

BODY SURFACE AREA (BSA)

Charts are used to determine the body surface area in square meters according to height and weight. Once the body surface area is determined, the following formula is used:

$$\frac{\text{surface area of the child in square meters}}{\text{surface area of an adult in square meters}} \times \text{usual adult dose} = \text{child dose}$$

The figure for the average area of an adult in square meters is 1.7.

EXAMPLE

The average adult dose of Nembutal is 100 mg.; how much Nembutal would be given to a child whose body surface area is 0.4 square meters?

$$\frac{0.4}{1.7} \times 100 \text{ mg.} = \frac{40}{1.7} = 23.5 \text{ mg.}$$

Note: The decimals could also be removed from the above fraction:

$$\frac{4}{17} \times 100 \text{ mg.} = \frac{400}{17} = 23.5 \text{ mg.}$$

Solutions

A **solute** is a substance dissolved in a **solvent**. A solvent can be water or some other liquid. Usually water is used for preparing a solution unless another liquid is specified.

Solutions are prepared by using a solid (powder, tablet, and so on) and a liquid or a liquid and a liquid.

TYPES OF SOLUTIONS

WEIGHT TO WEIGHT (W/W)—a given *weight* of *solute* is dissolved in a given *weight* of *solvent*.

WEIGHT TO VOLUME (W/V)—a given *weight* of *solute* is dissolved in the *amount* of *solvent* necessary to make the required amount of solution.

VOLUME TO VOLUME (V/V)—a given *volume* of *solute* is added to a given *volume* of *solvent*.

Weight to weight solutions are almost always prepared by a pharmacist, as scales are needed to measure the weight of the solvent and solute.

SOLUTIONS FROM LIQUID DRUGS

There are several facts that must first be known before a solution can be prepared from a liquid drug.

1. the *amount* of solution finally required, e.g., 500 ml., 1 Liter.
2. the *strength* of the solution, e.g., 5%, 10%.
3. the *strength* of the drug available.

A proportion can be set up to determine the amount of drug (solute) to be used:

$$\text{strength desired} : \text{strength on hand} : : \text{amount of solute} : \text{amount of solution desired}$$

EXAMPLE

A 100% strength drug is available; the strength desired is 10%; the amount of solution desired is 1 Liter (1000 ml.); the unknown factor is: How much solute is needed to make 1 Liter (1000 ml.) of a 10% (strength) solution?

Setting up this problem as a proportion:

$$10\% : 100\% : : x : 1000 \text{ ml.}$$
$$100x = 10{,}000$$
$$x = 100 \text{ ml.}$$

Therefore 100 ml. of the 100% drug is needed to make a 10% solution of 1 Liter (1000 ml.).

Another formula can also be used:

$$\frac{\text{strength desired}}{\text{strength on hand}} \times \frac{\text{quantity of solution}}{\text{desired}} = \text{amount of solute}$$

$$\frac{10\% \text{ (strength desired)}}{100\% \text{ (strength on hand)}} \times 1000 \text{ ml. (quantity)}$$
$$= x \text{ (amount of solute)}$$

$$\frac{1}{10} \times 1000 = x$$

$$x = 100 \text{ ml.}$$

Sometimes the strength desired and the strength on hand may be expressed in unlike terms, for example:

strength desired—1 : 10 ⎫
strength on hand—50% ⎬ UNLIKE TERMS
amount of solute—x ⎭
amount of solution desired—1 Liter (1000 ml.)

In this type of problem, the ratio (1 : 10) can be changed to a percent, or the percent (50%) can be changed to a ratio. 1 : 10 converted to a percent is 10%. 50% converted to a ratio is 1 : 2.

Using the formula:

$$\frac{\text{strength desired}}{\text{strength on hand}} \times \text{quantity of solution desired}$$

$$= x \text{ (amount of solute)}$$

$$\frac{10\%}{50\%} \times 1000 = x$$

$$\frac{1}{5} \times 1000 = 200 \text{ ml.}$$

Thus 200 ml. of a 50% strength solute in 1 Liter of solution will give a 1 : 10 (or 10%) solution.

Therefore add 200 ml. of the drug to 800 ml. of solvent to make 1000 ml. of a 1 : 10 solution.

If both terms are expressed in ratios:

$$\frac{1/10}{1/2} \times 1000 = x$$

$$\frac{1}{10} \div \frac{1}{2} = \frac{1}{10} \times \frac{2}{1} = \frac{1}{5}; \frac{1}{5} \times 1000 = x$$

$$x = 200 \text{ ml.}$$

Some solutions are prepared on a volume to volume basis. For example, the stock solution is a 50% solution and the strength of the solution to be used is 10%. Note that the stock solution is *stronger* than the desired solution.

EXAMPLE
Prepare 500 ml. of a 10% solution from a stock solution of 50%.

Using the same formula:

$$\frac{\text{strength desired}}{\text{strength on hand}} \times \text{quantity of solution desired}$$

$$= \text{amount used (from stock)}$$

$$\frac{10\%}{50\%} \times 500 \text{ ml.} = x \text{ (amount of 50\% stock solution used)}$$

$$\frac{1}{5} \times 500 = x$$

$$x = 100 \text{ ml. (used from stock)}$$

Since 500 ml. of solution (quantity) is desired, measure 100 ml. of the 50% stock solution and then add the amount of diluent necessary to make the desired amount (500 ml.). The amount of diluent is:

500 ml. (the quantity desired)
− 100 ml. (amount used from the stock solution of 50% strength)
_____
400 ml. (amount of diluent)

The same type of problem can also be presented in *unlike terms*.

EXAMPLE

Prepare 1000 ml. of a 1:10 solution from a stock solution of 100%.

1 : 10 converted to a percent is 10%. 100% converted to a ratio is 1 : 1.

Either set of figures can be used in the problem as long as the numerator and denominator are in *like terms*.

$$\frac{\text{strength desired}}{\text{strength on hand}} \times \text{quantity of solution desired}$$
$$= \text{amount of stock solution used}$$

$$\frac{10\%}{100\%} \times 1000 \text{ ml.} = 100 \text{ ml. of stock solution}$$

$$\frac{1/10}{1/1} \times 1000 \text{ ml.} = 100 \text{ ml. of stock solution}$$

Therefore, 100 ml. of stock solution is used. Since the quantity desired is 1000 ml., the 100 ml. of stock solution is placed in a container and 900 ml. of diluent (usually water unless specified otherwise) is added. The result will be a 1 : 10 (or 10%) solution.

Some solutions may be expressed as ratios and the strength desired expressed as a ratio.

EXAMPLE

Prepare 1000 ml. of a 1 : 5000 solution from a stock solution of 1 : 1000.

$$\frac{\text{strength desired}}{\text{strength on hand}} \times \text{quantity of solution desired}$$
$$= \text{amount of stock solution used}$$

The ratios are converted to fractions before they are used in the formula.

$$\frac{1/5000}{1/1000} \times 1000 \text{ ml.} = \frac{1}{5000} \div \frac{1}{1000} \times 1000 = \frac{1}{5000} \times$$

$$\frac{1000}{1} \times 1000 = \frac{1}{5} \times 1000 = 200 \text{ ml.}$$

Therefore, 200 ml. of stock solution is used. Since the desired amount is 1000 ml., 800 ml. of diluent is added to the 200 ml. of stock solution to make 1000 ml. of a 1 : 5000 strength solution.

In order to prepare a solution from a stock solution, the stock solution is removed from its container and placed in *another container*. Then, the prescribed amount of diluent is added to obtain the desired strength and volume of solution.

SOLUTIONS FROM SOLIDS (TABLETS, CRYSTALS, POWDER)

Some solutions are made from tablets of a known strength. When such solutions are prepared, there is a weight/volume relationship. The number of ml. of (liquid) solute per 100 ml. *or* the number of Grams of (solid) solute per 100 ml. can be read as *percent*.

For example, a solution that contains 4 Grams of a solute in 100 ml. of solution is a 4% solution. If 6 ml. of (liquid) solute is in 100 ml. of solution, this is a 6% solution.

EXAMPLE

How many 5-grain (also expressed as grains v̄) tablets are required to make 1000 ml. of a 1 : 7000 solution?

$$\frac{\text{strength desired}}{\text{strength on hand}} \times \text{quantity of solution desired}$$
$$= \text{amount (here, the number of tablets) used}$$

1 : 7000 is converted to a fraction: 1/7000.

$$\frac{1/7000}{5 \text{ gr.}} \times 1000 \text{ ml.} = x$$

Since the numerator and denominator are unlike terms, the apothecaries' (grains v̄) measurement is changed to the metric equivalent.

$$15 \text{ gr.} : 1 \text{ Gm.} : : 5 \text{ gr.} : x \text{ Gm.}$$

or

$$\frac{15 \text{ gr.}}{1 \text{ Gm.}} = \frac{5 \text{ gr.}}{x \text{ Gm.}}$$

$$15 x = 5$$

$$x = 0.33 \text{ or } \frac{1}{3}$$

(The decimal is changed to a fraction):

$$\frac{33}{100} = \frac{1}{3}$$

Then the formula is applied:

$$\frac{1/7000}{1/3} \times 1000 \text{ ml.} = x$$

$$\frac{1}{7000} \div \frac{1}{3} \times 1000 = \frac{1}{7000} \times \frac{3}{1} \times 1000 = \frac{3}{7000} \times 1000$$

$$= \frac{3000}{7000} = \frac{3}{7}$$

Therefore 3/7ths of a 5-grain tablet is used to make 1000 ml. of a 1 : 7000 solution. As it is not possible to break one into 3/7ths, the following must be done:

1. if the *whole* tablet is placed into a given amount of solution and dissolved, and then 3/7ths of the total amount of solution is removed, the amount removed contains 3/7ths of the tablet, and the amount remaining, 4/7ths of the tablet. The first step then is to find the amount of solution in which to dissolve the tablet.
2. find the number of milliliters or ounces divisible by the denominator of the fraction. In most instances it is best to use ounces as there must be a sufficient amount

of solution to dissolve the tablet as well as insure accuracy.

$$\frac{3}{7} \times 7 \text{ (ounces)} = \frac{21}{7} = 3 \text{ ounces}$$

Therefore, if the tablet is dissolved in 7 ounces and 3 ounces are removed, the solution removed contains 3/7ths of the (dissolved) tablet.

Therefore, 3 ounces (of the 7 ounces of solution in which was dissolved a 5-grain tablet of the drug) is put into a container, to which a diluent (usually water) is added to make 1000 ml. of a 1 : 7000 solution.

1000 ml.	(the quantity desired)	
− 90 ml.	(3 ounces)	
910 ml.	(amount of diluent)	

RATIO OF A SOLUTION

If a solution is labeled in percent, it can be converted to a ratio in the same manner that any percent is converted to a ratio:

$$\frac{\text{percent of solution}}{100}$$

EXAMPLE
A 10% solution is converted to a ratio.

$$\frac{10}{100} = \frac{1}{10} \text{, which, expressed as a ratio, is } 1:10$$

Therefore a 10% solution is a 1 : 10 solution.

FINDING THE PERCENTAGE OF A SOLUTION

EXAMPLE NO. 1
If 1 Liter (1000 ml.) contains 8 Grams of a drug, what is the *percentage* of the solution?

For practical purposes in solving weight/volume problems, it can be assumed that 1 ml. of solution is approximately equivalent to 1 Gram. In order to find the percentage of a solution, change the ml. to Grams. In the problem stated above, 1000 ml. of solution now becomes 1000 Grams.

$$\frac{\text{known amount of drug (in Grams) in solution}}{\text{amount of solution (in Grams)}}$$
$$= \text{percent of solution}$$

$$\frac{8 \text{ Gm.}}{1000 \text{ Gm.}} = \frac{1}{125}$$

The resulting fraction is converted to a percentage by dividing the denominator into the numerator:

$$125 \overline{)1.000} 0.008$$

and converting the decimal to a percent:

$$0.008 \times 100 = 0.8\%$$

Therefore a 1000-ml. solution containing 8 Grams of a drug is an 0.8% solution.

EXAMPLE NO. 2
If 500 ml. contains 7 1/2 grains (grains $\overline{\text{viiss}}$), what is the strength of the solution?

First, the apothecaries' weight is converted to the metric equivalent.

$$15 : 1 : : 7.5 : x$$
$$15x = 7.5$$
$$x = 0.5 \text{ Gram}$$

As in Example No. 1, ml. is converted to Grams. Since 1 ml. equals approximately 1 Gram, 500 ml. equals 500 Grams. Using the formula:

$$\frac{0.5 \text{ Gm.}}{500 \text{ Gm.}} = \frac{5}{5000} = \frac{1}{1000}$$

Convert the fraction to a decimal:

$$1000 \overline{) 1.000}^{\;0.001}$$

and convert the decimal to a percent:

$$0.001 \times 100 = 0.1\%$$

Therefore a 500-ml. solution containing 7 1/2 grains of a drug is a 0.1% solution.

*Note: *t* following page number refers to tables

Absorbable gelatin sponge, 305-306
Acenocoumarol, 86*t*, 91*t*
Acetaminophen, 48, 50, 51-52, 53*t*, 265*t*
Acetazolamide, 104, 110*t*
Acetohexamide, 122*t*, 129*t*, 320
Acetophenazine, 242*t*, 251*t*
Acetylcholine (ACh), 23-24, 107
    inhibition of, 30 (*see also* Cholinergic blocking
      agents)
Acetylcholinesterase (AChE), 23, 24
Acetylcysteine, 262
Acetyldigitoxin, 80*t*
Acetylsalicylic acid. *See* Aspirin
ACh. *See* Acetylcholine
AChE. *See* Acetylcholinesterase
Acid (hallucinogen). *See* LSD
Acidosis, treatment of, 99
Acids, antiseptic, 301
Acidulin. *See* Glutamic acid hydrochloride
Acrisorcin, 146*t*, 156*t*
ACTH (adrenocorticotropic hormone), 178-182, 187*t*
Acthar. *See* ACTH
Actidil. *See* Triprolidine
Actifed, constituents, 265*t*
Acylanid. *See* Acetyldigitoxin
Adenohypophysis, 177
ADH (antidiuretic hormone). *See* Vasopressin
Adrenal cortex hormones. *See* Corticosteroids
Adrenal gland, 7, 18
Adrenalin, 11*t*, 14*t*
Adrenaline. *See* Epinephrine
Adrenergic blocking agents, 17-22
  as antihypertensives, 107, 108, 113*t*
Adrenergic drugs, 7-16, 18
Adrenocorticosteroids. *See* Corticosteroids
Adrenocorticotropic hormone. *See* ACTH
Aerosporin. *See* Polymyxin B
Agoral, constituents, 277*t*
Akineton. *See* Biperiden

Index*

Akrinol. *See* Acrisorcin
Alcohol:
    as antiseptic, 302
    interaction with drugs, 59, 108
Alcopara. *See* Bephenium hydroxy-
    naphthoate
Aldactone A. *See* Spironolactone
Aldomet. *See* Methyldopa
Aldosterone, 182
Aldosterone antagonist, 104, 105, 110t
Alkalosis, 100
Alka-Seltzer, 269-270
Alkavervir, 114t
Alkeran. *See* Melphalan
Alkylating agents, 215, 216t, 221-222t
Allergic reactions, 2-3
    to penicillin, 136-138
    to sulfonamides, 132
Allopurinol, 318, 320, 322, 323t
Aloe, 276t
Alpha adrenergic blocking agents, 17,
    18, 19, 20, 93. *See also* Adrenergic
    blocking agents
Alpha adrenergic receptors, 8, 10-11, 17
Alphaprodine, 38, 39, 44t
Alseroxylon, 113t
Aludrox, constituents, 275t
Aluminum hydroxide, 268, 272, 275t,
    276t
Aluminum phosphate, 268t
Alurate. *See* Aprobarbital
Amantadine, 236-237, 238t
Ambenonium, 24, 27t
Amcill. *See* Ampicillin trihydrate
Amcill-GC, constituents, 148t
Amcill-S. *See* Sodium ampicillin
Amebacides, 171-172, 175-176t
Amebiasis, 165, 170-172
Aminophylline U.S.P.:
    as CNS stimulant, 116, 117-118, 119t
    as diuretic, 104, 112t
Aminosalicylic acid, 159, 160-161, 163t
Amitriptyline, 243t, 244, 256t, 257t
Ammoniated mercury ointment, 303

Ammonium chloride, 261
Amobarbital, 56t, 60t
Amodiaquin, 167t, 171, 173t, 175t
Amphetamines, abuse of, 67, 70t
Amphogel. *See* Aluminum hydroxide
Amphotericin B, 146, 147, 156t
Ampicillin trihydrate, 148t
Amylase, 278t, 306
Amyl nitrite, 94, 96t
Amytal. *See* Amobarbital
Anacin, constituents, 116
Analeptic agents, 115
Analgesics:
    narcotic, 35-41, 44-45t, 58, 108
    neurolept, as anesthetics, 313-314
    non-narcotic, 41-42, 45t, 47-53
Anaphylactic reactions, 3
Ancobon. *See* Flucytosine
Androgens, 191-192, 195, 197-198t
    as antineoplastic agents, 217
Anectine. *See* Succinylcholine chloride
Anemia, drugs used in treatment of, 288-
    290, 292t
Anesthetic agents, 309-316
    dissociative, 314
    gaseous, 311-312
    intravenous, 311
    local, 315-316
    neurolept analgesics, 313-314
    neuromuscular blocking agents, 314-
    315
    preparation for, 30, 309-310
    volatile, 312-313
Anileridine, 38, 39, 44t
Anisindione, 86t, 91t
Ansolysen. *See* Pentolinium
Antacids, 267-268, 272, 273-274, 275-
    276t
Antepar. *See* Piperazine
Anthelmintic drugs, 169-170, 174-175t
Antiarrhythmic drugs. *See* Cardiac de-
    pressants
Antibacterial agents, 132. *See also* Sul-
    fonamides

Antibiotics, broad spectrum, 139-145,
    150-156t. *See also* Penicillin
    with anticoagulants, 90t
    antiparasitic use, 171, 176t
Antibodies, 293-294
Anticoagulant drugs, 85-92
Anticonvulsant drugs, 227-233
Antidepressant agents, 243-244, 245,
    247, 249, 255-257t
Antidepressant antianxiety agents, 244,
    249, 257t
Antidiarrheal agents, 271, 273, 274, 280t
Antidiuretic hormone (ADH). *See* Vaso-
    pressin
Antiemetics, 268-269, 272, 279-280t
Antifungal agents, 146-147, 156-157t
Antigens, 293-294
Antihistamines, 109, 259, 260, 261, 263-
    265t
Antihypertensive agents, 18, 19-20, 107-
    110, 113-114t
Antimalarial drugs, 167-168, 173-174t
Antimetabolites, 215, 217t, 222-223t
Antiminth. *See* Pyrantel pamoate
Antineoplastic agents, 215-225
Antiparasitic drugs, 165-176. *See also*
    Amebacides; Anthelmintic drugs
Antiparkinsonism agents, 235-240
Antipyretics, 47-48. *See also* Analgesics,
    non-narcotic
Antiseptics and disinfectants, 301-308
Antithyroid agents, 205-207, 208t
Antitoxins, 294
Antitubercular agents, 159-162, 163-164t
Antitussives, 261-263, 265t
Antivert. *See* Meclizine
Anturane. *See* Sulfinpyrazone
Anxiety, treatment of, 18, 41, 249, 257t
Apomorphine, 37, 38, 46t, 278t
Aprobarbital, 56t, 60t
Aralen. *See* Chloroquine
Aramine. *See* Metaraminol
Arfonad. *See* Trimethaphan
Aristocort. *See* Triamcinolone

Aristospan. *See* Triamcinolone hexacetonide
Arsenic, 281
Artane. *See* Trihexyphenidyl
Ascorbic acid. *See* Vitamin C
Ascriptin, 268
Aspidium oleoresin, 169, 174*t*
Aspirin (acetylsalicylic acid):
    analgesic action, 48, 49, 53*t*
    for arthritis, 317, 322, 323*t*
    precautions, 90*t*
Atabrine. *See* Quinacrine hydrochloride
Ataractic agents. *See* Tranquilizers
Athrombin-K. *See* Warfarin potassium
Atropine, 29-32, 33*t*
    antidiarrheal use, 271, 280*t*
    as cholinergic antagonist, 25, 26
    in Parkinson's disease, 235
    preanesthetic use, 310*t*
Atropine methylnitrate, 30
Attenuvax. *See* Measles virus vaccine
Aureomycin. *See* Chlortetracycline
Aurothioglucose, 282, 284*t*, 318, 323*t*
Autonomic nervous system, 7, 8-11
Aventyl. *See* Nortriptyline
Azo-Mandelamine, constituents, 308*t*

Bacid. *See* Lactobacillus acidophilus
Bacitracin, 140, 142, 150*t*
Baking soda. *See* Sodium bicarbonate
BAL. *See* Dimercaprol U.S.P.
Banthine. *See* Methantheline
Barbiturates, 55-56, 57, 60-61*t*. *See also*
    Sedatives and hypnotics
    abuse of, 67-68, 70*t*
    anesthetic use, 310*t*, 311
    anticonvulsant use, 228-229
    overdose treatment, 116
    precautions, 90*t*, 108
BCG vaccine, 296*t*
Belladonna, 29, 33*t*
Benadryl. *See* Diphenhydramine
Bendroflumethiazide, 111*t*

Benemid. *See* Probenecid
Bentyl. *See* Dicyclomine
Benylin expectorant, constituents, 265*t*
Benzalkonium chloride, 304
Benzathine penicillin G, 135-136, 148*t*
Benzocaine, 316*t*
Benzodiazepine tranquilizers, 243*t*
Benzonatate, 262
Benzoquinonium chloride, 314*t*
Benzthiazide, 111*t*
Benztropine, 236*t*, 239*t*
Bephenium hydroxynaphthoate, 169*t*, 174*t*
Beta adrenergic blocking agents, 17, 18, 19, 20. *See also* Adrenergic blocking agents
Beta adrenergic receptors, 8, 10-11, 17
Betadine. *See* Povidone-iodine
Betamethasone, 188*t*
Betamethasone acetate, 188*t*
Betamethasone sodium phosphate, 188*t*
Betapar. *See* Meprednisone
Bethanechol, 23, 24, 27*t*
Bicillin Long-Acting. *See* Benzathine penicillin G
Biguanides, 122*t*
Bile salts, 269, 278*t*
Biotin, 288
Biperiden, 236*t*, 239*t*
Bisacodyl, 276*t*
Blenoxane. *See* Bleomycin sulfate
Bleomycin sulfate, 217*t*, 224*t*
Blood clots, prevention of. *See* Anticoagulant drugs
Blood vessels, 9*t*, 116. *See also* Vasodilating agents
Body fluids, management of, 97-102
Body size, and drug action, 2
Bonine. *See* Meclizine
Boric acid, 301, 304
Botulism antitoxin, 296*t*
Brevital. *See* Methohexital
Brompheniramine, 263*t*

Bromsulphalein. *See* sulphobromophthalein
Buerger's disease, 95
Bufferin, constituents, 268
Bupivacaine hydrochloride, 316*t*
Busulphan, 216*t*, 221*t*
Butabarbital, 56*t*, 60*t*
Butaperazine, 242*t*, 251*t*
Butazolidin. *See* Phenylbutazone
Butisol. *See* Butabarbital

C. *See* Cocaine
Caffeine, 104, 115, 116-117, 119*t*
Calcium, 98, 99
Calcium carbonate, 275*t*
Calcium chloride, 98, 99
Calcium disodium edetate, 282, 283, 284*t*
Calcium disodium versenate. *See* Calcium disodium edetate
Calcium gluconate, 98, 102*t*
Calcium lactate, 102*t*
Camoquin. *See* Amodiaquin
Camphorated opium tincture. *See* Paregoric
Cancer, treatment of. *See* Antineoplastic agents
Candeptin. *See* Candicidin
Candicidin, 146*t*, 157*t*
Cannabis, 66
Cantil. *See* Mepenzolate
Capastat. *See* Capreomycin
Capreomycin, 159, 161, 163*t*
Carbarsone, 171, 175*t*
Carbenicillin indanyl sodium, 148*t*
Carbetapentane, 261
Carbocaine. *See* Mepivacaine hydrochloride
Carbolic acid. *See* Phenol
Carbonic anhydrase inhibitors, 104, 105, 110*t*
Carcinoma, treatment of. *See* Antineoplastic agents

Cardiac arrhythmias, treatment of, 18, 20, 31. *See also* Cardiac depressants; Cardiotonic drugs
Cardiac depressants, 71, 76-79, 82-83*t*
Cardiac output, defined, 72
Cardiac stimulants. *See* Cardiotonic drugs; Catecholamines
Cardilate. *See* Erythrityl tetranitrate
Cardiotonic drugs, 71-75, 80-81*t*
Cardrase. *See* Ethoxyzolamide
Carisoprodol, 319, 324*t*
Carotene, 287
Casanthranol, 271, 277*t*
Cascara sagrada, 276*t*
Castor oil, 270, 277*t*
Catecholamines, 7-8, 11, 14*t*
Cathartics and laxatives, 270-278
Cation-exchange resins, 98, 99, 100
Cedilanid. *See* Lanatoside C
Cedilanid-D. *See* Deslanoside
Celestone. *See* Betamethasone
Celestone Soluspan, constituents, 188*t*
Celontin. *See* Methsuximide
Celsus, Aurelius Cornelius, 121
Central nervous system (CNS), effect on:
    of adrenergic drugs, 8
    of cholinergic blocking agents, 30
    of sulfonamides, 132
    of thyroid dysfunction, 204*t*
Central nervous system (CNS) stimulants, 115-119
Cephalexin, 140*t*, 142-143, 151*t*
Cephaloglycin, 140*t*, 143, 151*t*
Cephaloridine, 140*t*, 143, 151*t*
Cephalosporins, 138, 140, 142-143
Cephalothin, 140*t*, 143, 151*t*
Chloral hydrate, 57, 59, 61*t*
Chlorambucil, 216*t*, 221*t*
Chloramphenicol, 139, 142, 151*t*
Chlorazepate, 243*t*, 246, 253*t*
Chlordantoin, 146*t*, 157*t*
Chlordiazepoxide, 243, 246, 253*t*
Chlormerodrin, 110*t*
Chlormezanone, 243*t*, 253*t*

Chloroform, 309, 312
Chloromycetin. *See* Chloramphenicol
Chloroprocaine hydrochloride, 316*t*
Chloroquine, 167*t*, 171, 173*t*, 176*t*
Chlorothiazide, 111*t*
Chlorotrianisene, 198*t*
Chlorphenesin, 319, 324*t*
Chlorpheniramine, 264*t*
Chlorpromazine:
    as antiemetic, 279*t*
    preanesthetic use, 310*t*
    psychotherapeutic use, 241, 242, 252*t*
Chlorpropamide, 122*t*, 129*t*, 320
Chlorprothixene, 242*t*, 243, 244, 246, 253*t*
Chlortetracycline, 139*t*, 152*t*
Chlor-Trimeton. *See* Chlorpheniramine
Cholera vaccine, 297*t*
Cholinergic blocking agents, 29-34
    antidiarrheal use, 271
    effect of, on uterus, 210
    preanesthetic use, 310*t*
Cholinergic drugs, 23-28
Chymoral, 306
Chymotrypsin, 306
Citanest. *See* Prilocaine hydrochloride
Citrate of magnesia, 270
Cleocin. *See* Clindamycin
Clindamycin, 140, 143, 152*t*
Clinistix, 127, 304
Coal-tar derivatives. *See* Nonsalicylates
Cocaine, 65, 316*t*
Codasa, 39
Codeine, 35, 37, 39, 44*t*
    abuse of, 65
    as antitussive, 261
Cogentin. *See* Benztropine
Coke. *See* Cocaine
Colace. *See* Dioctyl sodium sulfosuccinate
Colchicine, 318, 320, 321, 324*t*
Colistimethate, 140, 143, 152*t*
Colistin sulfate, 140, 143, 152*t*
Coly-Mycin M. *See* Colistimethate

Coly-Mycin S. *See* Colistin sulfate
Combistix, 127
Compazine. *See* Prochlorperazine
Compocillin-VK. *See* Potassium phenoxymethyl penicillin
Contraceptives, oral. *See* Oral contraceptives
Convulsants, 115
Convulsive disorders, treatment of. *See* Anticonvulsant drugs
Copper poisoning, 282
Coramine. *See* Nikethamide
Cortef. *See* Hydrocortisone
Corticosteroids, 104, 178-189, 318-319
Corticotropin. *See* ACTH
Cortisol. *See* Hydrocortisone
Cortisone, 180-181
Cortisone acetate, 188*t*
Coryban-D cough syrup, constituents, 265*t*
Cosmegen. *See* Dactinomycin
Cotazym. *See* Pancreatic enzymes
Cottonseed oil, 270-271
Coughing, treatment of. *See* Antitussives
Coumadin. *See* Warfarin sodium
Coumarin derivatives, 85, 86*t*, 88. *See also* Anticoagulant drugs
Cresol, 304
Cretinism, 203-204
Crystalluria, 133
Crystodigin. *See* Digitoxin
Crystoids. *See* Hexylresorcinol
Cuprimine. *See* Penicillamine
Curare, 314
Cushing's disease, 182
Cyanocobalamin. *See* Vitamin B_{12}
Cyclandelate, 93, 94, 96*t*
Cyclizine, 264*t*
Cyclomethycaine, 316*t*
Cyclophosphamide, 216*t*, 221*t*
Cyclopropane, 312
Cycloserine, 159, 160, 163*t*
Cyclospasmol. *See* Cyclandelate
Cycrimine, 236*t*, 239*t*

Cytarabine, 217t, 222t
Cytomel. *See* Liothyronine
Cytosar. *See* Cytarabine
Cytoxan. *See* Cyclophosphamide

Dactinomycin, 217t, 220, 224t
Dalmane. *See* Flurazepam
Danthron, 277t
Daraprim. *See* Pyrimethamine
Darbid. *See* Isopropamide
Daricon. *See* Oxyphencyclimine
Darvon, 49. *See also* Propoxyphene hydrochloride
Darvon-N. *See* Propoxyphene napsylate
Davy, Sir Humphry, 309
DBI. *See* Phenformin
D-calcium pantothenate, 277t
Deaner. *See* Deanol
Deanol, 116, 119t
Decadron. *See* Dexamethasone
Decamethonium bromide, 314t
Decholin. *See* Dehydrocholic acid
Declomycin. *See* Demeclocycline
Dehydrocholic acid, 278t
Delirium tremens (D.T.'s), treatment of, 57
Delta-Cortef. *See* Prednisolone
Deltasone. *See* Prednisone
Demeclocycline, 139t, 152t
Demerol. *See* Meperidine
Demulen, constituents, 200t
Depo-Provera. *See* Medroxyprogesterone
Depressants:
    abuse of, 67-68
    cardiac (*see* Cardiac depressants)
    general (*see* Parbiturates)
Depression, treatment of. *See* Antidepressant agents
DES. *See* Diethylstilbestrol U.S.P.
Desenex, constituents, 157t
Desipramine, 243t, 256t
Deslanoside, 80t
Desoxycorticosterone, 182, 188t
DET (diethyltryptamine), 67

Dexamethasone, 188t, 319
Dextran, 97, 98, 99, 100
Dextroamphetamine, 8
Dextromethorphan, 261, 265t
Diabetes mellitus, treatment of, 121-129
Diabinese. *See* Chlorpropamide
Diamox. *See* Acetazolamide
Dianabol. *See* Methandrostenolone
Diapid. *See* Lypressin
Diarrhea, treatment of. *See* Antidiarrheal agents
Diazepam:
    for muscular skeletal disorders, 319, 324t
    psychotherapeutic use, 243, 246, 254t
Dibenzyline. *See* Phenoxybenzamine
Dibucaine hydrochloride, 316t
Dicarbosil, constituents, 275t
Dick test, 294, 296
Dicumarol, 85, 86t, 91t
Dicyclomine, 33t, 276t
Dienestrol, 193
Diethylstilbestrol U.S.P. (DES), 193, 198t
Diethyltryptamine (DET), 67
Digestants, 268-269, 272, 278t
Digitalis, 71, 72, 73, 80t
Digitalis purpurea glycosides, 80t
Digitalization, 74-75
Digitoxin, 72, 81t
Digoxin, 72, 74, 81t
Dihydrostreptomycin, 160, 161, 164t
Diiodohydroxyquin, 171, 176t
Dilantin. *See* Diphenylhydantoin
Dilaudid. *See* Hydromorphone
Dimenhydrinate, 264t, 272t, 279t
Dimercaprol U.S.P. (BAL), 171, 281, 282, 284t
Dimethoxymethylamphetamine (STP, DOM), 67
Dimethylamine phenothiazines, 242t
Dimethyltryptamine (DMT), 67
Dimethyl tubocurarine chloride, 314t
Dimethyl tubocurarine iodide, 314t

Dimetane. *See* Brompheniramine
Dioctyl calcium sulfosuccinate, 273, 277t
Dioctyl sodium sulfosuccinate, 270, 277t
Diodoquin. *See* Diiodohydroxyquin
Dipaxin. *See* Diphenadione
Diphemanil, 34t
Diphenadione, 86t
Diphenhydramine, 264t, 265t
Diphenoxylate, 271, 280t
Diphenylhydantoin:
    anticonvulsant use, 227, 228, 230, 231t
    as cardiac depressant, 76, 77, 78, 82t
    and folic acid, 289
Diphenylmethane tranquilizer, 243t
Diphtheria test, 294
Diphtheria toxoid, 297t, 300t
Dipyridamole, 93, 94, 96t
Discharge teaching:
    amebacides, 172
    anthelmintic drugs, 169-170
    anticoagulants, 90
    anticonvulsants, 230
    antifungal agents, 147
    antihistamines, 261
    antihypertensives, 109-110
    antimalarial drugs, 168
    and body fluid management, 101
    broad spectrum antibiotics, 145
    cardiac depressants, 79
    cardiotonics, 75
    cholinergic blocking agents, 32-33
    cholinergic drugs, 26
    corticosteroids, 185-186
    diuretics, 107
    gastrointestinal agents, 274-275
    insulin and oral hypoglycemics, 127-128
    musculoskeletal disorders, 321-323
    Parkinson's disease, 238
    penicillin, 138-139
    psychotherapeutic agents, 250
    salicylates, 52
    sedatives and hypnotics, 59
    sulfonamides, 133

Discharge teaching (*continued*)
thyroid and antithyroid agents, 206-207
Disinfectants. *See* Antiseptics and disinfectants
Disipal. *See* Orphenadrine
Disodium carbenicillin, 149*t*
Diuretics, 103-107, 110-112*t*
Diuril. *See* Chlorothiazide
DMT (dimethyltryptamine), 67
Doca acetate. *See* Desoxycorticosterone
Dolophine. *See* Methadone
DOM (dimethoxymethylamphetamine), 67
Donnagel, constituents, 271, 280*t*
Donnagel-PG, 38
Dopamine, 236
Dopar. *See* Levodopa
Dopram. *See* Doxapram
Doriden. *See* Glutethimide
Dornavac. *See* Pancreatic dornase
Doxapram, 117, 119*t*
Doxepin, 244, 247, 249, 257*t*
Doxidan, constituents, 277*t*
Doxycycline, 139*t*, 142, 152*t*
D.P.T., 300*t*
Dramamine. *See* Dimenhydrinate
Drolban. *See* Dromostanolone
Dromostanolone, 197*t*
Droperidol, 39, 313-314
Drug abuse, 63-70
of cocaine, 65
of hallucinogens, 65-67
of heroin, 64-65
of stimulants and depressants, 67-68
of volatile hydrocarbons, 68
Drug addiction, defined, 64
Drug allergy, defined, 2-3
Drug dependence, 57, 63
Drug habituation, defined, 64
Drug idiosyncrasy, 3, 30, 32
Drug interaction, defined, 4

Drugs:
absorption of, 4-5
action of, 1-2
adverse reactions to, 2-3
effects of, 3-4
Drug synergism, defined, 4
Drug tolerance, defined, 3
Dulcolax. *See* Bisacodyl
Duphaston. *See* Dydrogesterone
Durabolin. *See* Nandrolone
Dust. *See* Cocaine
Dwarfism, treatment of, 178
Dydrogesterone, 199*t*
Dyes, antiseptic, 302, 305
Dymelor. *See* Acetohexamide
Dynapen. *See* Sodium dicloxacillin

Edecrin. *See* Ethacrynic acid
Edema, 104. *See also* Diuretics
Edrophonium, 27*t*, 315
Elavil. *See* Amitriptyline
Electrolyte balance:
and body fluids, 97-102
and corticosteroids, 182, 189*t*
Emetics, 268, 272, 278*t*. *See also* Apomorphine
Emetine, 171, 172, 176*t*
Emetrol. *See* Levulose
Emivan. *See* Ethamivan
Empirin Compound, 39, 48, 49, 116
Endocrine system, and corticosteroids, 182, 189*t*
Enduron. *See* Methyclothiazide
Enovid, constituents, 201*t*
Entozyme, constituents, 278*t*
Enzymes, absorbable, 305, 306, 307
Ephedrine, 14*t*
Epilepsy:
diagnosis of, 116, 118
treatment of, 76, 104 (*see also* Anticonvulsant drugs)
Epinephrine, 14*t*
administration of, 11*t*, 13
blocking of, 18

Epinephrine (*continued*)
as histamine antagonist, 261
and nervous system, 7, 8, 24
Epsom salts, 270
Equilenin, 192
Equilin, 192
Ergonovine maleate, 209, 211, 213*t*
Ergot derivatives, 209, 210, 211
Ergotrate. *See* Ergonovine maleate
Erythrityl tetranitrate, 94, 96*t*
Erythrocin ethyl succinate. *See* Erythromycin ethylsuccinate
Erythrocin lactobionate. *See* Erythromycin lactobionate
Erythrocin stearate. *See* Erythromycin stearate
Erythromycin:
antiparasitical use, 171, 172, 176*t*
as broad spectrum antibiotic, 139, 142, 153*t*
Erythromycin estolate, 139*t*
Erythromycin ethylsuccinate, 139*t*, 153*t*
Erythromycin gluceptate, 139*t*, 153*t*
Erythromycin lactobionate, 139*t*, 153*t*
Erythromycin stearate, 139*t*, 153*t*
Eserine. *See* Physostigmine
Esidrix. *See* Hydrochlorothiazide
Estradiol, 192, 193, 199*t*
Estriol, 192, 193
Estrogenic substances, conjugated, 199*t*
Estrogens, 192-193, 194, 198-199*t*, 217
Estrone, 192
Ethacrynic acid, 90*t*, 104, 105, 112*t*
Ethambutol, 160, 161, 163*t*
Ethamide. *See* Ethoxyzolamide
Ethamivan, 116, 117, 119*t*
Ethchlorvynol, 56, 59, 61*t*, 90*t*
Ether, 309, 312
Ethinamate, 57, 61*t*
Ethinyl estradiol, 200*t*, 201*t*
Ethionamide, 160, 161, 163*t*
Ethopropazine, 236*t*, 239*t*
Ethosuximide, 228, 231*t*
Ethotoin, 228, 231*t*

Ethoxyzolamide, 110*t*
Ethyl alcohol, 302
Ethynodiol diacetate, 200*t*
Etrafon, constituents, 257*t*
Euthroid. *See* Liotrix
Eutonyl. *See* Pargyline
Evipal. *See* Hexobarbital
Exna. *See* Benzthiazide
Extended Insulin Zinc Suspension
U.S.P., 122*t*, 126*t*, 129*t*
Eyes:
and autonomic nervous system, 9*t*
effect on, of drugs, 30, 37, 182, 189*t*
examination of, drugs for, 30-31

Female hormones, 192-194, 198-200*t*.
See also Oral contraceptives
Fentanyl, 38-39, 44*t*, 313-314
Feosol. *See* Ferrous sulfate
Fergon. *See* Ferrous gluconate
Ferrocholinate, 292*t*
Ferrolip. *See* Ferrocholinate
Ferrous fumarate, 193, 292*t*
Ferrous gluconate, 292*t*
Ferrous sulfate, 292*t*
Festal, constituents, 278*t*
Fibrin, 86
Fibrinogen, 86
5-FU. *See* Fluorouracil
Flaxedil. *See* Gallamine triethiodide
Fleet Brand, constituents, 270, 278*t*
Fleming, Sir Alexander, 135
Florinef. *See* Fludrocortisone acetate
Floxuridine, 217*t*, 222*t*
Flucytosine, 146, 147, 157*t*
Fludrocortisone acetate, 182, 188*t*
Fluorescein, 302
Fluorouracil, 217*t*, 222*t*
Fluothane. *See* Halothane
Fluoxymesterone, 197*t*
Fluphenazine, 242*t*, 252*t*
Flurazepam, 56, 61*t*
Folic acid, 289, 290, 292*t*
Follicle stimulating hormone. *See* FSH

Folvite. *See* Folic acid
FSH (follicle stimulating hormone), 177,
178
FUDR. *See* Floxuridine
Fulvicon. *See* Griseofulvin
Fungizone. *See* Amphotericin B
Fungus, 146. *See also* Antifungal agents
Furacin. *See* Nitrofurazone
Furadantin. *See* Nitrofurantoin
Furan antiseptics, 302-303
Furazolidone, 302-303, 304-305, 307*t*
Furosemide, 104, 105, 112*t*
Furoxone. *See* Furazolidone

Galen, 121
Gallamine triethiodide, 314*t*
Gammacorten. *See* Dexamethasone
Ganglionic blocking agents, 107, 108,
113*t*
Gantanol. *See* Sulfamethoxazole
Gantrisin. *See* Sulfisoxazole
Gantrisin diolamine. *See* Sulfisoxazole
diolamine
Garamycin. *See* Gentamicin
Gaseous anesthetics, 311-312
Gas gangrene antitoxin, 300*t*
Gastrointestinal agents, 267-280
Gastrointestinal system, effect on:
of cholinergic blocking agents, 30, 31
of corticosteroids, 182, 189*t*
of morphine, 37, 38
of sulfonamides, 132
Gelfoam. *See* Absorbable gelatin sponge
Gelusil, constituents, 276*t*
Gemonil. *See* Metharbital
Gentamicin, 140, 143-144, 153*t*
Gentian violet. *See* Methylrosaniline
Gentlax S, constituents, 277*t*
Geocillin. *See* Carbenicillin indanyl
sodium
Geopen. *See* Disodium carbenicillin
Gitaligin. *See* Gitalin
Gitalin, 81*t*
Glaucoma, treatment of, 25, 104

Globin Zinc Insulin U.S.P., 122*t*, 129*t*
Glucagon, 125
Glucocorticoids, 178, 180-181, 182,
188*t*, 189*t*
Glucose, 97, 98, 99
Glue-sniffing, 68
Glutamic acid hydrochloride, 268-269,
278*t*
Glutethimide, 61*t*, 68, 90*t*
Glycerin, 270-271, 277*t*
Glyceryl trinitrate (nitroglycerin), 94-95,
96*t*
Glycobiarsol, 171, 176*t*
Glycosides. *See* Cardiotonic drugs
Glycyrrhiza, 262
Gold:
poisoning, 281, 282
treatment, 282, 283
Gold sodium thiomalate, 318, 324*t*
Gonadotropins, 177
Gout, treatment of, 48, 318
Grass. *See* Marijuana
Griseofulvin, 146, 147, 157*t*
G-Strophanthin. *See* Ouabain
Guanethidine, 18, 21*t*, 113*t*

H. *See* Heroin
Haldol. *See* Haloperidol
Haldrone. *See* Paramethasone acetate
Hallucinogens, abuse of, 65-67, 69*t*
Halogen antiseptics, 303
Haloperidol, 242*t*, 244, 246, 253*t*
Haloprogin, 146*t*, 157*t*
Halotestin. *See* Fluoxymesterone
Halotex. *See* Haloprogin
Halothane, 312
Harry. *See* Heroin
Hashish, abuse of, 66
Heart, effect on:
of adrenergic drugs, 10
of cholinergic blocking agents, 30
of xanthines, 116
(*see also* Cardiac depressants; Cardio-
tonic drugs)

Heavy metals and heavy metal antago-
nists, 281-284, 303
Hedulin. See Phenindione
Helminthiasis, 165, 168-170. See also
Anthelmintic drugs
Hemicellulose, 278t
Hemostatics, absorbable, 305
Heparin, 85, 86, 87, 88-89
Heparin sodium, 91t
Heroin, 35, 39, 64-65, 69t
Hetacillin, 149t
Hexachlorophene, 304
Hexobarbital, 311t
Hexocyclium, 34t
Hexylresorcinol, 169, 174t, 304
Hippocrates, 47, 121
Histamine, 259-260, 261, 263t
Histamine phosphate U.S.P., 263t
Histamine reaction, 261
Homatropine, 34t
Hookworms. See Helminthiasis
Hormones:
    as antineoplastic agents, 216-217
    pituitary (see Pituitary hormones)
    sex (see Androgens; Female hormones)
Horse. See Heroin
Hospital Formulary, 2
Humatin. See Paromomycin
Hyaluronidase, 306
Hydeltra. See Prednisolone
Hydrea. See Hydroxyurea
Hydrochloric acid, 267, 268-269, 272,
278t
Hydrochlorothiazide, 111t
Hydrocortisone, 180-181, 188t
Hydrocortone. See Hydrocortisone
HydroDIURIL. See Hydrochlorothiazide
Hydrogen peroxide, 303
Hydromorphone, 39, 44t
Hydroxychloroquine, 167t, 173t
Hydroxyurea, 217t, 223t
Hydroxyzine:
    for gastrointestinal disorders, 272t,
    279t

Hydroxyzine (continued)
    preanesthetic use, 310t
    psychotherapeutic use, 243t, 254t
Hykinone. See Menadione sodium bisul-
fite
Hyoscine, 271, 280t
Hyoscyamine, 271, 280t
Hyperkalemia, 98, 99
Hyperkinesis, treatment of, 116, 118
Hypertension, treatment of, 18, 19-20.
See also Antihypertensive agents
Hypertensive crisis, symptoms, 247t
Hyperthyroidism, 203, 204, 205
Hypnotics. See Sedatives and hypnotics
Hypocalcemia, 98
Hypoglycemia, 123, 124, 125-126
Hypoglycemic agents, oral, 122, 123,
124, 128, 129t. See also Insulin
Hypokalemia, 98, 99, 106t
Hyponatremia, 99, 106t
Hypoprothrombinemia, defined, 86
Hypotension, 19
Hypothalamus, 48
Hypothyroidism, 203-204, 205

Ibuprofen, 324t
Ilosone. See Erythromycin estolate
Ilotycin. See Erythromycin
Ilotycin gluceptate. See Erythromycin
gluceptate
Imferon. See Iron dextran
Imipramine, 243t, 257t
Immunological agents, 293-300
Inapsine. See Droperidol
Indandione derivatives, 85, 86t, 88. See
also Anticoagulant drugs
Inderal. See Propranolol
Indocin. See Indomethacin
Indomethacin, 318, 320, 322-323, 324t
Influenza vaccine, 297t
INH. See Isoniazid
Innovar, 313
Inositol, 288
Insecticide poisoning, treatment of, 31

Insulin, 121-122, 123-128, 126t, 129t
Insulin Injection U.S.P., 122t, 126t, 129t
Insulin Zinc Suspension U.S.P., 122t,
126t, 129t
Inversine. See Mecamylamine
Iodine, and thyroid function, 203-204,
206
Iodine, radioactive, 205, 207
Iodine solution, 303, 305
Iodine U.S.P., 205t, 208t
Iodism, symptoms of, 171t
Iodochlorhydroxyquin, 171, 176t
Ipecac U.S.P., 269, 278t
Ircon. See Ferrous fumarate
Iron, and anemia, 288-289, 290
Iron dextran, 290, 292t
Iron sorbitex, 290, 292t
Ismelin. See Guanethidine
Isoniazid, 159, 160, 161, 164t
Isophane Insulin Suspension U.S.P.,
122t, 126t, 129t
Isopropamide, 34t
Isopropyl alcohol, 302
Isoproterenol, 8, 13, 14t
Isordil. See Isosorbide dinitrate
Isosorbide dinitrate, 93, 96t
Isoxsuprine, 93, 94, 96t
Isuprel. See Isoproterenol

Jectofer. See Iron sorbitex
Jenner, Edward, 293

Kafocin. See Cephaloglycin
Kanamycin, 140, 144, 154t
Kantrex. See Kanamycin
Kaolin, 271, 280t
Kaon. See Potassium gluconate
Kayexalate. See Sodium polystyrene
Keflex. See Cephalexin
Keflin. See Cephalothin
Kemadrin. See Procyclidine
Kenacort. See Triamcinolone
Ketalar. See Ketamine
Ketamine, 314

Kidneys, and diuretics, 103-104
K-Lyte. *See* Potassium bicarbonate
Koch, Robert, 159
Kolantyl, constituents, 276t
Konakion. *See* Phytonadione

Lactinex, constituents, 271, 280t
Lactobacillus acidophilus, 271, 280t
Lactobacillus bulgaricus, 280t
Lanatoside C, 72, 81t
Lanoxin. *See* Digoxin
Laradopa. *See* Levodopa
Lasix. *See* Furosemide
Laxatives. *See* Cathartics and laxatives
Lead poisoning, 282, 283
Lente Iletin. *See* Insulin Zinc Suspension
    U.S.P.
Lente Insulin. *See* Insulin Zinc Suspen-
    sion U.S.P.
Leritine. *See* Anileridine
Letter. *See* Levothyroxine
Leukeran. *See* Chlorambucil
Levallorphan, 42t, 43, 46t
Levarterenol, 8, 11t, 12-13, 14t, 18
Levodopa, 235, 236, 237, 238, 240t
Levo-Dromoran. *See* Levorphanol
Levophed. *See* Levarterenol
Levoprome. *See* Methotrimeprazine
Levorphanol, 38, 44t
Levothyroxine, 204t, 207t
Levulose, 279t
LH (luteinizing hormone), 177, 178
Librium. *See* Chlordiazepoxide
Lidocaine, 76, 77, 78, 79, 82t, 316t
Lincocin. *See* Lincomycin
Lincomycin, 140-141, 144, 154t
Liothyronine, 203, 204t, 207t
Liotrix, 204t, 207t
Lipase, 269, 278t
Lister, Joseph, 301
Lithane. *See* Lithium
Lithium, 243, 245, 246-247, 249, 255t
Liver extract, 289
Lomotil, constituents, 271, 280t

Lorfan. *See* Levallorphan
Loridine. *See* Cephaloridine
Lotusate. *See* Talbutal
LSD (lysergic acid diethylamide), 66-67
LTH (luteotropic hormone), 177
Lugol's solution. *See* Iodine U.S.P.
Luminal. *See* Phenobarbital
Luteinizing hormone. *See* LH
Luteotropic hormone. *See* LTH
Lutrexin. *See* Lututrin
Lututrin, 210, 211, 213, 214t
Lypressin, 178, 187t
Lysergic acid diethylamide (LSD), 66-67
Lysodren. *See* Mitotane

Maalox, 268, 275t
Macrodantin. *See* Nitrofurantoin
Mafenide, 131, 132
Magaldrate, 268t, 275t
Magnesia, citrate of, 270
Magnesia magna. *See* Milk of magnesia
Magnesium carbonate, 268t, 275t, 276t
Magnesium hydroxide, 268t, 272, 275t,
    276t
Magnesium oxide, 268t
Magnesium trisilicate, 268t, 275t, 276t
Malaria, 76, 165-168. *See also* Antima-
    larial drugs
Male fern. *See* Aspidium oleoresin
Male hormones. *See* Androgens
Mandelamine. *See* Methenamine mande-
    late
Mandelic acid, 301-302
Mannitol, 103, 104, 105, 111t
Mantoux test, 296
MAO inhibitors:
    as antidepressants, 243, 244, 245, 247,
        249, 255t
    as antihypertensives, 108-109, 114t
Maolate. *See* Chlorphenesin
Marcaine. *See* Bupivacaine hydrochlo-
    ride
Marezine. *See* Cyclizine
Marijuana, 65-66, 69t

Matulane. *See* Procarbazine
Measles virus vaccine, 297t
Mebaral. *See* Mephobarbital
Mecamylamine, 113t
Mechlorethamine, 216t, 219-220, 221t
Meclizine, 264t, 272t, 279t
Mecostrin. *See* Dimethyl tubocurarine
    chloride
Medrol. *See* Methylprednisolone
Medroxyprogesterone, 200t
Mellaril. *See* Thioridazine
Melphalan, 216t, 221t
Menadiol sodium diphosphate, 92t, 291t
Menadione sodium bisulfate, 88, 89, 92t,
    291t
Meningitis, treatment of, 132
Menotropins, 177, 179, 180, 187t
Mepenzolate, 280t
Meperidine, 35, 36, 37, 38, 39, 44t
    abuse of, 65
    preanesthetic use, 310t
Mephentermine, 8, 11t, 15t
Mephenytoin, 228, 232t
Mephobarbital, 228-229, 232t
Mephyton. *See* Phytonadione
Mepivacaine hydrochloride, 316t
Meprednisone, 188t
Meprobamate, 243t, 246, 254t, 319
Merbromin, 303
Mercaptomerin, 110t
Mercaptopurine, 217t, 223t
Mercurial compounds, antiseptic, 303
Mercurial diuretics, 104, 105, 110t
Mercurochrome. *See* Merbromin
Mercury ointment, ammoniated, 303
Mercury poisoning, 281
Merthiolate. *See* Thimerosal
Mesantoin. *See* Mephenytoin
Mescaline, 67
Mestinon. *See* Pyridostigmine
Mestranol, 200t, 201t
Metamucil. *See* Psyllium
Metaphen. *See* Nitromersol
Metaraminol, 8, 11t, 13, 14t

Methacycline, 139*t*, 154*t*
Methadone, 38, 39, 44*t*
Methamphetamines, 8, 67, 70*t*
Methandrostenolone, 197*t*
Methantheline, 34*t*
Methaqualone, 61*t*, 68
Metharbital, 228-229, 232*t*
Methenamine mandelate, 301-302, 304, 307*t*
Methergine. *See* Methylergonovine maleate
Methiacil. *See* Methylthiouracil
Methimazole, 205*t*, 206, 208*t*
Methocarbamol, 325*t*
Methohexital, 56*t*, 60*t*, 311*t*
Methotrexate, 217*t*, 223*t*
Methotrimeprazine, 41-42, 45*t*
Methoxamine, 8, 11*t*, 14*t*
Methoxyflurane, 312
Methscopolamine, 34*t*
Methsuximide, 228, 232*t*
Methyclothiazide, 112*t*
Methylatropine nitrate, 34*t*
Methylcellulose, 270
Methyldopa, 18, 20, 21*t*, 113*t*
Methylergonovine maleate, 209-210, 211, 213*t*
Methylphenidate, 116, 117, 119*t*
Methylprednisolone, 188*t*
Methylprednisolone sodium succinate, 188*t*
Methylrosaniline, 146*t*, 157*t*
Methylrosaniline chloride, 169, 174*t*
Methyl salicylate, 47
Methyltestosterone, 198*t*
Methylthiouracil, 205*t*, 208*t*
Methyprylon, 61*t*
Meticorten. *See* Prednisone
Metrazol. *See* Pentylenetetrazol
Metropine. *See* Methylatropine nitrate
Metubine. *See* Dimethyl tubocurarine iodide
Milibis. *See* Glycobiarsol
Milk of magnesia, 268*t*, 275*t*, 277*t*

Milontin. *See* Phensuximide
Miltown. *See* Meprobamate
Mineralocorticoids, 178, 180, 182, 183, 184-185, 188*t*, 189*t*
Mineral oil, 90*t*, 270, 273, 277*t*
Minocin. *See* Minocycline
Minocycline, 139*t*, 154*t*
Mintezol. *See* Thiabendazole
Miradon. *See* Anisindione
Mithracin. *See* Mithramycin
Mithramycin, 217*t*, 224*t*
Mitotane, 216, 225*t*
Modane, constituents, 277*t*
Moderil. *See* Rescinnamine
Monoamine oxidase inhibitors. *See* MAO inhibitors
Morphine, 35-38, 39
  abuse of, 65
  as antitussive, 37, 261
  preanesthetic use, 310*t*
Morphine sulfate, 45*t*
Morton, W. T. G., 309
Motrin. *See* Ibuprofen
Mucolytics, 261, 262
Mucomyst. *See* Acetylcysteine
Mumps vaccine, 298*t*
Muripsin, constituents, 278*t*
Musculoskeletal system:
  corticosteroid effect on, 182, 189*t*
  disorders of, drugs used in management of, 317-325
  xanthine effect on, 116
Mustargen. *See* Mechlorethamine
Myambutol. *See* Ethambutol
Myasthenia gravis, treatment of, 24, 25
Mycifradin. *See* Neomycin
Mycostatin. *See* Nystatin
Mycotic infections, treatment of. *See* Antifungal agents
Mylanta, constituents, 276*t*
Myleran. *See* Busulfan
Myochrysine. *See* Gold sodium thiomalate
Mysoline. *See* Primidone

Mysteclin F, constituents, 146
Mytelase. *See* Ambenonium
Mytolon. *See* Benzoquinonium chloride
Myxedema, 204

Nalidixic acid, 302, 304, 307*t*
Nalline. *See* Nalorphine
Nalorphine, 42*t*, 43, 46*t*
Naloxone, 42*t*, 43, 46*t*
Nandrolone, 198*t*
Naqua. *See* Trichlormethiazide
Narcan. *See* Naloxone
Narcolepsy, treatment of, 8, 116, 118
Narcotic analgesics. *See* Analgesics, narcotic
Narcotic antagonists, 42-43, 46*t*
Nardil. *See* Phenelzine
Naturetin. *See* Bendroflumethiazide
Navane. *See* Thiothixene
Nebs. *See* Acetaminophen
NegGram. *See* Nalidixic acid
Nembutal. *See* Pentobarbital
Neohydrin. *See* Chlormerodrin
Neomycin, 140, 144, 155*t*
Neostigmine, 23, 24, 27*t*, 315
Neo-Synephrine. *See* Phenylephrine
Nesacaine. *See* Chloroprocaine hydrochloride
Neurohormones. *See* Acetylcholine; Acetylcholinesterase; Epinephrine; Norepinephrine
Neurohumoral transmitters, 24
Neurohypophysis, 177
Neuroleptanalgesia, 39
Neuromuscular blocking agents, 314-315
Neutral Protamine Hagedorn (NPH) Insulin. *See* Isophane Insulin Suspension U.S.P.
Neutrapen. *See* Penicillinase
Niacin, 286
Nicotinic acid. *See* Niacin
Nikethamide, 116, 117, 119*t*
Nisentil. *See* Alphaprodine
Nitrofurantoin, 302, 304, 308*t*

Nitrofurazone, 302-303, 308*t*
Nitroglycerin. *See* Glyceryl trinitrate
Nitroglyn. *See* Glyceryl trinitrate
Nitromersol, 303
Nitrous oxide, 309, 311
Noludar. *See* Methyprylon
Nonbarbiturates, 55, 56, 57, 61*t*
 abuse of, 67-68, 70*t*
 (*see also* Sedatives and hypnotics)
Noncatecholamines, 7-8, 11, 14-15*t*
Non-narcotic analgesics. *See* Analgesics, non-narcotic
Nonsalicylates, 48, 50-51. *See also* Analgesics, non-narcotic
Noradrenaline. *See* Norepinephrine
Norepinephrine, 7, 8, 18, 24
Norethindrone, 200*t*, 201*t*
Norflex. *See* Orphenadrine
Norgestrel, 201*t*
Norinyl, constituents, 201*t*
Norlestrin, constituents, 201*t*
Norlutate. *See* Norethindrone
Norpramin. *See* Desipramine
Norquen, constituents, 200*t*
Nortriptyline, 243*t*, 257*t*
Novatrin. *See* Homatropine
Novocain. *See* Procaine hydrochloride
NPH Iletin. *See* Isophane Insulin Suspension U.S.P.
NPH Insulin. *See* Isophane Insulin Suspension U.S.P.
Numorphan. *See* Oxymorphone
Nupercaine. *See* Dibucaine hydrochloride
Nystatin, 146, 147, 157*t*

Ogen. *See* Piperazine estrone sulfate
Oil of wintergreen, 47
Oleum ricini. *See* Castor oil
Oliguria, treatment of, 103, 104
Olive oil, 270-271
Oncovin. *See* Vincristine
Opiates, abuse of, 65, 69*t*
Opium, 35, 36, 39

Opium, powdered, U.S.P., 38
Opium alkaloids, 36, 39, 45*t*
Oral contraceptives, 193, 194, 195-196, 200-201*t*
Oreton. *See* Testosterone
Oreton methyl. *See* Methyltestosterone
Orinase. *See* Tolbutamide
Orphenadrine, 236*t*, 240*t*, 325*t*
Ortho-Novum, constituents, 201*t*
Ortho-Novum SQ, constituents, 200*t*
Osmitrol. *See* Mannitol
Osmotic diuretics, 104-105, 111*t*. *See also* Diuretics
Ouabain, 82*t*
Ovral, constituents, 201*t*
Ovulen, constituents, 200*t*
Oxazepam, 243*t*, 254*t*
Ox bile extract, 278*t*
Oxidized cellulose, 305-306
Oxidizing agents, antiseptic, 303
Oxycel. *See* Oxidized cellulose
Oxycodone, 39, 45*t*
Oxymorphone, 39, 45*t*
Oxyphenbutazone, 318, 319, 320-321, 325*t*
Oxyphencyclimine, 30, 34*t*
Oxytetracycline, 139*t*, 156*t*
 antiparasitical use, 171, 172, 176*t*
Oxytocin, 178, 209, 210, 211-213, 213-214*t*
Oxytoxics, 209

PABA. *See* Para-aminobenzoic acid
Pagitane. *See* Cycrimine
Pamine. *See* Methscopolamine
Pancreatic dornase, 262, 306, 307
Pancreatic enzymes, 269, 278*t*
Pancreatin, 278*t*
Panheprin. *See* Heparin sodium
Pantopon. *See* Opium alkaloids
Pantothenic acid, 286, 287
Panwarfin. *See* Warfarin sodium
Papaverine, 38, 46*t*, 93, 94
Para-aminobenzoic acid (PABA), 288

Para-aminophenol derivatives. *See* Nonsalicylates
Paradione. *See* Paramethadione
Paral. *See* Paraldehyde
Paraldehyde, 57, 59, 61*t*
Paralysis agitans (Parkinson's disease), treatment of. *See* Antiparkinsonism agents
Paramethadione, 229, 233*t*
Paramethasone acetate, 188*t*
Parasal. *See* Aminosalicylic acid
Parasympathetic nervous system, 7, 24
Parasympathomimetic blocking agents. *See* Cholinergic blocking agents
Parasympathomimetic drugs. *See* Cholinergic drugs
Paratyphoid vaccine, 300*t*
Paregoric, 38, 45*t*, 271, 273, 274, 280*t*
Parest. *See* Methaqualone
Pargyline, 108, 114*t*
Parkinson, James, 235
Parkinson's disease, treatment of. *See* Antiparkinsonism agents
Parnate. *See* Tranylcypromine
Paromomycin, 171, 172, 176*t*
Parsidol. *See* Ethopropazine
PAS. *See* Aminosalicylic acid
Pectin, 271, 280*t*
Pecto-Kaolin, 38
Peganone. *See* Ethotoin
Penicillamine, 282, 284*t*
Penicillin, 135-137, 148-150*t*
Penicillinase, 137
Penicillin G, 135-136, 148*t*
Pentaerythritol tetranitrate, 96*t*
Pentazocine, 41, 45*t*
Penthrane. *See* Methoxyflurane
Pentids. *See* Potassium penicillin G
Pentobarbital, 56*t*, 60*t*, 310
Pentolinium, 113*t*
Pentothal. *See* Thiopental
Pentylenetetrazol, 116, 117, 118, 119*t*
Pepsin, 269, 278*t*
Pepto-Bismol, 269

Percodan, 39. *See also* Oxycodone
Percoten acetate. *See* Desoxycortico-
   sterone
Pergonal. *See* Menotropins
Peri-Colace, constituents, 271, 277*t*
Peripheral vascular disease, treatment of,
   18, 20, 94-95
Peritrate. *See* Pentaerythritol tetranitrate
Permitil. *See* Fluphenazine
Perphenazine:
   for gastrointestinal disorders, 272*t*,
      279*t*
   preanesthetic use, 310*t*
   psychotherapeutic use, 242, 244, 252*t*,
      257*t*
Persantine. *See* Dipyridamole
Pertussis vaccine, 298*t*, 300*t*
Peyote, 67
Phenacemide, 229, 233*t*
Phenacetin, 48-49, 50
Phenazopyridine hydrochloride, 302,
   304, 305, 308*t*
Phenelzine, 243*t*, 255*t*
Phenergan. *See* Promethazine
Phenformin, 122*t*, 123, 124, 129*t*
Phenindione, 86*t*, 91*t*
Phenobarbital, 56*t*, 60*t*, 228-229, 233*t*
Phenol, 304
Phenolphthalein, 277*t*
Phenolsulfonphthalein (P.S.P.), 302
Phenothiazines, 235, 242, 244, 245-246,
   251-252*t*, 272
Phenoxybenzamine, 17, 21*t*
Phensuximide, 228, 233*t*
Phentolamine, 17, 18, 21*t*
Phenurone. *See* Phenacemide
Phenylbutazone, 90*t*, 318, 319, 321-322,
   325*t*
Phenylephrine, 8, 11*t*, 14*t*
Pheochromocytoma, 18
Physicians' Desk Reference (PDR), 2
Physostigmine, 25, 27*t*
Phytonadione, 88, 89, 92*t*, 292*t*
Picrotoxin, 115, 116, 117

Pilocarpine, 25, 26, 27*t*
Pinworms. *See* Helminthiasis
Pipenzolate, 30, 34*t*
Piperacetazine, 242*t*, 252*t*
Piperazine, 169, 174*t*
Piperazine estrone sulfate, 199*t*
Piperazine phenothiazines, 242*t*, 244
Piperidyl phenothiazine, 242*t*
Piptal. *See* Pipenzolate
Pitocin. *See* Oxytocin
Pitressin. *See* Vasopressin tannate
Pituitary hormones, 177-180, 181-182,
   187*t*
Placidyl. *See* Ethchlorvynol
Plantago seed, 270
Plaquenil. *See* Hydroxychloroquine
Plasma, 97-98, 99, 100
Plasmodium, 166, 167
Poisoning, treatment of, 38. *See also*
   Heavy metals and heavy metal an-
   tagonists
Poliomyelitis vaccines, 298*t*
Polycillin. *See* Ampicillin trihydrate
Polycillin-N. *See* Sodium ampicillin
Polymyxin B, 141, 144, 155*t*
Polythiazide, 112*t*
Pontocaine. *See* Tetracaine hydrochlo-
   ride
Pot. *See* Marijuana
Potassium, 98, 99, 100-101, 106*t*
Potassium bicarbonate, 98, 102*t*
Potassium chloride, 98
Potassium gluconate, 98, 102*t*
Potassium hetacillin, 149*t*
Potassium penicillin G, 135, 148*t*
Potassium permanganate, 303, 305
Potassium phenoxymethyl penicillin,
   150*t*
Povan. *See* Pyrvinium pamoate
Povidone-iodine, 303
PPD test, 296
Prantal. *See* Diphemanil
Preanesthetics, 309-310
Prednisolone, 181, 188*t*

Prednisone, 181, 188*t*
Premarin. *See* Estrogenic substances,
   conjugated
Pressonex. *See* Metaraminol
Priestley, Joseph, 309
Prilocaine hydrochloride, 316*t*
Primaquine, 167*t*, 173*t*
Primidone, 229, 233*t*
Priscoline. *See* Tolazoline
Pro-Banthine. *See* Propantheline
Probenecid, 318, 320, 322, 325*t*
Procainamide, 76-77, 78-79, 82*t*
Procaine hydrochloride, 316*t*
Procaine penicillin G, 135, 148*t*
Procarbazine, 217*t*, 223*t*
Prochlorperazine:
   for gastrointestinal disorders, 272*t*,
      279*t*
   preanesthetic use, 310*t*
   psychotherapeutic use, 242, 244, 252*t*
Procyclidine, 236*t*, 240*t*
Progesterone, 192-194, 200*t*
Progestogens, 192, 193-194, 199-200*t*
Prognon. *See* Estradiol
Proloid. *See* Thyroglobulin
Prolutin. *See* Progesterone
Promethazine:
   for gastrointestinal disorders, 272*t*,
      279*t*
   preanesthetic use, 310*t*
   psychotherapeutic use, 260, 264*t*
Prompt Insulin Zinc Suspension U.S.P.,
   122*t*, 126*t*, 129*t*
Pronestyl. *See* Procainamide
Propanediol tranquilizer, 243*t*
Propantheline, 34*t*
Prophythiouracil, 205*t*, 208*t*
Propionate compound, 146*t*, 157*t*
Propion Gel. *See* Propionate compound
Propoxyphene hydrochloride, 48, 50-51,
   53*t*
Propoxyphene napsylate, 48, 50-51, 53*t*
Propranolol, 17, 18, 19, 21*t*
   as cardiac depressant, 76, 77, 78, 83*t*

Prostaphlin. *See* Sodium oxacillin
Prostigmin. *See* Neostigmine
Protamine sulfate, 88, 92*t*
Protamine Zinc Insulin Suspension
  U.S.P., 122*t*, 126*t*, 129*t*
Protease, 278*t*
Protein hydrolysate, 97, 98, 99
Prothrombin, 86, 89
Protriptyline, 243*t*, 257*t*
Provera. *See* Medroxyprogesterone
Pseudoephedrine, 265*t*
Psychomotor stimulants, 115
Psychotherapeutic agents, 241-257
Psychotropic agents, defined, 241
Psyllium, 270, 277*t*
Pteroylglutamic acid. *See* Folic acid
Ptyalin, 306
Purinethol. *See* Mercaptopurine
Purodigin. *See* Digitoxin
Pyopen. *See* Disodium carbenicillin
Pyrantel pamoate, 169, 175*t*
Pyrazolone derivatives, 318, 320-321
Pyridium. *See* Phenazopyridine hydro-
  chloride
Pyridoxine (vitamin B₆), 237, 286
Pyrimethamine, 167*t*, 173*t*
Pyrodostigmine, 24, 25, 27*t*
Pyrvinium pamoate, 169, 175*t*
PZI. *See* Protamine Zinc Insulin Suspen-
  sion U.S.P.

Quaalude. *See* Methaqualone
Quide. *See* Piperacetazine
Quinacrine hydrochloride, 175*t*, 216
Quinidine, 76-77, 78, 83*t*, 90*t*
Quinine, 76, 167*t*, 174*t*

Rabies vaccine, 298*t*
Raudixin. *See* Rauwolfia serpentina
Rau-Sed. *See* Reserpine
Rautina. *See* Rauwolfia
Rauwiloid. *See* Alscroxylon
Rauwolfia, 18, 20, 21*t*

Rauwolfia alkaloids, 109, 242, 244, 245,
  250*t*
Rauwolfia serpentina, 242, 250*t*
Raynaud's disease, 18, 95
Regitine. *See* Phentolamine
Renese. *See* Polythiazide
Repoise. *See* Butaperazine
Rescinnamine, 22*t*
Reserpine, 22*t*, 242, 250*t*
Resorcinol, 304
Respiratory depression, treatment of,
  116, 118
Riboflavin (vitamin B₂), 286
Ricinoleic acid, 270
Rifampin, 160, 161, 164*t*
Rimactane. *See* Rifampin
Riopan. *See* Magaldrate
Ritalin. *See* Methylphenidate
Robaxin. *See* Methocarbamol
Robitussin, 265*t*
Rocky Mountain spotted fever vaccine,
  299*t*
Rondomycin. *See* Methacycline
Roundworms. *See* Helminthiasis
Rubramin. *See* Vitamin B₁₂

Salicylates, 47-48, 49-50, 51-52
  in musculoskeletal disorders, 317-318,
    320, 321, 322
Salicylism, 50*t*
Scarlet fever test, 294
Schick test, 294, 296
Scopolamine, 29, 30, 31, 32, 34*t*, 310*t*
Secobarbital, 56*t*, 60*t*, 310*t*
Seconal. *See* Secobarbital
Sedatives and hypnotics, 55-62
  as antihypertensives, 108, 109
Semilente Iletin. *See* Prompt Insulin Zinc
  Suspension U.S.P.
Semilente Insulin. *See* Prompt Insulin
  Zinc Suspension U.S.P.
Senna concentrate, 277*t*
Septra, constituents, 134*t*
Serax. *See* Oxazepam

Seromycin. *See* Cycloserine
Serpasil. *See* Reserpine
Serum albumin, 97, 98, 99, 100
Setrol. *See* Oxyphencyclimine
Sex hormones, 178, 180. *See also* Andro-
  gens; Female hormones
Silain-Gel, constituents, 276*t*
Silver nitrate solution, 281-282, 283,
  284*t*
  antiseptic use, 303, 305
Silver poisoning, 282
Simethicone, 276*t*
Simpson, James Young, 309
Sinequan. *See* Doxepin
Singoserp. *See* Syrosingopine
Sintron. *See* Acenocoumarol
6-MP. *See* Mercaptopurine
Skeletal muscle relaxants, 319, 321, 323
Smack. *See* Heroin
Smallpox vaccine, 299*t*
Snow. *See* Cocaine
Sodium, 99, 100, 106*t*
Sodium ampicillin, 148*t*
Sodium benzoate, 119*t*
Sodium bicarbonate, 98-99, 100, 101,
  102*t*, 267, 272
Sodium biphosphate, 270
Sodium chloride, 99, 100, 101, 102*t*
Sodium cloxacillin, 149*t*
Sodium dicloxacillin, 149*t*
Sodium methicillin, 149*t*
Sodium nafcillin, 150*t*
Sodium oxacillin, 150*t*
Sodium phosphate, 270
Sodium polystyrene, 98, 102*t*
Sodium salicylate, 47, 317, 325*t*
Solanaceae (nightshade) family, 29
Solganal. *See* Aurothioglucose
Solu-Medrol. *See* Methylprednisolone
  sodium succinate
Soma. *See* Carisoprodol
Somatotropic hormone. *See* STH
Sonilyn. *See* Sulfachloropyridazine
Sopor. *See* Methaqualone

Sparteine, 209, 210, 211, 213, 214*t*
Spartocin. *See* Sparteine
Spectinomycin, 141, 144
Speedball, 65
Spironolactone, 110*t*
Sporostacin. *See* Chlordantoin
Staphcillin. *See* Sodium methicillin
Stelazine. *See* Trifluoperazine
Steroids. *See* Corticosteroids
Stevens-Johnson syndrome, 133, 229
STH (somatotropic hormone), 178
Stimulants:
    abuse of, 67-68
    cardiac (*see* Cardiotonic drugs;
        Catecholamines)
    central nervous system (*see* Central
        nervous system [CNS] stimulants)
STP (dimethoxymethylamphetamine),
    67
Streptokinase-streptodornase, 306
Streptomycin, 160, 161, 164*t*
Strychnine, 116, 117
Sublimaze. *See* Fentanyl
Succinylcholine chloride, 314*t*
Sulfabenzamide, 132, 134*t*
Sulfacetamide, 131, 132, 134*t*
Sulfachloropyridazine, 134*t*
Sulfameter, 131, 134*t*
Sulfamethizole, 132, 134*t*
Sulfamethoxazole, 132, 134*t*
Sulfamylon. *See* Mafenide
Sulfathiazole, 132, 134*t*
Sulfinpyrazone, 318, 320, 325*t*
Sulfisoxazole, 131, 132, 134*t*
Sulfisoxazole diolamine, 134*t*
Sulfobromophthalein (B.S.P.), 302
Sulfonamides, 131-134
Sulfonylureas, 122*t*, 123, 124
Sulla. *See* Sulfameter
Sultrin Triple Sulfa, constituents, 132,
    134*t*
Surfacaine. *See* Cyclomethycaine
Surfak. *See* Dioctyl calcium sulfosucci-
    nate

Surital. *See* Thiamylal
Symmetrel. *See* Amantadine
Sympathetic nervous system, 7, 24
Sympathomimetic blocking agents. *See*
    Adrenergic blocking agents
Sympathomimetic drugs. *See* Adrenergic
    drugs
Syncurine. *See* Decamethonium bromide
Synkayvite. *See* Menadiol sodium di-
    phosphate
Syntocinon. *See* Oxytocin
Syrosingopine, 22*t*

Tace. *See* Chlorotrianisene
Talbutal, 56*t*, 60*t*
Talwin. *See* Pentazocine
Tandearil. *See* Oxyphenbutazone
TAO. *See* Troleandomycin
Tapazole. *See* Methimazole
Tapeworms. *See* Helminthiasis
Taractan. *See* Chlorprothixene
Tea. *See* Marijuana
Tegopen. *See* Sodium cloxacillin
TEM. *See* Triethylenemelamine
Temaril. *See* Trimeprazine
Tensilon. *See* Edrophonium
Terramycin. *See* Oxytetracycline
Teslac. *See* Testolactone
Tessalon capsules, 262, 265*t*
Tes-Tape, 127, 304
Testolactone, 217
Testosterone, 191, 198*t*
Tetanus antitoxin, 299*t*, 300*t*
Tetanus toxoid, 299*t*, 300*t*
Tetracaine hydrochloride, 316*t*
Tetracycline, 139, 141-142, 146, 156*t*
Tetracyn. *See* Tetracycline
Tetrahydrocannabinol (THC), 66
Tetraiodothyronine, 203
Tetrex F, constituents, 146
THC. *See* Tetrahydrocannabinol
Theobromine, 104, 115, 117
Theophylline, 104, 115, 117

Theophylline ethylenediamine. *See*
    Aminophylline U.S.P.
Thiabendazole, 169*t*, 175*t*
Thiamine (vitamin B_1), 286
Thiamylal, 56*t*, 61*t*
Thiazide diuretics, 104, 105, 107, 111-
    112*t*
Thiethylperazine, 272*t*, 280*t*
Thimerosal, 303
Thioguanine, 217*t*, 223*t*
Thiomerin. *See* Mercaptomerin
Thiopental, 56*t*, 61*t*, 311*t*
Thioridazine, 242*t*, 252*t*
Thiosulfil. *See* Sulfamethizole
Thiotepa U.S.P., 216*t*, 221*t*
Thiothixene, 242*t*, 243, 244, 246, 253*t*
Thiouracils, 205, 206
Thorazine. *See* Chlorpromazine
Thrombin, 86, 305, 306
Thromboplastin, 86
Thyroglobulin, 204*t*, 207*t*
Thyroid agents, 90*t*, 203-205, 206, 207*t*
Thyroid stimulating hormone. *See* TSH
Thyroid U.S.P., 204*t*, 207*t*
Thyroxine, 178, 203, 204*t*. *See also*
    Levothyroxine
Tigan. *See* Trimethobenzamide
Tinactin. *See* Tolnaftate
Tindal. *See* Acetophenazine
Tine test, 296
Tofrānil. *See* Imipramine
Tolazamide, 122*t*, 129*t*, 320
Tolazoline, 17, 22*t*
Tolbutamide, 122*t*, 129*t*, 320
Tolinase. *See* Tolazamide
Tolnaftate, 146*t*, 157*t*
Torecan. *See* Thiethylperazine
Toxin, defined, 294
Toxoids, defined, 294
Tral. *See* Hexocyclium
Trancopal. *See* Chlormezanone
Tranquilizers, 241-254
    abuse of, 68, 70*t*
    antihypertensive use, 108, 109

Tranquilizers (*continued*)
  major, 242-243, 244, 245-246, 248, 250-252*t*
  minor, 243, 244, 246, 249, 253-254*t*
  preanesthetic use, 310*t*
  as skeletal muscle relaxants, 319, 323
Tranxene. *See* Chlorazepate
Tranylcypromine, 243*t*, 255*t*
Trecator. *See* Ethionamide
Triamcinolone, 188*t*
Triamcinolone diacetate, 188*t*
Triamcinolone hexacetonide, 188*t*
Triavil, constituents, 247, 257*t*
Trichlormethiazide, 112*t*
Trichloroethylene, 313
Tridione. *See* Trimethadione
Triethylenemelamine, 216*t*, 222*t*
Trifluoperazine, 242*t*, 252*t*
Triflupromazine, 242*t*, 252*t*, 310*t*
Trihexylphenidyl, 236*t*, 240*t*
Triiodothyronine, 178, 203, 204*t*. *See also* Liothyronine
Trilafon. *See* Perphenazine
Trilene. *See* Trichloroethylene
Trimeprazine, 265*t*
Trimethadione, 229, 233*t*
Trimethaphan, 113*t*
Trimethobenzamide, 280*t*
Trimethoprim, 134*t*
Triprolidine, 265*t*
Trobicin. *See* Spectinomycin
Troleandomycin, 141, 144
Trypsin, 306
TSH (thyroid stimulating hormone), 178, 203, 204
Tubarine. *See* Tubocurarine chloride
Tuberculosis, treatment of. *See* Antitubercular agents
Tuberculosis test, 296
Tubocurarine chloride, 314*t*
Tylenol. *See* Acetaminophen
Typhoid vaccine, 299*t*, 300*t*
Typhus vaccine, 299*t*

Ultralente Iletin. *See* Extended Insulin Zinc Suspension U.S.P.
Ultralente Insulin. *See* Extended Insulin Zinc Suspension U.S.P.
Undecylenic acid, 146*t*, 157*t*
Unipen. *See* Sodium nafcillin
Uracil mustard, 216*t*, 222*t*
Urea, 105, 111*t*
Urecholine. *See* Bethanechol
Urevert. *See* Urea
Uterus, drugs acting on, 209-214

Vaccines, 294, 296-300*t*. *See also* Immunological agents
Valium. *See* Diazepam
Valmid. *See* Ethinamate
Vancocin. *See* Vancomycin
Vancomycin, 141, 144-145, 156*t*
Varidase. *See* Streptokinase-streptodornase
Vasodilan. *See* Isoxsuprine
Vasodilating agents, 17, 93-96. *See also* Papaverine
Vasopressin (ADH), 37, 179, 180, 187*t*
Vasopressin tannate, 187*t*
Vasopressors. *See* Adrenergic drugs
Vasoxyl. *See* Methoxamine
Velban. *See* Vinblastine
Veratrum alkaloids, 107-108, 114*t*
Veriloid. *See* Alkavervir
Versapen. *See* Hetacillin
Versapen-K. *See* Potassium hetacillin
Vesprin. *See* Triflupromazine
Vibramycin. *See* Doxycycline
Vinblastine, 216, 217*t*, 224*t*
Vincristine, 216, 217*t*, 225*t*
Vinethene. *See* Vinyl ether
Vinyl ether, 312-313
Vioform. *See* Iodochlorhydroxyquin
Vistaril. *See* Hydroxyzine
Vitamins, 285-288, 291-292*t*
Vitamin A, 287, 288, 291*t*
Vitamin B complex, 286-287, 291*t*

Vitamin B$_6$. *See* Pyridoxine
Vitamin B$_{12}$, 289, 290, 292*t*
Vitamin C, 285-286, 291*t*
Vitamin D, 287, 288, 291*t*
Vitamin E, 287, 288, 291*t*
Vitamin K, 86, 88, 89, 287-288, 291*t*, 292*t*
Vivactil. *See* Protriptyline
Volatile anesthetics, 312-313
Volatile hydrocarbons, abuse of, 68, 70*t*
Vomiting:
  agents to induce (*see* Emetics)
  agents to prevent (*see* Antiemetics)

Warfarin potassium, 86*t*, 91*t*
Warfarin sodium, 86*t*, 91*t*
Whipworms. *See* Helminthiasis
Whooping cough vaccine. *See* Pertussis vaccine
WinGel, constituents, 275*t*
Wintergreen oil, 47
Withering, William, 71
Worms. *See* Helminthiasis
Wyamine. *See* Mephentermine
Wycillin. *See* Procaine penicillin G
Wydase. *See* Hyaluronidase

Xanthines:
  as CNS stimulants, 115-117
  as diuretics, 104, 105, 112*t*
Xylocaine. *See* Lidocaine

Yellow fever vaccine, 299*t*

Zarontin. *See* Ethosuximide
Zephiran. *See* Benzalkonium chloride
Zinc oxide, 303
Zinc peroxide, 303
Zinc undecylenate, 146*t*, 157*t*
Zyloprim. *See* Allopurinol